The 5-Minute Veterinary Consult

Clinical Companion

Canine and Feline Infectious Diseases and Parasitology

The 5-Minute Veterinary Consult
Clinical Companion

Canine and Feline Infectious Diseases and Parasitology

Stephen C. Barr, BVSc, MVS, PhD
Diplomate, American College of Veterinary Internal Medicine
Professor of Medicine
Department of Clinical Sciences
College of Veterinary Medicine
Cornell University
Ithaca, New York

Dwight D. Bowman, MS, PhD
Professor of Parasitology
Department of Microbiology and Parasitology
College of Veterinary Medicine
Cornell University
Ithaca, New York

Blackwell Publishing

©2006 Blackwell Publishing

Blackwell Publishing Professional
2121 State Avenue, Ames, Iowa 50014, USA

Orders:	1-800-862-6657
Office:	1-515-292-0140
Fax:	1-515-292-3348
Web site:	www.blackwellprofessional.com

Blackwell Publishing Ltd
9600 Garsington Road, Oxford OX4 2DQ, UK
Tel.: +44 (0)1865 776868

Blackwell Publishing Asia
550 Swanston Street, Carlton, Victoria 3053, Australia
Tel.: +61 (0)3 8359 1011

First edition, 2006

Library of Congress Cataloging-in-Publication Data

Barr, Stephen C.
    The 5-minute veterinary consult clinical companion : canine and feline infectious diseases and parasitology / Stephen C. Barr, Dwight D. Bowman.
        p. cm.
    Includes index.
    ISBN 0-7817-4766-X
        Dogs—Infections. 2. Cats—Infections. 3. Dogs—Parasites. 4. Cats—Parasites. 5. Veterinary medicine. I. Bowman, Dwight D. II. Title. III. Title: Five-minute veterinary consult clinical companion.
SF991.B287 2005
636.7'089'69—dc22

The last digit is the print number: 9 8 7 6 5 4 3 2 1

To my wife, Beryl, and my daughters, Jacqueline and Alexandria,
who give reason to all enterprises!
Stephen C. Barr

Preface

The 5-Minute Veterinary Consult Clinical Companion: Canine and Feline Infectious Diseases and Parasitology is a quick-reference text designed mainly for clinicians, but also for students of veterinary medicine. It assumes a basic knowledge of infectious and parasitic diseases. There are several excellent texts available in infectious diseases of both cats and dogs and also many detailing the parasites of these species. The infectious disease texts offer detailed information regarding the epidemiology and pathophysiology of disease, clinical manifestations, diagnostic techniques, pathology, and therapeutic regimens, and most parasitology texts detail life cycles, parasite morphology, and pathology, with little emphasis on diagnosis and therapy. Although these are excellent reference texts with a place in veterinary libraries and on the shelves of the clinical veterinarian, there are few if any texts that include both infectious and parasitic diseases in one volume. This text was written to make clinically relevant information on both infectious and parasitic diseases of cats and dogs available for quick reference in the workplace.

The 5-Minute Veterinary Consult Clinical Companion: Canine and Feline Infectious Diseases and Parasitology is designed to help the reader recognize various infectious and parasitic diseases common in North America and identify appropriate diagnostic tests to perform. Drug dosages have been presented in table format to allow the busy clinician to access therapeutic information quickly between appointments. Many of the chapters have been adapted from the Infectious Disease section of the third edition of *The 5-Minute Veterinary Consult: Canine and Feline,* for which I served as section editor. Chapters from other sections in that text were also used, as were several from *The 5-Minute Veterinary Consult Clinical Companion: Small Animal Dermatology,* by Karen Helton Rhodes. Most of the parasitology chapters are unique to this book and include diagnostic images provided by my friend, colleague, and coeditor, Dr. Dwight Bowman.

ORGANIZATION AND FORMAT

Like *The 5-Minute Veterinary Consult: Canine and Feline,* the organization of this book is based on an alphabetic listing of, in most instances, the etiologic agent. Sometimes the more common version of a disease entity is used as a heading (e.g., Tick Bite Paralysis, Ear Mites) instead of the name of the etiologic agent. Although this might aggravate the purist, we have adhered to this format to aid the fundamental principle of the text—that of a quick reference.

Each chapter in the text is organized into sections of Definition/Overview, Etiology/Pathophysiology, Signalment/History, Clinical Features, Differential Diagnosis, Diagnostics, Therapeutics with Drugs of Choice, Precautions/Interactions, and

Comments. This latter section often alludes to the zoonotic potential of the agent in question and occasionally includes comments by the authors based on their experience of the disease. Each section is intentionally kept short, with the information presented in bullet format and usually in incomplete sentences, similar to how one might take notes from a lecture. The purpose of this writing style was to present information as concisely as possible for quick reference. This also allowed us to present the book in a manageable size and at a reasonable cost.

KEY FEATURES

In most cases, color images emphasizing the major diagnostic feature of the disease are presented. The key diagnostic feature itself, where applicable, is highlighted in blue in the text. Where there are a number of drugs involved in treating the disease, the dosage, route of administration, and therapy length are presented in table format for quick reference. A short list of Suggested Readings at the end of each chapter offers the reader the current or most important references for the topic. This reference list is by no means exhaustive.

APPENDICES

Appendices, including core vaccination schedules, antiparasitic products for the treatment of gastrointestinal parasites in dogs, parasiticides for cats, canine heartworm preventives, and canine products with efficacy against arthropods, have been included. A drug formulary extracted from *The 5-Minute Veterinary Consult: Canine and Feline,* third edition, with emphasis on those agents used against infectious and parasitic diseases, is provided. Several new drugs, particularly in regard to those used in treating parasitic infections, have also been added.

Stephen C. Barr

Acknowledgments

To my colleagues who participated in the writing of this book, who provided many color images and expertise along the way, I extend my gratitude. My thanks to Frank Smith and Larry Tilley for their support and guidance for both *The 5-Minute Veterinary Consult* and this spinoff project.

Table of Contents

chapter 1

Amebiasis

DEFINITION/OVERVIEW

- Facultative parasitic ameba that infects people and non-human primates (including dogs and cats)
- Found primarily in tropical areas throughout the world, although still occurs in North America.

ETIOLOGY/PATHOPHYSIOLOGY

- *Entamoeba histolytica*—dogs and cats become infected by ingesting cysts from human feces.
- Encystment of trophozoites seldom occurs in dogs or cats so they are not a source of infection.
- One of the few organisms transmitted from man to pets but rarely from pets to man.
- Trophozoites (the pathogenic stage)—inhabit the colonic lumen as commensals or invade the colonic wall, but can disseminate to other organs (rare) including lungs, liver, brain, and skin.
- Trophozoites damage intestinal epithelial cells by secreting enzymes that lyse cells and disrupt intercellular connections.
- Certain bacteria and a diet deficient in protein increase the virulence of the ameba.
- The host's immune response to invasion exacerbates pathology.
- Colonic ulceration results when trophozoites in the submucosa undermine the mucosa.
- *Acanthamoeba castellani* and *A. culbertsoni*—free-living species found in freshwater, saltwater, soil, and sewage; can infect dogs.
- *Acanthamoeba* spp.—infection thought to be by inhalation of organisms from contaminated water or colonization of the skin or cornea; hematogenous spread or direct spread from the nasal cavity through the cribiform plate to the central nervous system may occur resulting in a granulomatous amebic meningoencephalitis.

SIGNALMENT/HISTORY

- Mainly young and/or immunosuppressed animals are infected.

CLINICAL FEATURES

Dogs

- *E. histolytica* infections are usually asymptomatic
- Severe infections—result in ulcerative colitis to cause dysentery (may be fatal).
- Hematogenous spread—results in failure states of the organs (invariably fatal).
- Granulomatous amebic meningoencephalitis (caused by *Acanthamoeba* spp.)—causes signs similar to distemper (anorexia, fever, lethargy, oculonasal discharge, respiratory distress, and diffuse neurologic abnormalities).
- Syndrome of inappropriate secretion of antidiuretic hormone has been reported in a young dog with Acanthamoebisis causing granulomatous meningoencephalitis with invasion of the hypothalamus.

Cats

- Colitis—causing chronic intractable diarrhea (similar to dogs).
- Systemic amebiasis—not been reported in the cat.
- *Acanthamoeba*—not been reported in the cat.

DIFFERENTIAL DIAGNOSIS

Dogs

- Causes of bloody diarrhea or tenesmus including: constipation; food intolerance/allergy; parasitism (whip worms, Leishmaniasis, Balantidiasis); HGE; foreign body; irritable bowel syndrome; inflammatory bowel disease; diverticula; infectious (parvovirus, Clostridial enteritis, bacterial overgrowth and other bacterial causes, fungal such as histoplasmosis or blastomycosis); neoplasia; ulcerative colitis; endocrinopathy (Addison's disease); toxic (lead, fungal, or plant); occasionally major organ disease causing colonic ulceration such as renal failure.
- Other causes of diffuse neurologic disease in young animals including: Infectious (distemper, fungal such as *Cryptococcus, Blastomyces, Histoplasma*, bacterial, protozoal such as *Toxoplasma* and *Neospora*); toxic (lead, organophosphate); trauma; GME; extracranial (hypoglycemia; hepatic encephalopathy); inherited epilepsy; neoplasia.

Cats

- Other causes of diarrhea including: food intolerance/allergy; inflammatory bowel disease; parasitism (giardiasis, parasites such as hookworms, roundworms, tritrichomonas); infectious (panleukopenia, FIV, FeLV producing panleukopenia-like syndrome, bacterial including *Salmonella*, rarely *Campylobacter*); drug (acetaminophen); neoplasia; pancreatitis; and major organ dysfunction.

DIAGNOSTICS

Diagnostic Feature
- **Microscopic examination—colonic biopsies (H&E) obtained via endoscopy is the most reliable method.**
- Trophozoites in feces—very difficult to detect although methylene blue staining improves chances *(Fig. 1-1)*.
- Trichrome and iron-hematoxyline—the ideal fecal stains but require a reference laboratory to perform.
- Fecal concentration techniques—of little help.
- Brain biopsy—may be required to definitively diagnose neurologic forms antemortem.
- A dog reported with granulomatous amebic meningoencephalitis due to *Acanthamoeba* showed elevated WBC counts (70% mononuclear cells), protein, and xanthochromia in CSF.

 THERAPEUTICS

- Colitis (caused by *E. histolytica*)—responds to metronidazole although dogs continue to shed organisms.
- Systemic forms (particularly neurologic disease)—invariably fatal despite treatment.

■ **Fig. 1-1** Trophozoite of *Entamoeba histolytica* in the feces of a dog. Note the size (about 20 μm) in comparison to the 2 RBC in the same image. (Wright's-Giemsa stain, 1500×).

Drugs of Choice

■ Metronidazole (20 mg/kg, PO, q12h, for 7 days)

Precautions/Interactions

■ High doses of metronidazole (usually > 30 mg/kg) for extended periods may cause neurologic signs in dogs.

 COMMENTS

■ Dogs and cats are an unlikely source of infection in people.
■ Pets usually acquire infections from the same source as their owners; veterinarians must warn owners of possible risk.
■ People and pets are at risk of exposure to free-living amebiasis from the same environmental sources.
■ Immunocompetency often determines whether infection will become established.

Abbreviations

CSF, cerebrospinal fluid; FeLV, feline leukemia virus; FIV, feline immunodeficiency virus; GME, granulomatous meningoencephalopathy; HGE, hemorrhagic gastroenteritis; H&E, hematoxylin and eosin; WBC, white blood cells.

Suggested Reading

Brofman PJ, Knostman KAB, Dibartola SP. Granulomatous amebic meningoenchephalitis causing the syndrome of inappropriate secretion of antidiuretic hormone in a dog. *J Vet Int Med* 2003;17: 230–234.
Barr SC. Amebiasis. In: Greene CE, ed. *Infectious Diseases of the Dog and Cat*. Philadelphia: WB Saunders, 1998;487–488.

Author: Stephen C. Barr
Consulting Editor: Stephen C. Barr

chapter 2

Anaerobic Infections

DEFINITION/OVERVIEW

- Caused by bacteria that require low oxygen tension, and elaborate toxins and enzymes leading to extension of the infection into adjacent healthy tissue.

ETIOLOGY/PATHOPHYSIOLOGY

- Most common genera—*Bacteroides, Fusobacterium, Actinomyces, Clostridium,* and *Peptostreptococcus.*
- Pathogenesis determined by the body system involved.
- Body areas involved—usually those near a mucosal surface.
- Usually caused by normal flora of body—a break in protective barriers allows bacterial invasion.
- Anaerobes—often overlooked as involved in an infectious process.

SIGNALMENT/HISTORY

- Predisposing factors—bite wounds; dental disease; open fractures; abdominal surgery; foreign bodies.

CLINICAL FEATURES

- A foul odor associated with a wound or exudative discharge.
- Gas in the tissue or associated exudates.
- Peritonitis.
- Pyothorax.
- Pyometra.
- Severe dental disease.
- Bite wounds with considerable trauma (*Fig. 2-1*).
- Wounds or deep abscesses that do not heal as anticipated.

■ **Fig. 2-1** Deep bite wounds with considerable tissue damage are likely sources of anaerobic infections.

DIFFERENTIAL DIAGNOSIS

- Wounds that fail to respond to appropriate medical therapy—aerobic cultures may be negative; suspect anaerobic organisms.
- Cats with non-healing wounds—test for FeLV and FIV.
- Middle-aged and old animals—tumor invasion (e.g., in the GIT) may be responsible for establishing infection.

DIAGNOSTICS

- CBC—neutrophilic leukocytosis and monocytosis common.
- Biochemical panel—abnormalities depend on specific organ involvement.

Diagnostic Feature
- **Microbiological culture—collect appropriate samples such as pus (1–2 ml in stoppered syringe) and tissue (minimum 1 g sample).**
- Minimize exposure to air when collecting and transporting.
- Appropriate transport devices should be on hand before the sample is collected and include screw-top glass vials with media that accept a Culturette swab and syringes evacuated of all air and capped with a rubber stopper.

THERAPEUTICS

- Surgical intervention should not be delayed.
- Surgical removal of devitalized tissue, cleaning of wound, and drainage of pus with the provision for continuous drainage combined with systemic antimicrobial therapy usually gives the best chance of a positive outcome.

TABLE 2-1. Drug Therapy for Anaerobic Infections

Drug	Dose (mg/kg)	Route	Interval (Hours)
Penicillin G	20,000–40,000[a]	IM, IV	6–8
Amoxicillin/clavulanic acid	20	PO, IV	8–12
Cefoxitin	10–20	IM, IV	8
Clindamycin	5–10	PO, IV	12
Metronidazole	10	PO, IV	8

[a] U/kg

- Surgical removal of foreign body—essential if positive outcome to be achieved.
- Pyothorax—thoracic drainage via chest tube placement.
- Removal of swelling to help re-establish local blood flow and increase oxygen tension will help limit spread of tissue damage.

Drugs of Choice

- Antibiotic of choice (except for *Bacteroides* strains)—penicillin G
- Amoxicillin—comparable to penicillin G in spectrum of activity.
- Amoxicillin combined with clavulanic acid—effective against *Bacteroides*.
- Cefoxitin—the only cephalosporin with reliable activity against anaerobes but expensive.
- Clindamycin—useful for respiratory tract infections.
- Metronidazole—effective against all anaerobes except *Actinomyces* (*Table 2-1*).
- Aminoglycosides—ineffective against anaerobes.
- Trimethoprim-sulfa combinations—ineffective and poor penetration.

Precautions/Interactions

- Determine renal and hepatic function to understand how excretion of antibiotics will occur in debilitated patient.
- Support patient appropriately with fluid therapy and nutrition.

 COMMENTS

- Antimicrobial therapy alone—unlikely to be successful due to poor drug penetration into exudates and poorly vascularized tissue.
- Antibiotic selection—initially largely empirical (delay in return of culture results).
- Use antibiotics against anaerobes if mixed population of aerobes and anaerobes are suspected because of the symbiotic nature of the infection.

Abbreviations

FeLV, feline leukemia virus; FIV, feline immunodeficiency virus; GIT, gastrointestinal tract.

Suggested Reading

Hirsh DC, Jang SS. Anaerobic infections. In: Greene CE, ed. *Infectious Diseases of the Dog and Cat.* Philadelphia: WB Saunders, 1998:258–263.

Author: Sharon Fooshee Grace
Consulting Editor: Stephen C. Barr

Angiostrongylus Infection

DEFINITION/OVERVIEW

- Nematode parasite of the pulmonary arterial tree of dogs in Europe, Ireland, Uganda, Australia, and South America.
- Recently reported in a dog from Newfoundland, Canada.
- Important to North American veterinarians as may be an emerging parasite.

ETIOLOGY/PATHOPHYSIOLOGY

- *Angiostrongylus vasorum*—adult worms (2.5 cm) reside in the pulmonary arteries of dogs.
- L1 enter airways—are carried up the tracheobronchial tree and swallowed and shed in the feces.
- LI in feces—invade molluscan intermediate hosts where they develop to infective L3.
- Molluscan intermediate hosts—eaten by dogs and L3 migrate to pulmonary artery.
- Pulmonary artery obstruction, endarteritis, and pulmonary thrombosis are caused by the adult worms, as well as parenchymal lung damage due to migration of the larvae into the airways.
- Infected dogs develop thrombocytopenia probably as a result of DIC or (as in one dog) immune mediated thrombocytopenia leading to.
- PPP = 40 days.

SIGNALMENT/HISTORY

- Mainly in rural and stray dogs (due to ingestion of mollusks).

CLINICAL FEATURES

- Clinical signs—vary markedly from asymptomatic to DIC.
- Cough.
- Exercise intolerance.
- Weight loss.
- Hemoptysis.

- Subcutaneous edema consistent with congestive heart failure and parenchymal lung disease.
- Respiratory difficulty—increased respiratory rate and tachycardia.
- Thrombocytopenia and DIC—spontaneous hemorrhage into subcutaneous tissues.

DIFFERENTIAL DIAGNOSIS

A general differential diagnosis for cough includes such categories as:
- **C**ardiovascular and congestive heart failure (pulmonary edema, enlarged heart especially the left atrium, left heart failure, pulmonary emboli, mitral valve insufficiency).
- **A**llergic (bronchial asthma, eosinophilic pneumonia or granulomatosis, pulmonary infiltrate with eosinophilia).
- **T**rauma (foreign body, irritating gases, collapsing trachea, hypoplastic trachea).
- **N**eoplasia (not only of respiratory tree but associated structures such as ribs, lymph nodes, muscles).
- **I**nflammatory (pharyngitis, tonsillitis, kennel cough from such agents as *Bordetella bronchoseptica*, parainfluenza virus, infectious laryngotracheitis virus, and mycoplasma, systemic fungal pneumonia, bacterial bronchopneumonia, aspiration, chronic pulmonary fibrosis, pulmonary abscess or granuloma, chronic obstructive pulmonary disease).
- **P**arasites (*Capillaria aerophila*, *Oslerus [Filaroides] osleri*, *Filaroides hirthi*, *F. milksi*, *Paragonimus kellicotti*, *Dirofilaria immitis*—heartworm disease).
- Differentiated from canine heartworm disease (causes by *D. immitis*) based on L1 of *A. vasorum* in feces, absence of *D. immitis* antigen or microfilaria in blood in a dog with radiographic signs consistent with heartworm disease.

■ **Fig. 3-1** Lateral (**A**) and DV (**B**) thoracic radiograph showing typical changes of severe angiostrongylus infestation including increased prominence of the main pulmonary artery, enlarged lobar and peripheral pulmonary arteries, perivascular parenchymal disease, and right ventricular enlargement. These signs must be distinguished from those caused by heartworm disease (*Dirofilaria immitis*).

DIAGNOSTICS

- CBC—anemia of chronic disease, thrombocytopenia.
- Thoracic radiographs—show similar signs as heartworm disease *(Figs. 3-1a and 1b)* and may include increased prominence of the main pulmonary artery, enlarged lobar and peripheral pulmonary arteries, and perivascular parenchymal disease especially in the caudal lung lobes.
- Right ventricular enlargement may be seen in severe cases.

Diagnostic Feature
- **L1 larvae—identified in transtracheal wash samples and fecal samples using the Baermann technique** *(Fig. 3-2).*
- L1 larvae have a cephalic button and a kink at the end of the tail that distinguishes it from other L1 larvae found in dog's feces.
- L1 larvae of *A. vasorum* are extremely similar to the lungworm parasite of cats, *Aelurostrongylus abstrusus*; it is possible for larvae of the latter to appear in dog feces after coprophagy.

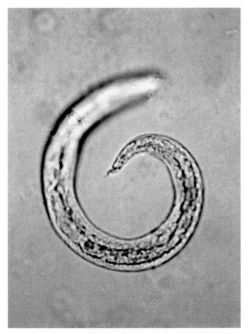

■ **Fig. 3-2** L1 larva of *A. vasorum* in the fecal sample of a dog. Note the kink in the tail making this larva similar to *Oslerus (Filaroides) osleri*. Clinical cases of *A. vasorum* invariably show abnormalities on thoracic radiographs similar to heartworm disease but not found in *Oslerus* infestations.

THERAPEUTICS

- If right sided heart failure exists, stabilize cardiac function before treating the parasite.

Drugs of Choice

- Levamisole (7.5 mg/kg, SC, or 10 mg/kg, PO, q24h for 2 days)

Precautions/Interactions

- Levamisole—not registered for use in the dog.
- Do not use levamisole with pyrantel (both are cholinergic agonist).
- Above doses should not cause toxic signs but signs of toxicity include vomiting, diarrhea, hypersalivation, increased lacrimation, miosis, frequent urination, dyspnea (due to increased respiratory secretions), muscle fasciculation, nervousness, ataxia, apprehension progressing to seizures.

COMMENTS

Abbreviations

CBC, complete blood count; DIC, disseminated intravascular coagulation; FeLV, feline leukemia virus; FIV, feline immunodeficiency virus; GIT, gastrointestinal tract; PPP, prepatent period.

Suggested Reading

Bourque A, Conboy G, Miller L, *et al. Angiostrongulus vasorum* infection in 2 dogs from Newfoundland. *Can Vet J* 2002;43:876–879.

Chapman PS, Boag AK, Guitian J, et al. Angiostrongylus vasorum infection in 23 dogs (1999–2002). *J Sm Anim Pract* 2004;45:435–440.

Author: Stephen C. Barr
Consulting Editor: Stephen C. Barr

Aspergillosis

chapter 4

DEFINITION/OVERVIEW

- An opportunistic fungal infection causing localized (nasal cavity and frontal sinuses) or disseminated disease in both dogs and cats.

ETIOLOGY/PATHOPHYSIOLOGY

- *Aspergillus* spp.—common spore-forming molds ubiquitous in the environment, especially in dust, straw, grass clippings, and hay.
- *A. fumigatus*—causes nasal aspergillosis, but *A. flavus*, *A. niger*, and *A. nidulans* have also been isolated.
- Infection—thought to occur by direct inoculation of the nasal mucosa.
- *A. terreus*—causes disseminated disease, although *A. deflectus* and *A. fumigatus* reported.
- Portal of entry unknown—possibly respiratory tract or GI tract followed by hematogenous spread.

SIGNALMENT/HISTORY

Dogs

- More commonly affected than cats, with the nasal form more common than the disseminated form.

Nasal
- Dolichocephalic and mesaticephalic breeds.
- No sex predilection.
- Outdoor dogs and farm dogs—higher prevalence.

Disseminated
- Higher prevalence in German shepherd dogs (average age: 3 years).
- More females affected than males.
- Immune defect proposed in German shepherd dogs (and their crosses).
- Geographic distribution—more commonly reported in California, Louisiana, Michigan, Georgia, Florida, and Virginia, as well as in Western Australia, Barcelona, and Milan.

Cats

- Marginally higher prevalence in Persian cats.

Disseminated
- Main category of disease in cats.
- Involves mainly the respiratory tract and/or GI tract.
- Associated with FIP, FPV, FeLV, FIV, diabetes mellitus, and chronic corticosteroid and antibiotic administration.

Nasal
- Small number of cases reported.
- Usually involves frontal (occasionally orbital) sinuses as well.

 # CLINICAL FEATURES

Dogs

Nasal
- Chronic unilateral or bilateral sanguinopurulent (occasionally serous early or mucopurulent) nasal discharge unresponsive to antibiotics—most common sign.
- Sneezing.
- Nasal pain.
- Epistaxis.
- Inappetance.
- Lethargy.
- Depigmentation or ulceration—common around external nares (but not pathognomonic).
- CNS signs—if cribriform plate involved.

Disseminated
- Usually acute onset.
- May develop gradually over several months.
- Often spinal pain (fungal diskospondylitis).
- Lameness (fungal osteomyelitis).
- Neurologic signs (brain or spinal cord involvement).
- Polyuria/polydipsia.
- Hematuria (renal involvement).
- Uveitis (ocular involvement).
- Nonspecific signs of systemic infection—fever, weight loss, vomiting, lymphadenopathy, anorexia.

Cats

Nasal
- Mucopurulent nasal discharge.
- Sneezing.
- Stertor.

Disseminated
- Nonspecific signs—lethargy, depression, vomiting, diarrhea.
- Ocular signs—exophthalmos.

 DIFFERENTIAL DIAGNOSIS

Nasal

- Neoplasia; foreign body; bacterial rhinitis/sinusitis; penicilliosis; *Pneumonyssoides caninum* (nasal mite—dogs); nasopharyngeal polyps (cats); nasal cryptococcosis (cats); dental disease.

Disseminated

- Bacterial osteomyelitis/diskospondylitis (due mainly to *Staphylococcus* or *Brucella* spp.—dogs); spinal neoplasia; intervertebral disk disease; skeletal neoplasia; bacterial pyelonephritis; bacterial pneumonia; and other causes of uveitis (toxoplasmosis, leptospirosis); and other systemic fungal diseases (blastomycosis, histoplasmosis).

 DIAGNOSTICS

Nasal

- CBC—neutrophilic leukocytosis and monocytosis.
- Nasal radiographs—increased radiolucency in affected rostral and maxillary nasal turbinate area (turbinate lysis), especially on open-mouth ventrodorsal and skyline views of frontal sinuses; mixed densities seen due to turbinate destruction and soft tissue dense fungal granulomas or accumulated nasal discharge.
- CT and MRI—accurately define extent of disease and allow assessment of the integrity of the cribriform plate; important when considering treatment with local infusion of antifungal agents (*Fig. 4-1*).
- Rhinoscopy—directly visualize fungal granulomas (*Fig. 4-2*); appreciate destruction of nasal turbinates (cavernous appearance in severe cases); collect material for culture and cytologic (*Fig. 4-3*) and histopathologic examination.
- Fungal culture—should be taken from specific lesions or may give false positive results because the organism is a common contaminant.
- Positive culture results—should be confirmed by histopathologic or cytologic examination.
- Serologic findings (agar gel double diffusion, counterimmunoelectrophoresis, ELISA)—support a diagnosis if made in conjunction with culture and evidence of disease (consistent radiographic changes in nares).
- False positive results and cross-reactivity with *Penicillium* spp. reported.

■ **Fig. 4-1** A CT scan of a dog with nasal aspergillosis beginning most rostrally (*panel 1*—level of the premolars) and moving caudally (*panel 4*—level of the frontal lobe of the brain). Note the extensive loss of turbinates, especially on the left; involvement of both frontal sinuses; an intact cribriform plate (*panel 3*); and a compressed fracture over the left frontal sinus (*panel 4*), probably the initiating cause of infection in this dog.

Diagnostic Feature

- **Histopathologic findings, or positive titer plus culture, or positive titer plus appropriate radiographic signs, or consistent cytologic findings with fungal plaques identified at rhinoscopic examination.**

Disseminated

- CBC and biochemical panel—often nonspecific and reflect organ involvement.
- Mature leukocytosis and lymphopenia (dogs) or nonregenerative anemia with leucopenia (cats).
- Test cats—for FeLV, FPV, FIP, and FIV.

■ **Fig. 4-2** *Aspergillus* fungal granulomas as viewed during rhinoscopy.

■ **Fig. 4-3** Budding heads and microconidia of *Aspergillus* as viewed on cytology.

- Hyperglobulinemia—chronic cases.
- Elevated BUN, creatine, and phosphorus with isosthenuria, hematuria, and pyuria in renal involvement.
- Fungal hyphae—in urine sediment.
- Urine sediment yield—improve detection by allowing sample to incubate at room temperature for 24 to 48 hours.
- Examine urine sediment—as a wet prep or with Diff-Quik.
- Identify hyphae—stain purple and hyphae branch at a 45-degree angle.
- Radiology—may show proliferative lesions in bones such as spine *(Fig. 4-4).*

 THERAPEUTICS

Nasal

- Systemic antifungal agents (fluconazole, itraconazole)—of limited success unless cribriform plate is breached (as shown on CT or MRI).

■ **Fig. 4-4** Lateral radiographic view of proliferative lesions on the ventral body of thoracic vertebrae in a dog with systemic aspergillosis.

- Topical therapy—clotrimazole infused into the nasal and sinus cavities for 1 hour under general anesthesia is method of choice (although some still prefer enilconazole).

Method of Nasal Antifungal Therapy
- Prepare patient—general anesthesia with well-fitting cuffed endotracheal tube in place.
- Occlude caudal nares by placement of an appropriate-sized Foley catheter (24 French for average-sized dog) in caudal nasopharynx dorsal to soft palate.
- Author prefers using 2 × 2 gauze sponges held in place by monofilament nylon thread placed as follows:
  - Pass the tip of a 1-meter length of nylon suture (no. 3 Supramid Extra II) into the holes of a RRF tube (8 French, 16 inch), which acts as a carrier for the nylon suture material.
  - Pass the RRF tube into the nares on the medioventral floor of the nasal cavity until it can be visualized using a laryngoscope in the oropharynx.
  - Snare the nylon suture with forceps and pull out through the mouth; there is now nylon thread passing from the nares, around the soft palate, and out the mouth.
  - In the center of the nylon thread, tie two 2 × 2 dry gauze sponges and pull them back into the nasophaynx until they are firmly lodged. They are held in place by clamping the nylon thread extending out of the nares in place.
  - The nylon thread exiting the mouth is used to pull the gauze sponges out of the nasopharynx once the procedure is completed.
  - The back of the pharynx may be packed with more gauze sponges (to catch leaks) tied together with nylon thread that protrudes from the mouth for easy retrieval.
- Lavage both nasal cavities (via a 10 French RRF tube)—use warmed saline (sometimes with 1% Lugol's iodine added) to physically remove mucopurulent material and mildly irritate nasal mucosa.
- Drain well—air can be gently blown into the nares to dry.
- Place dog in dorsal recumbancy with the nasal opening uppermost (pointing to the ceiling).
- Fill nasal cavities and sinuses with clotrimazole solution and maintain full for 1 hour.
- Average dog requires 50 to 60 ml clotrimazole for each side.
- Once the nasal cavity is full, obstruct the nostril (using Foley catheters—12 French, dental swabs, or tampons) and rotate the head to improve the distribution of the clotrimazole to all nasal and sinus surfaces.
- Once treatment completed, after 1 hour drain clotrimazole by placing the patient in sternal recumbency, open nares to allow solution to drain rostrally, and irrigate with saline to ensure no clotrimazole remains to be swallowed when the dog wakes.
- Remove pharyngeal and nasopharyngeal gauzes through the mouth and ensure that no clotrimazole is left in the pharynx or nasopharynx.
- Treat pharyngeal or laryngeal irritation postrecovery—one dose of corticosteroids (prednisone 0.5 mg/kg).
- More than one treatment may be required.

■ **Fig. 4-5** Placement of bone marrow needles into frontal sinuses for irrigation with clotrimazole in a dog with intractable nasal aspergillosis.

- Should extensive sinus involvement be appreciated on CT or radiologic examination, irrigation of the sinuses may be indicated via needles (the author uses Jamshidi bone marrow needles) placed directly into the frontal sinuses (*Fig. 4-5*) to improve contact of clotrimazole with sinuses should nasal infusions fail.
- Surgical placement of catheters is associated with more complications.
- Enilconazole infusion can be used in place of clotrimazole (as above) or twice daily for 7 to 14 days via surgically placed frontal sinus catheters (results of single infusion do not appear to be as good as those with clotrimazole).
- Consider enilconazole for treatment failures with clotrimazole—may be associated with greater complication rate (discomfort, aspiration, dislodgement of tubes).

Drugs of Choice

Local Infusion
- Clotrimazole (Lotrimin [Schering-Plough Animal Health, Union, NJ])—30-ml bottles of 1% solution in PG.

Systemic
- Fluconazole (Diflucan [Pfizer, Exton, PA]).
- Itraconazole (Sporanox [Janssen, Titusville, NJ]) (*Table 4-1*).

Precautions/Interactions

- Lotrimin contains PG and isopropyl alcohol, which can irritate mucus membranes (larynx and ocular membranes) and has been associated with megaesophagus in some dogs if swallowed.
- Ensure that all clotrimazole has been drained out of nares before recovering dog from general anesthesia.

TABLE 4-1. Drug Therapy for Systemic Aspergillosis					
Drug	**Formulations (mg)**	**Dose (mg/kg)**	**Route**	**Interval (Hours)**	**Duration (Weeks)[a]**
Fluconazole (Diflucan)	50, 100, 200 tabs powder for oral suspension	1.25–2.5	PO	12	8
Itraconazole (Sporanox)	100 capsules Solution–100 mg/10 ml	5	PO	12	8

[a] Continue at least 2 weeks after clinical recovery.

- Protect eyes during procedure using a generous coating of Paralube or antibiotic ointment in each eye.
- If Lotrimin enters subcutaneous tissues during infusion via needles or catheters placed into the frontal sinuses, facial tissues will swell dramatically and be painful for 24 hours, after which resorption and recovery is uncomplicated.
- Clotrimazole may prolong the recovery from pentobarbital anesthesia, possibly due to hepatic microsomal enzyme inhibitory effects.
- Nasal topical infusion with any drug is contraindicated if the CT shows a damaged cribriform plate; systemic therapy should be attempted.
- Monitor liver enzymes in animals receiving long-term itraconazole and fluconazole.

 # COMMENTS

- Local infusion with clotrimazole—approximately 90% success rate.
- Success rate can be improved—perform second clotrimazole infusion 2 weeks after the first if severe extensive nasal and sinus involvement is identified at the first visit.
- Persistent cases in which the cribriform plate remains intact should be infused every 2 weeks for four treatments.
- Rhinotomy and turbinectomy should be considered in persistent cases.
- Cats with nasal aspergillosis are best treated with rhinotomy and turbinectomy followed by itraconazole or fluconazole systemic therapy.
- Topical application of clotrimazole has not been reported in the cat but may be contraindicated because the PG carrier could be toxic to cats.
- Prognosis of disseminated aspergillosis (especially in German shepherd dogs) is poor.
- Long-term systemic therapy with itraconazole or fluconazole may alleviate clinical signs in disseminated cases but seldom results in a cure.

Abbreviations

BUN, blood urea nitrogen; CBC, complete blood count; CNS, central nervous system; CT, computed tomography; ELISA, enzyme-linked immunosorbent assay; FeLV, feline leukemia virus; FIP, feline infectious peritonitis; FIV, feline immunodeficiency virus; FPV, feline panleukopenia virus; GI, gastrointestinal; MRI, magnetic resonance imaging; PG, propylene glycol; RRF, red rubber feeding.

Suggested Reading

Davidson A, Mathews KG. Nasal aspergillosis: treatment with clotrimazole. *J Am Anim Hosp Assoc* 1997;33:475–476.

Kelly SE, Shaw SE, Clark WT. Long-term survival of four dogs with disseminated *Aspergillus terreus* treated with itraconazole. *Aust Vet J* 1995;72:311–313.

Mathews KG, Davidson AP, Koblik PD, et al. Comparison of topical administration of clotrimazole through surgically placed versus non-surgically placed catheters for treatment of nasal aspergillosis in dogs: 60 cases (1990–1996). *J Am Vet Med Assoc* 1998;213:501–506.

Author: Stephen C. Barr
Consulting Editor: Stephen C. Barr

chapter 5

Astrovirus Infection

DEFINITION/OVERVIEW

- A rare intestinal viral infection of cats causing enteritis and diarrhea.

ETIOLOGY/PATHOPHYSIOLOGY

- *Astrovirus*—a small non-enveloped, RNA virus
- More than one serotype may infect cats.
- Probably causes disease by killing the enterocytes on the villus tips.

SIGNALMENT/HISTORY

- No sex, breed, or age predilection, although kittens show more severe disease when infected.
- May affect both adults and kittens in a cattery situation.
- EM of feces from normal cats (irrespective of age)—suggests that astrovirus may be present in 5% to 10% of fecal samples of normal cats.
- Disease incidence—extremely low.

CLINICAL FEATURES

- Small bowel diarrhea often green and watery, may persist from 4 to 14 days.
- Diarrhea (with or without vomiting) may be severe and acute enough to produce dehydration, and anorexia.

DIFFERENTIAL DIAGNOSIS

- Other causes of acute small bowel diarrhea including the following:
  - Dietary indiscretion.
  - Inflammatory bowel disease.
  - Food intolerance and allergy.
  - Neoplasia (especially GI lymphoma).

- Drugs (antibiotics).
- Toxins (lead).
- Parasites (giardiasis, cryptosporidiosis, tritrichomoniasis).
- Infectious agents (panleukopenia, FIP, salmonellosis, enteric calici virus, rotavirus).
- Systemic organ dysfunction (renal, hepatic, pancreatic, cardiac).
- Metabolic (hyperthyroidism).

DIAGNOSTICS

- CBC—is normal.
- Serum biochemical profile—see mild acidosis from dehydration.
- EM of negatively stained preparations of diarrheic feces—reveals characteristic viral particles (5- to 6-pointed star-shaped surface pattern—30 nm diameter) *(Fig. 5-1)*.

THERAPEUTICS

- Aim of therapy—to control dehydration while seroconversion occurs to eliminate viral infection.
- If vomiting present—NPO with parenteral fluids (some cases are mild enough that subcutaneous fluids (0.9% saline with KCl added to 30 U/L) will suffice.
- Antibiotic therapy—not usually indicated unless fever develops, in which case use broad-spectrum coverage, and investigate other causes.

Drugs of Choice

- N/A.

■ **Fig. 5-1** Electron microscopy image of *Astrovirus* in the feces of a cat. Note the distinctive star-shaped surface pattern of each viral particle (bar = 100 nm).

Precautions/Interactions

- No vaccine is available.
- Affected cats should be isolated from others to prevent spread.

 COMMENTS

- Diarrhea—usually not severe enough to warrant treatment, and most healthy cats recover quickly without the need for veterinary care.
- If diarrhea persists—investigate exacerbating conditions or other causes (FIV, FeLV, inflammatory bowel disease, concurrent GI infections such as giardiasis).
- Recent sequence analysis of human and mammalian astroviruses suggests that animal-to-human transmission does not occur.

Abbreviations

CBC, complete blood count; EM, electron microscopy; FeLV, feline leukemia virus; FIP, feline infectious peritonitis; FIV, feline immunodeficiency virus; GI, gastrointestinal; NPO, nothing per os; RNA, ribonucleic acid.

Suggested Reading

Harbour DA, Ashley CR, Williams PD, et al. Natural and experimental astrovirus infection of cats. *Vet Rec* 1987;120:555–557.

Lukashov VV, Goudsmit J. Evolutionary relationships among Astroviridae. *J Gen Virol* 2002;83:1397–1405.

Marshall JA, Kennett ML, Rodger SM, et al. Virus and virus-like particles in the feces of cats with and without diarrhea. *Aust Vet J* 1987;64:100–105.

Author: Fred W. Scott
Consulting Editor: Stephen C. Barr

chapter 6

Babesiosis

DEFINITION/OVERVIEW

- A protozoal disease (genus *Babesia*) of dogs and cats in which merozoites (piroplasms) infect RBCs.
- Degree of illness usually dependent on the severity and rate of anemia development.
- Anemia mainly as a result of immune-mediated hemolysis but also due to direct piroplasm damage to RBCs.

ETIOLOGY/PATHOPHYSIOLOGY

- Infection (by tick transmission, transplacental, or by blood transfusion) followed by 2-week incubation period during which piroplasms infect and multiply in RBCs, resulting in RBC damage mainly from immune-mediated processes but also direct RBC lysis.

Dogs

- Large (4 to 7 μm).
- *B. canis* distributed worldwide; three subspecies based on biologic, genetic, and geographic distribution.
  - *B. canis vogeli*—United States, Africa, Asia, Australia.
  - *B. canis rossi*—Africa (most virulent subspecies).
  - *B. canis canis*—Europe, areas of Asia.
- Small (2 to 5 μm); three genetically distinct subspecies.
  - *B. gibsoni*—worldwide distribution (especially Asia), but an emerging disease in the United States.
  - *B. gibsoni* (California: genetically distinct form)—infects only dogs and reported only in California.
  - *Theileria annae* (Spanish dog piroplasm)—reported in Spain and Europe.

Cats

- Small (2 to 5 μm)—*B. felis* reported in Africa.

SIGNALMENT/HISTORY

- History of tick attachment.
- History of recent dog bite wound may be a risk for *B. gibsoni* (Asia) infection.
- Any age or breed of dog can be infected.
- Severity of disease—depends on the strain of the organism and the age and breed of the animal.
- *B. canis* infections—more prevalent in greyhounds (United States).
- *B. gibsoni* (Asia) infections—more prevalent in American pit bull terriers (United States).
- Southern Asia and Africa—any age or breed dog or cat can be infected.
- United States—cats often infected with a closely related organism (*Cytauxzoon felis*).

 CLINICAL FEATURES

Dogs

- Peracute, acute, chronic, or asymptomatic (in some carrier animals).
- Splenectomy and immunosuppression—severely worsen disease (*B. canis rossi*) or makes it apparent (*B. canis* in the United States).
- Immunosuppression—may result in an increase in parasitemia and manifestation of clinical signs in chronically infected dogs (*B. canis* in the United States).
- Most severe disease—caused by *B. gibsoni* in the United States and *B. canis rossi* in Africa.
- *B. canis*—rarely causes clinical disease in the United States.
- Signs include the following:
  - Lethargy.
  - Anorexia.
  - Weight loss.
  - Pale mucous membranes *(Fig. 6-1)*.
  - Fever.
  - Splenomegaly.
  - Lymphadenopathy.
  - Hemoglobinemia/uria.
  - Icterus *(Fig. 6-2)*.
  - GI signs—some dogs develop vomiting, diarrhea, dark feces (from increased bilirubin excretion).
  - Cerebral babesiosis—weakness, disorientation, collapse (*B. canis rossi* in Africa).
  - Renal/urologic disease—results in renal failure (*B. canis rossi* in Africa).

Cats

- Similar to dogs.
- Lethargy.
- Anorexia.

■ **Fig. 6-1** Pale mucous membranes typical of anemia is often found in dogs with *Babesia gibsoni* infections.

- Pale mucus membranes.
- Icterus.

 DIFFERENTIAL DIAGNOSIS

- Immune-mediated diseases—hemolytic anemia, ITP, ehrlichiosis, RMSF, haemobartonellosis, cytauxzoonosis, SLE.

■ **Fig. 6-2** Icterus in a dog with *Babesia gibsoni* usually indicates acute infection with marked intravascular hemolysis.

- Non–immune-mediated diseases—hemolytic anemia; heartworm caval syndrome, zinc toxicity, splenic torsion, Heinz body anemia, DIC, PK deficiency, PFK deficiency.
- Causes of jaundice—hepatic or posthepatic disease (obstruction or rupture of biliary tract).

 DIAGNOSTICS

Complete Blood Count

- Mild to severe (packed cell volume <10%) regenerative anemia.
- Peracute—animal may present before a regenerative response has time to occur.
- Anemia—may not be present in all cases (e.g., carriers: greyhounds with *B. canis* in the United States).
- Thrombocytopenia—usually moderate to severe, and can occur without anemia).
- Variable leukocytosis or leukopenia.

Biochemical Profile/Urinalysis

- Hyperbilirubinemia/uria—if hemolysis acute and severe (African rather than U.S. cases).
- Hyperglobulinemia—common in chronic cases (sometimes the only blood chemistry abnormality in these cases).
- Mildly elevated liver enzymes—due to anemia/hypoxia.
- Renal failure and metabolic acidosis (*B. canis rossi* in Africa).
- Bilirubinuria—common.
- Hemoglobinuria—detected less commonly in the United States than in Africa.

Other Tests

- Microscopic examination of stained thin or thick blood smears—can provide definitive diagnosis, but sensitivity depends on experience of microscopist; modified Wright's stain best for viewing organism; blood from peripheral capillary (ear prick) may improve sensitivity; does not differentiate subspecies using microscopy.
  - *B. canis*—large piriforms within RBCs but also ring forms *(Fig. 6-3)*.
  - *B. gibsoni*—smaller and often single forms are found per RBC *(Fig. 6-4)*.
- Serologic examination—IFA; false negative results in young dogs; does not differentiate species and subspecies; use if microscopic examination negative with high clinical suspicion of disease.
- PCR—tests for the presence of *Babesia* DNA in a biologic sample (usually EDTA-anticoagulated whole blood), and can differentiate subspecies and species
  - More sensitive than microscopy.
  - Only available from one place in the United States (North Carolina State University, School of Veterinary Medicine, 4700 Hillsborough Street, Raleigh, NC).

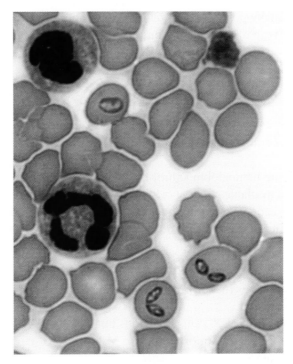

■ **Fig. 6-3** Red blood cells containing the typical piriform and ring forms of *Babesia canis* (Wright's stain).

■ **Fig. 6-4** Red blood cells (RBCs) containing the typical piriform and ring forms of *Babesia gibsoni*. Note the nucleated RBC and polychromasia typical of a regenerating anemia often seen in dogs with *B. gibsoni* (Wright's-Giemsa stain, 1500×).

■ Coombs' test—usually positive result in dogs with babesiosis, making it necessary to perform other tests to distinguish it from other causes of anemia.

 THERAPEUTICS

■ Anemic patients—transfusion of whole blood or packed RBCs (for loss of RBC mass).
■ Polymerized bovine hemoglobin solution—may be used in some anemic animals if fresh blood is not available.
■ Severely affected patients—require aggressive fluid therapy for hypovolemic shock from blood loss (usually as a result of thrombocytopenia with bleeding).

Drugs of Choice

■ Imidocarb dipropionate (Imizol [Schering-Plough]).
  • Preferred therapy.
  • May completely clear *B. canis* infections but usually not *B. gibsoni* (Asia).
  • Decrease morbidity and mortality.
■ Diminazine aceturate.
  • Not readily available in the United States and not FDA approved.
  • Efficacy similar to that of imidocarb dipiropionate.
■ Metronidazole, clindamycin, and doxycycline.
  • Decrease clinical signs but do not clear infection.
■ Azithromycin—give in combination with atovaquone.
  • Effective in treating *Babesia* infections in humans and mice.
■ Primaquine phosphate—preferred treatment of cats with *B. felis*.
■ Prednisone—treat immune-mediated component of anemia (*Table 6-1*).

TABLE 6-1. Drug Therapy for Babesiosis in Dogs

Drug	Dose (mg/kg)	Route	Interval (Hours)	Duration (Days)
Imidocarb dipropionate	5.0–6.6	IM or SC	14 days	2 doses
Diminazine aceturate	3.5–7.0	IM or SC	14 days	2 doses
Metronidazole	25–50	PO	12	7
Clindamycin	12.5–25	PO	12	7–10
Doxycycline	10	PO	12	7–10
Azithromycin	10	PO	24	10
Atovaquone[a]	13.3	PO	8	10
Primaquine phosphate	1	IM	Once	
Prednisone	1	PO	12	5

[a] Give in combination with azithromycin.

Precautions/Interactions

- Imidocarb and diminazene.
  - May cause pain and swelling at injection site, hypersalivation, nasal drip, shivering, increased lacrimation, diarrhea, vomiting, periorbital edema similar to that with organophosphate toxicity (has inherent anticholinesterase activity).
  - Do not use these drugs simultaneously with other anticholinesterase agents; side effects can be minimized by administering atropine pretreatment.
  - High doses of antibabesial drugs may cause liver and renal damage.
- Metronidazole—higher doses, >30 mg/kg, can be associated with neurologic toxicity.

 COMMENTS

- Imidocarb—current treatment of choice for babesiosis in dogs; few side effects when treated.
- It is particularly important to warn owners that the treatment may not completely remove the parasite from the body.

Abbreviations

DIC, disseminated intravascular coagulation; DNA, deoxyribonucleic acid; EDTA, ethylenediamine tetra-acetic acid; GI, gastrointestinal; IFA, immunofluorescent antibody assay; ITP, idiopathic thrombocytopenic purpura; PCR, polymerase chain reaction; PFK, phosphofructokinase; PK, pyruvate kinase, RBCs, red blood cells; RMSF, Rocky Mountain spotted fever; SLE, systemic lupus erythematosus.

Suggested Reading

Birkenheuer AJ, Neel J, Ruslander D, et al. Detection and molecular characterization of a novel large *Babesia* species in a dog. *Vet Parasitol* 2004;124:151–160.

Birkenheuer AJ, Levy MG, Breitschwert EB. Development and evaluation of a seminested PCR for detection and differentiation of *Babesia gibsoni* (Asian genotype) and *B. canis* DNA in canine blood samples. *J Clin Microbiol* 2003;41:4172–4177.

Boozer AL, Macintire DK. Canine babesiosis. *Vet Clin North Am Small Anim Pract* 2003;33:885–904.

Meinkoth JH, Kocan AA, Loud SD, et al. Clinical and hematologic effects of experimental infections with recently identified *Babesia gibsoni*-like isolates from Oklahoma. *J Am Vet Med Assoc* 2002;220:185–189.

Author: Adam J. Birkenheuer
Consulting Editor: Stephen C. Barr

chapter 7

Balantidiasis

DEFINITION/OVERVIEW

- A protozoal infection usually of pigs that occasionally infects the colon of dogs (and humans) to produce a hemorrhagic diarrhea.

ETIOLOGY/PATHOPHYSIOLOGY

- *Balantidium coli*—large ciliated protozoan found throughout the world, infecting mainly pigs.
- *B. coli* trophozoites—inhabit the colon, producing cysts that are passed in the feces to infect other species, including dogs but not cats.
- Invasion of the layer between the mucosa and submucosa results in colonic ulceration with hemorrhagic diarrhea.
- Certain colonic bacteria and infection with whipworms (*Trichuris vulpis*) may predispose commensal *B. coli* infection to become pathogenic.
- Extraintestinal invasion of *B. coli* is very rare, unlike that of amebiasis.

SIGNALMENT/HISTORY

- History of contact of dogs with swine (which are usually asymptomatic).

CLINICAL FEATURES

- Clinical signs of hemorrhagic colitis:
  - Mucoid bloody diarrhea.
  - Increased frequency of defecation.
  - Chronic weight loss.

DIFFERENTIAL DIAGNOSIS

- Causes of bloody diarrhea or tenesmus, including constipation; food intolerance/allergy; parasitism (whipworms, leishmaniasis, amebiasis); HGE; foreign body; irritable bowel syndrome; inflammatory bowel disease; diverticula; infectious (parvovirus, clostridial enteritis, bacterial overgrowth and other bacterial causes, fungal such as histoplasmosis or blastomycosis); neoplasia; ulcerative colitis; endocrinopathy (Addison's disease); occasionally major organ disease such as renal failure causing colonic ulceration.

DIAGNOSTICS

- Fecal flotation (using ZSCT) may detect trophozoites *(Fig. 7-1)* and *B. coli* cysts *(Fig. 7-2)*.
- Staining to reveal the macronucleus of both cysts and trophozoites using acidic methyl green (1 g methyl green mixed with 1 ml glacial acetic acid and 100 ml water) is preferred.

Diagnostic Feature
- **Fresh fecal smear mixed with normal saline often show trophozoites.**

THERAPEUTICS

- Few reports of treatment of *B. coli* exist in the literature.
- In humans—metronidazole and tetracyclines have been effective.

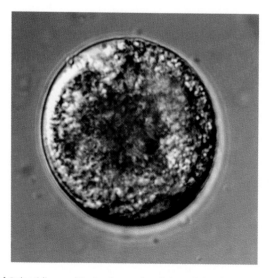

■ **Fig. 7-1** Trophozoite of *Balantidium coli* in the feces of an infected dog (Giemsa stain, 1500×).

■ **Fig. 7-2** Cyst of *Balantidium coli* in a fecal smear from an infected dog (1000×).

Drugs of Choice

- Metronidazole.
- Tetracycline *(Table 7-1).*

Precautions/Interactions

- High doses for extended periods of metronidazole may cause neurologic signs in dogs.

 COMMENTS

- Excreted *B. coli* cysts in the feces of infected dogs—source of infection to humans and other dogs.
- Unlike pigs, dogs do not constitute a significant reservoir of infection for humans.

TABLE 7-1. Drug Therapy for Balantidiasis in Dogs				
Drug	Dose (mg/kg)	Route	Interval (Hours)	Duration (Days)
Metronidazole (Flagyl)	15–30	PO	12	7
Tetracycline[a]	22	PO	8	10

[a] Many generic formulations.

Abbreviations

HGE, hemorrhagic gastroenteritis; ZSCT, zinc sulfate concentration technique.

Suggested Reading

Barr SC. Balantidiasis. In: Greene CE, ed. *Infectious Diseases of the Dog and Cat.* Philadelphia: WB Saunders; 1998:489–490.

Author: Stephen C. Barr
Consulting Editor: Stephen C. Barr

chapter 8

Bartonellosis

DEFINITION/OVERVIEW

- An intracellular bacterial infection of cats and dogs—various bacterial species cause different syndromes from bacteremia in cats to endocarditis in dogs.
- Human syndromes—includes CSD (regional lymphadenopathy after a cat scratch), bacillary peliosis, bacillary angiomatosis, relapsing fever with bacteremia, encephalitis, meningitis, neuroretinitis, and endocarditis.
- Distribution—worldwide.
- Estimated 25,000 human cases per year in the United States—but few fatalities.
- Seasonal in human cases—most reported in summer months.

ETIOLOGY/PATHOPHYSIOLOGY

- Fastidious hemotropic gram-negative rod bacterium.
- *Bartonella* is thought to invade and multiply within RBCs.
- At least one *Bartonella* species (and probably others) produces a factor that causes vascular endothelial proliferation, a feature of human syndromes—bacillary angiomatosis, bacillary splenic peliosis, and peliosis hepatis.

Cats

- Infected with four *Bartonella* species—*B. henselae*, *B. clarridgeiae*, *B. koehlerae*, and *B. bovis*.
- 10% of cats with *Bartonella* bacteremia—due to *B. clarridgeiae*.
- *B. koehlerae* and *B. bovis*—only a few case reports.
- Mixed infections—of *B. henselae* (which contains at least two subgroups) and *B. clarridgeiae* occur.
- Transmission—via cat fleas (*Ctenocephalides felis felis*), but exact role not yet determined.
- Transmission—does not occur without the presence of infected fleas.
- Bacteremia with *B. henselae* and *B. clarridgeiae*—chronic and recurrent.
- *Bartonella* organisms have been seen within RBCs, in blood and other tissues—but other locations within the body may occur.

Dogs

- Infected with four *Bartonella* species—*B. vinsonii* subsp. *berkhoffii*, *B. henselae*, *B. clarridgeiae*, and *B. elizabethae*.
- Ticks and fleas—may be vectors for transmission of *B. vinsonii* subsp. *berkhoffii* to dogs.
- *B. vinsonii* subsp. *berkhoffii*—experimentally, causes no clinical signs but mild immunosuppression and persistent bacteremias (up to 247 days).
- Natural cases—rare disease caused by *B. henselae* (peliosis hepatis) and *B. vinsonii* subsp. *berkhoffii* (endocarditis, granulomatous rhinitis, and granulomatous lymphadenitis).

 SIGNALMENT/HISTORY

Cats

- Seroprevalence highest for *B. henselae*—worldwide occurrence.
- Highest seroprevalence—in warm humid climates, older cats, and those most exposed to fleas.
- Prevalence of bacteremia in cats in the United States—5% to 40% (highest in warm humid climates).
- Flea infestation—appears to be necessary for the transmission of *B. henselae* from cats to humans, but direct transmission to humans via a flea bite is speculative.
- Until recently—was not thought to cause disease in the cat.

Dogs

- Seroprevalence of *B. henselae*—approximately 3% to 9% in the United States.
- High seroprevalence in coyotes for *B. vinsonii* subsp. *berkhoffii*—approximately 25% to 75%, suggesting they may be the reservoir host for this species.
- Endocarditis cases—variable, but often include weight loss, syncope, collapse, and sudden death.
- Hepatic disease—depression, weight loss, and vomiting.

 CLINICAL FEATURES

Cats

- In natural cases—clinical signs are rare and include uveitis and possibly lymphadenopathy.
- In experimentally infected cats—most remained asymptomatic for over a year, in spite of persistent infection.
- After intradermal inoculation of *B. henselae*—develop abscess at inoculation site, lymphadenomegaly, periodic fever, and mild neurologic signs (nystagmus, whole body tremors, focal motor seizures, and behavior changes).
- Histologic lesions—include peripheral lymph node hyperplasia, splenic follicular hyperplasia, lymphocytic cholangitis/pericholangitis, lymphocytic hepatitis, lymphoplasmacytic myocarditis, and interstitial lymphocytic nephritis.

- Reproductive failure—has occurred in some cats infected experimentally with *B. henselae*.
- Experimental infections with *B. koehlerae*—no clinical signs.
- Cats with FIV and bartonellosis—may have more lymphadenopathy and gingivitis than just cats with FIV alone.
- Bartonellosis may increase incidence of stomatitis and UTIs in cats.
- To date—*Bartonella* infections have not been verified to cause chronic illness in cats.

Dogs

- *B. vinsonii* subsp. *berkhoffii*—associated with endocarditis, cardiac arrhythmias, granulomatous rhinitis, and granulomatous lymphadenopathy.
- Dogs experimentally infected with *B. vinsonii* subsp. *berkhoffii*—show no clinical signs (transient fever in some).
- *B. henselae*—identified by PCR in the liver of a dog with peliosis hepatis; another with granulomatous hepatitis.

Humans

- Erythematous papule at inoculation site (scratch, bite)—then unilateral regional lymphadenopathy (painful, often suppurative) in 3 to 10 days (>90% of cases).
- Symptoms—mild fever, chills (infrequent), anorexia, myalgia, and nausea.
- Atypical manifestations (usually in immunosuppressed patients, in up to 25% of cases)—encephalopathy (1% to 7%), palpebral conjunctivitis (3% to 5%), meningitis, osteolytic lesions, granulomatous hepatitis, and pneumonia.

 # DIFFERENTIAL DIAGNOSIS

- Other causes of endocarditis—bacterial.
- Other causes of hepatic dysfunction—differentiate from other causes by ruling out other causes of dysfunction and demonstrating *Bartonella* organisms associated with pathology.

 # DIAGNOSTICS

- Diagnosis of a disease caused by *Bartonella* is not easy because so many healthy animals are seropositve and PCR-positive.
- CBC, serum biochemistry, urinalysis—noncontributory, although may show elevations of hepatic enzymes in dogs with liver syndromes.
- Serologic assays—IFA test and ELISA are available, but value is questionable given that 12% of cats with *B. henselae* bacteremia are seronegative, and many animals that have cleared the bacteremia are seropositive.
- The positive predictive value of a positive serologic test for bacteremia is low in cats (40% to 45%)—the positive predictive value of a negative serologic test is high (90% to 97%).

■ **Fig. 8-1** Aspirate from the lymph node of a human with cat scratch fever and local lymphadenophathy showing bacillus bacteria (Warthin-Starry silver stain, 1,000×).

- Predictive value for serology tests in dogs—not assessed, but in coyotes, negative (29%) and positive (73%) predictive values are lower than in cats.
- Blood or tissue culture—use 1 to 2 mL EDTA blood (freeze to release organisms from RBCs) in enriched blood containing media—positive in 1 to 3 weeks.

Diagnostic Feature
- **Blood culture—is the most reliable definitive test for detecting active infection in cats; may need to perform several due to relapsing nature of bacteremia.**
- Blood culture in dogs—considered insensitive because endocarditis cases are usually negative; need to culture heart valve.
- PCR assay of blood—no more sensitive than cultures.
- PCR assays—available through some laboratories (e.g., North Carolina State and UC Davis).
- PCR results—advantages over blood culture are that it is usually quicker and can detect species of *Bartonella* involved.
- In humans—may see bacillus in lymph node aspirates using Warthin-Starry silver stain (*Fig. 8-1*).

 THERAPEUTICS

Humans

- Supportive treatment, including bed rest and heat on swollen lymph nodes.
- Doxycycline, erythromycin, and rifampin are recommended.
- Treat for 2 weeks in immunocompetent, 6 weeks in immunocompromised, individuals.

TABLE 8-1. Drug Therapy for Bartonellosis in Dogs and Cats				
Drug	Dose (mg/kg)	Route	Interval (Hours)	Duration (Weeks)
Enrofloxacin (Baytril)	5	PO	12	4–6
Doxycycline (Vibramycin)	5–10	PO	12	4–6
Azithromycin (Zithromax)	5–15	PO	12	4–6

Cats

- Efficacy of antibiotics much worse in cats than in humans.
- Indication for treating infected cats with no clinical signs is questionable.
- Treat only those cats showing clinical signs of disease.
- If treated, follow-up blood cultures (taken 3 weeks after antimicrobial therapy had been discontinued) are needed to confirm treatment success.
- Control fleas.

Dogs

- Dogs with clinical signs and that are seropositive—treat with antibiotics.

Drugs of Choice

- Enrofloxacin (Baytril [Bayer, Shawnee Mission, KS]), doxycycline (Vibramycin [Pfizer, Exton, PA]) and azithromycin (Zithromax [Pfizer, Exton, PA]) are probably the drugs of choice, although there is little controlled data—treat for a minimum of 4 to 6 weeks (*Table 8-1*).

Precautions/Interactions

- In humans, thoroughly cleanse all cat scratches or bites.
- Prevent cats from contacting open wounds.
- Immunocompromised persons should avoid young cats.
- Enrofloxacin causes retinal degeneration and blindness in some cats.
- Doxycycline may cause esophagitis and stricture.
- Azithromycin—reduce dosage with hepatic or biliary dysfunction.
- Treat cats vigorously for fleas.

 COMMENTS

- The involvement of *Bartonella* spp. as a cause of significant disease in the cat is yet to be fully elucidated.
- Occasional case reports implicate some *Bartonella* spp. as causes of certain rare diseases in dogs.
- The zoonotic potential of *Bartonella* infection in dogs and cats is still uncertain.

Abbreviations

CBC, complete blood count; CSD, cat scratch disease; EDTA, ethylenediamine tetra-acetic acid; ELISA, enzyme-linked immunosorbent assay; FIV, feline immunodeficiency virus; IFA, immunofluorescent antibody test; PCR, polymerase chain reaction; RBCs, red blood cells; UTIs, urinary tract infections.

Suggested Reading

Breitschwerdt EB, Kordick DL. *Bartonella* infection in animals: carriership, reservoir potential, pathogenicity, and zoonotic potential for human infection. *Clin Micro Rev* 2000;13:428–438.

Guptill L. Bartonellosis. *Vet Clin North Am Small Anim Pract* 2003;33:101–110.

Mikolajczyk MG, O'Reilly KL. Clinical disease in kittens inoculated with a pathogenic strain of *Bartonella henselae. Am J Vet Res* 2000;61:375–379.

Windsor JJ. Cat-scratch disease: epidemiology, aetiology and treatment. *Br J Biomed Sci* 2001; 58:101–110.

Author: J. Paul Woods
Consulting Editor: Stephen C. Barr

chapter 9

Blastomycosis

DEFINITION/OVERVIEW

- A systemic mycotic infection affecting dogs, and rarely cats, most commonly in the Mississippi, Ohio, and Tennessee River basins.

ETIOLOGY/PATHOPHYSIOLOGY

- *Blastomyces dermatitidis*—small soil fungus.
- Small spores (conidia)—shed from the mycelial phase of the organism growing in soil.
- Conidia—inhaled and enter the terminal airway.
- At body temperature—spores become yeast, which initiate lung infection.
- From this focus of mycotic pneumonia—yeast disseminates hematogenously throughout the body.
- The immune response to the invading organism—pyogranulomatous infiltrate to control the organism, resulting in organ dysfunction.
- Of affected dogs—85% have lung disease.
- Eyes, skin, lymphatic system, and bones—commonly affected.
- CNS, testes, prostate, mammary gland, nasal cavity, gums, and vulva—less commonly affected.

SIGNALMENT/HISTORY

- Historically, most commonly reported complaints:
  - Weight loss.
  - Depressed appetite.
  - Cough or dyspnea.
  - Lameness.
  - Draining skin lesions.
- History of exposure to wet soil by rivers, streams, or lakes.
- Often history of construction or soil disturbance.

Dogs

- Breed predilection—large-breed dogs (>25 kg) most often affected, especially sporting breeds (probably reflects exposure rather than susceptibility).

- Age predilection—2 to 4 years (uncommon >7 years).
- Sex predilection—males.

Cats

- Age predilection—young to middle age.

 CLINICAL FEATURES

Dogs

- Fever up to 104°F (40°C)—approximately 50% of patients.
- Harsh, dry lung sounds associated with increased respiratory effort—common.
- Generalized or regional lymphadenopathy—with or without skin lesions.
- Uveitis—with or without secondary glaucoma and conjunctivitis, ocular exudates, corneal edema, retinal granulomas.
- Lameness—common because of fungal osteomyelitis.
- Testicular enlargement and prostatomegaly—occasionally seen.

Cats

- Increased respiratory effort.
- Granulomatous skin lesions.

 DIFFERENTIAL DIAGNOSIS

- Respiratory signs—a general differential diagnosis for respiratory signs and cough includes such categories as:
  - Cardiovascular (pulmonary edema; enlarged heart, especially the left atrium; pleural effusion; pulmonary emboli).
  - Allergic (bronchial asthma, chronic bronchitis, eosinophilic pneumonia, or granulomatosis, pulmonary infiltrate with eosinophilia).
  - Trauma (foreign body, irritating gases, collapsing trachea).
  - Neoplasia (not only of the respiratory tree but also associated structures such as ribs, lymph nodes, muscles).
  - Inflammatory (pharyngitis; tonsillitis; kennel cough from such agents as *Bordetella bronchiseptica*, parainfluenza virus, infectious laryngotracheitis virus, and mycoplasma; bacterial bronchopneumonia; chronic pulmonary fibrosis; pulmonary abscess or granuloma; chronic obstructive pulmonary disease).
  - Parasites (*Oslerus* [*Filaroides*] *osleri*, *Crenosoma vulpis*, *Capillaria aerophila*, *F. milksi*, *Paragonimus kellicotti*, *Dirofilaria immitis*—heartworm disease).
- Lymph node enlargement—similar to lymphosarcoma; differentiated by lymph node aspirate cytologic examination.
- Combination of fever and respiratory disease with eye, bone, or skin involvement in a young dog—suggests the diagnosis.

DIAGNOSTICS

- CBC—changes reflect mild to moderate inflammation (neutrophilic leukocytosis ± left shift, monocytosis).
- High serum globulins with borderline low albumin concentrations—dogs with chronic infections.
- Hypercalcemia—in some dogs, secondary to the granulomatous changes.
- *Blastomyces* yeasts—can be found in the urine of dogs with prostatic involvement.
- AGID—useful for making a diagnosis if organisms cannot be found on cytologic or histopathologic examination.
- Positive AGID—strongly supports diagnosis, with a specificity of >90%, but in endemic areas, dogs can be positive but not have disease.
- Negative AGID—common in dogs with early infection.
- Radiographic findings—lungs usually show generalized interstitial-to-nodular infiltrates *(Fig. 9-1)* with tracheobronchial lymphadenopathy (common).
- Chest radiographic findings—inconsistent with bacterial pneumonia but must be differentiated from metastatic neoplasia (especially hemangiosarcoma).
- Chylothorax secondary to blastomycosis—can occur in dogs.
- Focal lytic and proliferative radiographic bone lesions—must be differentiated from osteosarcoma.
- Cytologic findings—organisms usually (but not always) plentiful in lesions.

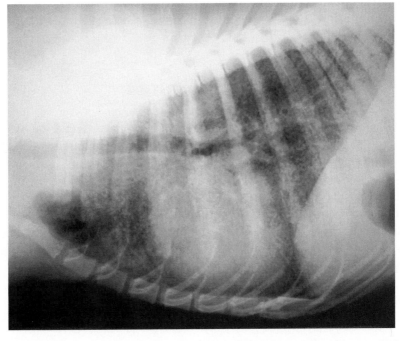

■ **Fig. 9-1** Lateral thoracic radiograph of a dog with blastomycosis showing diffuse fine interstitial-to-nodular infiltrates.

■ **Fig. 9-2** Cytologic findings of exudate from a skin lesion showing broad-based, thick-walled budding *Blastomyces* yeast cells on a background of degenerate neutrophils and red blood cells (Diff-Quik stain, 400×).

Diagnostic Feature

- **Cytology—most definitive method of diagnosis; aspirates from lymph nodes and lungs, impression smears of draining skin lesions, or tracheal wash fluid are often best sources of infective material *(Fig. 9-2)*.**
- Histopathologic findings—bone biopsies, enucleated eyes, or single firm skin pyogranulomas sometimes needed to confirm diagnosis if cytologic examination unsuccessful.
- **Do not attempt culture of lesions in-hospital, because cultures can be a source of infection to humans—send culture material out to diagnostic laboratory if culture needed.**

 ## THERAPEUTICS

- Usually outpatient—oral itraconazole treatment if patient is stable.
- Severely dyspneic dogs—require an oxygen cage for a minimum of 1 week before lung improvement is sufficient for comfort in room air.
- Many have worsening of lung disease during the first few days of treatment, owing to an increase in the inflammatory response after the *Blastomyces* organisms die and release their contents (inflammatory response may be dampened by judicious use of anti-inflammatory glucocorticoids with antifungals—use glucocorticoids judiciously).
- Removal of an abscessed lung lobe—may be required when medical treatment cannot resolve infection.

Drugs of Choice

Itraconazole
DOGS

- Give with a fat-rich meal, such as canned dog food, for the first 3 days to achieve a therapeutic blood concentration as soon as possible.

TABLE 9-1. Drug Therapy for Blastomycosis in Small Animals					
Drug	Species	Dose (mg/kg)	Route	Interval (Hours)	Duration (Days)[a]
Itraconazole	B	5	PO	12[b]	60
Fluconazole	B	5[c]	PO, IV	12	60
AMB deoxycholate	D	0.5	IV	3 times weekly	[d]
	C	0.25	IV	3 times weekly	[e]
AMB-lipid complex (Abelcet)	D	1–2.5	IV[f]	3 times weekly	[g]

[a] Continue treatment at least 30 days beyond resolution of clinical signs.
[b] Dogs—after 3 days, reduce dosing interval to q24h.
[c] Cats—up to a maximum total daily dose of 200 mg.
[d] To a total dose of 12 mg/kg.
[e] To a total dose of 4 to 10 mg/kg, or until renal toxicity occurs.
[f] IV infusion rate—2.5 mg/kg/hr.
[g] Use for 1 month or until renal toxicity occurs.
B, both cats and dogs; C, cats; D, dogs.

- Dogs with neurologic signs should be treated with amphotericin B or fluconazole.
- Treat for a minimum of 60 days or for 1 month after all signs of disease have disappeared.
- Avoid corticosteroid use unless life-threatening dyspnea is present (dexamethasone—0.2 mg/kg, q24h, for 2 to 3 days in conjunction with itraconazole treatment).

CATS
- Have drug compounded by an appropriate pharmacy or open the 100-mg capsules containing pellets and mix with palatable food.

Alternative Drugs
- Amphotericin B—use in dogs that cannot take oral medication or that do not respond to itraconazole (see Histoplasmosis).
- Lipid complex form of amphotericin B—less nephrotoxic than other forms; use in dogs with renal dysfunction that cannot take itraconazole.
- Ketoconazole (cheaper alternative to itraconazole)—lower response rate; higher rates of anorexia, malaise, and hepatopathy; and higher recurrence rate; not recommended.
- Fluconazole—more expensive but fewer side effects than other conazoles and better penetration into ocular and CNS tissues; IV preparation available.
- See *Table 9-1*.

Precautions/Interactions

Itraconazole Toxicity
- Anorexia—most common sign; attributed to liver toxicity; monitor serum ALT monthly (itraconazole induces ALT) for duration of treatment or when anorexia occurs; temporarily discontinue drug for patients with anorexia and ALT activities >200; after appetite improves, restart at half the previously used dose.
- Ulcerative dermatitis—seen in some dogs; the result of vasculitis; dose-related condition; temporarily discontinue drug; when ulcers have resolved, restart at half the previously used dose.

- Teratogenic effects of itraconazole—none reported at therapeutic doses in rats and mice; embryotoxicity found at high doses; no dog or cat studies; one dog started on itraconazole halfway through her pregnancy delivered a normal litter.

 COMMENTS

- Inform owner—treatment is costly and requires a minimum of 60 to 90 days.
- Determine duration of treatment—based on resolution of clinical signs and follow-up chest radiographs.
- Considerable permanent lung changes—may occur after the infection has resolved, making determination of persistent active disease difficult.
- At 60 days of treatment—if active lung disease is seen, continue treatment for 30 days.
- If lungs are normal—stop treatment and obtain repeat radiographs in 30 days.
- At 90 days of treatment—if condition is the same as at day 60, changes are residual.
- Fibrosis on radiographs—inactive disease; if condition is better than at day 60, continue treatment for 30 more days; if lesions are significantly worse than at 60 days, change treatment to amphotericin B and then obtain another radiograph.
- At 120 days of treatment—obtain another radiograph; continue treatment as long as there is improvement in the lungs; if there is no further improvement and no indication of active disease, the lesions are probably scarring.
- Prognosis—death; 25% of dogs die during the first week of treatment; early diagnosis improves chance of survival.
- Severity of lung involvement and invasion into the CNS affect prognosis.
- Recurrence—about 20% of dogs; usually within 3 to 6 months after completion of treatment, even with 60 to 90 days of treatment; may occur up to 15 months after treatment; a second course of itraconazole treatment will cure most patients; drug resistance to itraconazole has not been observed.
- Inform owners—there is no spread from animals to humans, except through bite wounds; inoculation of organisms from dog bites has occurred.
- Caution—avoid cuts during necropsy of infected dogs; avoid needle sticks when aspirating lesions.
- Warn clients—blastomycosis is acquired from an environmental source and that they may have been exposed at the same time as the patient; common source exposure has been documented in duck and raccoon hunters; the incidence in dogs is 10 times that in humans; encourage clients with respiratory and skin lesions to inform their physicians—they may have been exposed to blastomycosis.

Abbreviations

AGID, agar gel immunodiffusion; ALT, alanine aminotransferase; CBC, complete blood count; CNS, central nervous system.

Suggested Reading

Arceneaux KA, Taboada J, Hosgood G. Blastomycosis in dogs: 115 cases (1980–1995). *J Am Vet Med Assoc* 1998;213:658–664.

Krawiec DR, McKiernan BC, Twardock AR, et al. Use of amphotericin B lipid complex for treatment of blastomycosis in dogs. *J Am Vet Med Assoc* 1996;209:2073–2075.

Legendre AM. Blastomycosis. In: Greene CE, ed. *Infectious Diseases of the Dog and Cat*. Philadelphia: WB Saunders; 1998:371–377.

Legendre AM, Rohrbach BW, Toal RL, et al. Treatment of blastomycosis with itraconazole in 112 dogs. *J Vet Intern Med* 1996;10:365–371.

Author: Alfred M. Legendre
Consulting Editor: Stephen C. Barr

chapter 10

Bordetellosis: Cats

DEFINITION/OVERVIEW

- A contagious bacterial disease of cats (and dogs—see Infectious Canine Tracheobronchitis) primarily causing respiratory abnormalities.

ETIOLOGY/PATHOPHYSIOLOGY

- *Bordetella bronchiseptica*—a small, aerobic gram-negative coccobacillus *(Fig. 10-1)*.
- Infections spread rapidly—usually by direct contact from seemingly healthy cats to others in the same environment.
- Infected queens—may not shed organisms prepartum but serve as a source of infection to newborn kittens when shedding begins postpartum.
- Stress—may serve as a cause of shedding.

SIGNALMENT/HISTORY

- Most severe in kittens <6 weeks old, and kittens living in less than ideal hygienic conditions.
- Occurs at all ages and often with preexisting, subclinical airway disease (e.g., feline herpesvirus and calicivirus infections).
- Predisposition is seen in cats with coexisting subclinical airway disease such as congenital anomalies, chronic bronchitis, allergic bronchitis, and viral URI.
- No breed or gender predilection recognized.

CLINICAL FEATURES

- May be nonexistent, mild, or severe—for example, kittens with life-threatening pneumonia.
- Signs—usually begin ~5 days after exposure to infecting agent.
- Bacterial agent—spreads rapidly from apparently healthy cats to others in the same environment.
- Fever.

■ **Fig. 10-1** Gram stain of *Bordetella bronchiseptica.*

- Sneezing.
- Nasal discharge.
- Mandibular lymphadenopathy.
- Spontaneous or induced cough—characteristic of uncomplicated disease.

Severe Disease

- Fever—may note constant, low-grade, or fluctuating fever (39.4° to 40°C [103° to 104°F]).
- Cough—usually moist and productive.
- Nasal discharge.
- Lethargy.
- Anorexia.
- Dyspnea.
- Lung sounds—often normal, but may detect increased intensity of normal sounds, crackles, or (less frequently) wheezes.

DIFFERENTIAL DIAGNOSIS

- Specific diagnosis is difficult.
- Clinical signs mimic those seen with other respiratory disease agents.
- Several agents may be involved concurrently.
- Consider viral URI with secondary bacterial infections other than *Bordetella* (*Pasturella* spp.).
- In severe disease in the individual cat, historic exposure to point source of infection 5 days previously can help differentiate from other severe URIs.

DIAGNOSTICS

- CBC—neutrophilic leukocytosis with a left shift in cases of severe pneumonia.
- Serum chemistry profile and urinalysis—usually normal.
- Bacterial isolation from oropharyngeal swab specimens—relatively easy during active clinical disease.
- Bacterial isolation during chronic carrier state—difficult because few organisms are shed.
- Thoracic radiographs—unremarkable with uncomplicated disease.
- Radiologic examination—useful for ruling out noninfectious causes; may demonstrate an interstitial and alveolar lung pattern with a cranioventral distribution typical of bacterial pneumonia; a diffuse interstitial lung pattern typical of viral pneumonia; a mixed lung pattern (combination of alveolar, interstitial, and peribronchial lung patterns).
- Bacterial cultures by endotracheal wash or tracheobronchial lavage via bronchoscopy—helpful in ruling out other bacterial agents but is rarely indicated except in the case of chronic cough.

THERAPEUTICS

- Outpatient—strongly recommended for uncomplicated disease.
- Inpatient—strongly recommended for complicated disease or pneumonia.
- Isolation—essential to keep inpatients isolated from rest of hospital population.
- Fluid therapy—with complicated disease or pneumonia.
- Cage rest—for at least 14 to 21 days with uncomplicated disease or for at least the duration of radiographic evidence of pneumonia.

Drugs of Choice

- Antibiotic therapy—ideally, antibiotic should be selected based on culture and sensitivity results.
- Amoxicillin/clavulanic acid—good for kittens.
- Doxycycline—very effective.
- Tetracyclines—organism usually very susceptible (*Table 10-1*).
- Antimicrobial therapy—should continue for at least 10 days beyond resolution of radiographic abnormalities.

TABLE 10-1. Drug Therapy for Bordetellosis in Cats				
Drug	Dose (mg/kg)	Route	Interval (Hours)	Duration (Days)
Amoxicillin/clavulanic acid	10–20	PO	12	10–14
Doxycycline	3–5	PO, IV	12	10–14
Tetracycline	10	PO	8	10–14

Precautions/Interactions

- Tetracycline and related drugs—may cause drug-induced fever.
- Doxycycline—at high doses has been associated with esophageal stricture in cats; give with food or water.
- Amoxicillin—may cause anorexia in cats.

 COMMENTS

- Uncomplicated disease—should respond to treatment in 10 to 14 days.
- Diagnosis of uncomplicated disease—question if respiratory signs persist 14 days or more after initiating treatment.
- Severe disease—typical course of 2 to 6 weeks.
- Repeat thoracic radiography in severe cases—at least 14 days beyond resolution of all clinical signs.
- Affected cats—may shed organisms for at least 19 weeks postinfection.
- Shedding of *B. bronchiseptica* in respiratory secretions of asymptomatic carriers— accounts for the persistence of disease in catteries, animal shelters, boarding facilities, and veterinary hospitals.
- *Bordetella bronchiseptica*–infected dogs—can be a source of infection for cats.
- Cats—presumably can be a source of infection for dogs.
- Kittens in infected environment—seroconvert at 7 to 10 weeks of age.
- Mortality—mainly occurs in kittens <7 weeks of age.
- Modified live vaccine available (Protex-Bb [Intervet])—not recommended for routine use.
- Vaccination—consider for cats entering or residing in multiple-cat environments where *B. bronchiseptica* infections associated with clinical disease have been documented.

Abbreviations

CBC, complete blood count; URI, upper respiratory tract infection.

Suggested Reading

Coutts AJ, Dawson S, Binns S, et al. Studies on natural transmission of *Bordetella bronchoseptica* in cats. *Vet Microbiol* 1996;48:19–27.

Dawson S, Jones D, McCraken CM, et al. *Bordetella bronchiseptica* infection in cats following contact with infected dogs. *Vet Rec* 2000;146:46–48.

Hoskins JD, Williams J, Rohde KR, et al. The prevalence of feline *Bordetella bronchiseptica* in the respiratory tract [abstract]. *J Vet Intern Med* 1997;11:133.

Speakman AJ, Dawson S, Binns SH, et al. *Bordetella bronchiseptica* infection in the cat. *J Small Anim Pract* 1999;40:252–256.

Author: Johnny D. Hoskins
Consulting Editor: Stephen C. Barr

chapter 11

Botulism

DEFINITION/OVERVIEW

- Disease caused by ingestion of a preformed neurotoxin from a bacterium found in carrion and spoiled foodstuff (raw meat).

ETIOLOGY/PATHOPHYSIOLOGY

- *Clostridium botulinum* type C—obligate anaerobic spore-forming gram-positive rod.
- Found worldwide.
- Very resistant to disinfectants and environmental exposure.
- Botulinal neurotoxin—inhibits acetylcholine release at the neuromuscular junctions and autonomic cholinergic synapses.
- Results in diffuse neuromuscular blockade and autonomic dysfunction.

SIGNALMENT/HISTORY

- Natural cases—only described in dogs.
- Cats—experimentally susceptible, but no natural cases reported.
- Risk factor—ingestion of toxin (usually associated with eating dead decomposing birds, especially ducks).
- Clinical signs—occur within hours to 6 days of toxin ingestion.
- Several dogs within a kennel, household, or neighborhood—may be affected at once.
- Historically—may initially show vomiting/diarrhea, gastroenteritis from eating carrion.
- Acute hind limb weakness ascending to trunk—then front limb, neck, and muscles innervated by cranial nerves become involved.
- Gait—initially stiff or short-strided progressing to recumbency within 12 to 24 hours.

CLINICAL FEATURES

- Severity of signs depends on how much toxin ingested.
- Signs vary from mild paraparesis to tetraplegia and respiratory muscle paralysis leading to death.
- Patient usually presents with generalized lower motor neuron weakness to tetraplegia with hypotonia, and hyporeflexia *(Fig. 11-1)*.
- Tail tone and movements are preserved.
- Patient remains alert with normal pain perception.
- Cranial nerve dysfunction is present as dysphagia, voice change (weakness), droopy face with poor eyelid closure, poor jaw and tongue tone, megaesophagus.
- Autonomic abnormalities are mydriasis with decreased PLR, ileus or constipation, urine retention or frequent voiding of small volumes, decreased lacrimation (dry eye).
- Muscle atrophy is marked after 7 days.

 ## DIFFERENTIAL DIAGNOSIS

Three main conditions that botulism must be differentiated include:
- Idiopathic polyradiculoneuritis—may follow raccoon bite, systemic illness or vaccination; cranial nerve involvement usually limited to facial and pharyngeal/laryngeal paresis; no autonomic signs; hyperesthesia may be present; diffuse denervation potentials on EMG examination because of demyelination of peripheral nerves.
- Tick bite paralysis
  - North America—cranial nerve involvement unusual or mild; no autonomic signs; rapid recovery after tick removal.

■ **Fig. 11-1** Dog with botulism showing tetraparesis with profound lower motor neuron dysfunction, hypotonia, and hyporeflexia, but with normal pain perception (courtesy Dr. A. deLahunta, Cornell University).

- Australia—cranial nerve and autonomic signs present; more severe signs may develop after tick removal; EMG: few, if any fibrillation potentials and marked reduction in amplitude of evoked motor potentials.
- Myasthenia gravis—exercise-induced weakness; rapid improvement after short period of rest; megaesophagus common, but cranial nerve involvement often limited to moderate facial and pharyngeal/laryngeal paralysis; normal spinal reflexes if patient ambulatory.

 ## DIAGNOSTICS

- CBC and serum biochemical panel—usually normal.
- Identify toxin (in ingested material, serum, vomit, and feces)—by neutralization test in mice or in vitro tests measuring toxin antigenicity.
- Radiographic examination—may reveal megaesophagus with or without aspiration pneumonia.
- EMG examination—no or few denervation potentials (come back during recovery phase).
- Reduced amplitude of evoked motor potentials.

 ## THERAPEUTICS

- Those in respiratory distress—respiratory support in intensive care facility.
- Swallowing difficulties—placement of a PEG tube will alleviate complications of megaesophagus.
- Care of recumbent patient—frequent turning; good padding; attend to urine scald or place urinary catheter.
- Laxatives or enemas—if recent ingestion.
- Perform physical therapy (both passive and active)—to prevent tendon contraction and limit muscle atrophy.
- Antibiotics—unhelpful because intestinal colonization of organism does not occur.
- Antibiotics—indicated if secondary aspiration pneumonia or UTI present.
- Medicate dry eye if present.

Drugs of Choice

- Type C or polyvalent containing type C antitoxin—only effective before toxin has bound nerve endings (dosage: 10,000 to 15,000 U, IV or IM twice at 4-hr interval).

Precautions/Interactions

- Aminogycosides, procaine penicillin, tetracyclines, phenothiazines, and magnesium may potentiate neuromuscular blockade.
- Antitoxin—has the potential to cause anaphylaxis.
- Test for anaphylaxis before use—0.1 ml, ID, 20 minutes before systemic administration.

COMMENTS

- Maximum severity of signs—usually reached within 12 to 24 hours after signs first start to develop.
- Signs disappear in reverse order from the order in which they appeared, but more slowly.
- Complete recovery usually occurs within 1 to 3 weeks.

Abbreviations

CBC, complete blood count; EMG, electromyography; PEG, percutaneous endoscopic gastrostomy; PLR, pupillary light reflex; UTI, urinary tract infection.

Suggested Reading

Barsanti JA. Botulism. In: Greene CE, ed. *Infectious Diseases of the Dog and Cat,* 2nd ed. Philadelphia: WB Saunders; 1998;263–267.

Author: Andree D. Quesnel
Consulting Editor: Stephen C. Barr

chapter 12

Brucellosis

DEFINITION/OVERVIEW

- A contagious disease of dogs characterized by abortion and infertility in females; epididymitis and testicular atrophy in males; and occasionally diskospondylitis.

ETIOLOGY/PATHOPHYSIOLOGY

- *Brucella canis*—an intracellular gram-negative coccobacillus.
- Target tissues—include those high in gonadal steroids (gravid uterus, fetus, epididymis, and prostate gland) and lymphoid tissues (lymph nodes, spleen, and bone marrow).
- Occasionally grows in other tissues (intervertebral disks, anterior uvea, meninges).

SIGNALMENT/HISTORY

- Most common in beagle dogs, but no known genetic predisposition.
- Overall prevalence unknown.
- Highest in dogs from rural areas (particularly of the southern states), and certain kennels (Labrador retrievers over represented).
- Also high in stray dogs (strays in Mexico have a 25% to 30% seroprevalence).
- Pets are occasionally affected.
- No age preference, but it is more common in sexually mature dogs.
- Females are more commonly affected than males.

CLINICAL FEATURES

- Suspect disease—whenever a female dog aborts or has reproductive failures or males have genital disease.
- Affected dogs (especially females)—usually appear healthy or have vague signs of illness.
- Lethargy.
- Loss of libido.

- Lymphadenopathy.
- Back pain.
- Abortion—a consistent sign.
- Abortion—commonly occurs 6 to 8 weeks after conception (although pregnancy may terminate at any stage).
- Males—may have swollen scrotal sacs, scrotal dermatitis *(Fig. 12-1)*, enlarged and firm epididymis *(Fig. 12-2)*, unilateral or bilateral testicular atrophy.
- Anterior uveitis with corneal edema—rare.
- Diskospondylitis—spinal pain with ataxia.
- Glomerulonephritis—weight loss, elevated blood pressure; rare.

 ## DIFFERENTIAL DIAGNOSIS

- Abortions or chronic infertility—maternal, fetal, or placental abnormalities; systemic infections (canine distemper, herpesvirus, *Brucella abortus*, *Escherichia coli*, leptospirosis, toxoplasmosis, neosporosis); chronic endometritis; hypothyroidism.
- Epididymitis and scrotal edema—inguinal hernias, blastomycosis, RMSF.
- Diskospondylitis—most often caused by *Staphylococcus* but also fungal infections, actinomycosis, *Streptococcus* spp., nocardiosis, and others.

■ **Fig. 12-1** Scrotal dermatitis may develop in dogs with *Brucella canis* due to self-trauma (rubbing scrotum on ground, licking) as a result of pain from epidydimitis.

■ **Fig. 12-2** Epidydimitis is a common finding in dogs with *Brucella canis*.

 DIAGNOSTICS

- CBC and biochemical profile—usually normal.
- Urinalysis and biochemistry—may reflect protein-losing nephropathy if glomerulonephritis exists (hypoalbuminemia, proteinuria).
- Serology—three main tests (all susceptible to error):
  - RSAT—commercially available; becomes positive 3 to 4 weeks postinfection; rapid and very good at identifying true negative status; high rate of false positive results (50%), so positive results must be confirmed by other tests.
  - Mercaptoethanol tube agglutination test—semiquantitative test; similar to RSAT in its lack of specificity.
  - AGID—highly sensitive (if uses cell wall lipopolysaccharide antigen of *B. canis*), but can give false positive results in negative dogs; if soluble antigens (extracted from bacterial cytoplasm) are used, test is highly specific for antibodies against other *Brucella* spp. (*B. suis*, *B. abortus*) that infect dogs; may give false negative results if performed soon after infection.
- Procedure for serologically testing dogs—first use RSAT; if positive, confirm using an AGID.
- Organism—can be isolated from the blood (if no antibiotics have been used) 2 to 4 weeks postinfection, and persist for 8 months to 5 years.

■ **Fig. 12-3** Lateral radiograph of lumbar vertebrae of a dog with diskospondylitis caused by *Brucella canis.*

- Best results for blood culture—most likely to be positive 1 to 28 months post-infection.
- Cultures of vaginal discharges after abortion—usually positive.
- Culture of semen—usually positive if collected in a sterile manner.
- Semen examination—commonly reveals sperm abnormalities 5 to 8 weeks post-infection, aspermia in dogs with bilateral testicular atrophy.
- Lymph node biopsies—shows lymphoid hyperplasia with plasma cell hyperplasia, intracellular bacteria (special stain: Brown-Brenn).
- Imaging—may reveal diskospondylitis lesions *(Fig. 12-3),* as well as splenomegaly and osteomylitis in some dogs.

THERAPEUTICS

- Antibiotic treatment—recommended only for nonbreeding dogs or those that have been spayed or castrated.
- Antibiotic therapy outcome—uncertain at best.
- If attempting antibiotic treatment in intact dogs—be aware that the risk of transmission to other dogs still remains.
- Aim of antibiotic treatment—to have dogs seroconvert to negative and be abacteremic for at least 3 months.
- Best treatment efficacy—achieved by high-dose doxycycline in combination with injectable streptomycin.
- If streptomycin is not available—substitute gentamicin for streptomycin.
- Using gentamicin in combination with doxycycline—improves the overall efficacy of treatment (over doxycycline alone) but is not as efficacious as using doxycycline and streptomycin in combination.
- Dogs with diskospondylitis—often experience recurrence of hyperesthetic episodes, requiring repeated treatments with doxycycline.

TABLE 12-1. Drug Therapy for Brucellosis in Dogs				
Drug	Dose (mg/kg)	Route	Interval (Hours)	Duration (Weeks)
Doxycycline	12–15	PO	12	4
Gentamicin	5	SC	24	1[a]

[a] Repeat after 1 week.

Drugs of Choice

- Doxycycline.
- Gentamicin *(Table 12-1)*.

Precautions/Interactions

- Use of doxycycline is contraindicated—in pregnant or lactating bitches.
- Use doxycycline with caution in pups <6 months of age—risk of tooth discoloration.
- Avoid the development of esophagitis—give doxycycline with food or liquids.
- Gentamicin—nephrotoxic; monitor for casts in urine; avoid giving drug to animals with dehydration, renal disease, or cardiac failure or with other drugs that may exacerbate renal disease, including tetracyclines (but not including doxycycline).

    COMMENTS

- Control of brucellosis in a kennel—problematic.
- First confirm—by isolation of the organism before antibiotic treatments are initiated.
- Quarantine infected kennels—all confirmed infected animals should be eliminated.
- Animals should not be admitted or released from the kennel—until the disease has been eradicated.
- All dogs in the infected kennels—serotest for at least 3 months after seronegative status has been achieved, especially before each breeding.
- If infected dogs are to be treated with antibiotics—they should be neutered and moved to separate housing.
- Clean kennels—use quaternary ammonium compounds or iodophors.
- Identify carrier dogs—essential, because these are usually responsible for transmission to other kennels.
- New acquisitions into a kennel—only admit if serologically negative on testing on two occasions 1 month apart.
- Warn clients—*B. canis* is infectious to humans.
- Contact with aborting bitches—main source of infection to humans.
- Clinical signs in humans—relatively mild (fevers, fatigue, malaise, lymphadenopathy) and easily treated with tetracyclines.

Abbreviations

AGID, Agar gel immunodiffusion; CBC, complete blood count; RMSF, Rocky Mountain spotted fever; RSAT, rapid 2-ME slide agglutination test.

Suggested Reading

Carmichael LE, Shin SJ. Canine brucellosis: a diagnostician's dilemma. *Semin Vet Med Surg Small Anim* 1996;11:161–165.

Carmichael LE, Greene CE. Canine Brucellosis. In: Greene CE, ed. *Infectious Diseases of the Dog and Cat.* Philadelphia: WB Saunders; 1998;248–257.

Author: Leland Carmichael
Consulting Editor: Stephen C. Barr

chapter 13

Campylobacteriosis

DEFINITION/OVERVIEW

- A gastrointestinal bacterial infection of dogs and cats (and other mammals)—causes a superficial erosive enterocolitis resulting in diarrhea.

ETIOLOGY/PATHOPHYSIOLOGY

- *Campylobacter jejuni*—fastidious microaerophilic gram-negative curved bacteria often isolated from the feces of normal cats and dogs.
- Infection—occurs by the fecal-oral route from contaminated food, water, fresh meat, and environment.
- Localizes in mucus-filled crypts of small intestine—bacteria produce enterotoxin, cytotoxin, cytolethal-distending toxin, and invasin.
- May invade intestinal mucosa—leads to ulceration, edema, congestion of the intestine, resulting in hematochezia, leukocytes in the feces (occasionally septicemia) with bacteria shed in feces for weeks to months afterward.
- Young dogs (but not cats) with diarrhea—more animals shed organisms than non-diarrheic animals.

SIGNALMENT/HISTORY

- Found in dogs less commonly than in cats.
- Higher prevalence in puppies and kittens (birth to 6 months of age).
- Organism often found in dogs and cats with chronic diarrhea.
- Risk factors are kennels with poor hygiene, immunosuppression or GI parasitism, or other concurrent causes of diarrhea.

CLINICAL FEATURES

- Diarrhea—ranges from mucus-like and watery to blood-streaked, sometimes chronic.
- Tenesmus common.
- Fever (rare and usually mild).
- Anorexia.
- Intermittent vomiting may accompany diarrhea.
- Young animals (<6 months)—signs more severe.
- Adults—usually asymptomatic carriers.

DIFFERENTIAL DIAGNOSIS

- Other causes of acute enterocolitis—dietary indiscretion; IBD; neoplasia (especially GI lymphoma); drugs (antibiotics); toxins (lead); parasites (cryptosporidiosis, trichomoniasis, giardiasis, whipworms); infectious agents (parvovirus, FIP, salmonellosis, rickettsia, GI bacterial overgrowth, clostridia, histoplasmosis, leishmaniasis, pythiosis, other rare infections); systemic organ dysfunction (renal, hepatic, pancreatic, cardiac); metabolic (hypoadrenocorticism, feline hyperthyroidism).

DIAGNOSTICS

- CBC—leukocytosis only with septicemia.
- Biochemical panel—reflects effects of diarrhea and dehydration.
- Fecal smear—high leukocyte count.
- Gram stain of feces (leaving counterstain [safranin] on for longer than usual)—will demonstrate curved gram-negative "seagull" bacteria (Fig. 13-1).
- Wet mount of feces (1 drop mixed with 1 drop of saline, coverslip) viewed on phase (condenser down) at 40× magnification will show large numbers of curved, highly motile bacteria with characteristic darting motility.
- Transportation to laboratory—organisms remain viable in feces at room temperature for 3 days, 7 days if refrigerated.
- Fecal culture—grown for 48 hour on special *Campylobacter* blood-agar plates.

THERAPEUTICS

- Mild diarrhea—treated with antibiotics as outpatients.
- Self-limiting—usually.
- Severe neonatal diarrhea—may require oral fluid therapy if not vomiting.
- If dehydrated—IV fluid support, or plasma (if albumin <2.0 mg/dl).
- Antibiotics—recommended if signs of systemic illness or diarrhea persists beyond 5 days, also in immunosuppressed patient.

■ **Fig. 13-1** Campylobacter organisms in the feces of a dog. Note the large number of curved bacteria often referred to as "seagull" shaped (1,500×).

Drugs of Choice

- Erythromycin.
- Tylosin—Tylan soluble powder (Elanco, Indianapolis, IN; 100-g containers; ~3 g/tsp).
- Neomycin *(Table 13-1).*

Precautions/Interactions

- Erythromycin—may cause GI irritability, resulting in vomiting, anorexia, and diarrhea.
- If GI irritability occurs—stop until signs abate, then restart at half the dose; slowly, over 48 hours, work back up to full dose.

 COMMENTS

- Erythromycin is the drug of choice.
- Repeat fecal culture—after completion of treatment.

TABLE 13-1. Drug Therapy for Campylobacteriosis in Dogs and Cats				
Drug	Dose (mg/kg)	Route	Interval (Hours)	Duration (Days)
Erythromycin	10–20	PO	8	5
Tylosin	11	PO	8	7
Neomycin	10–20	PO	8	5

- Zoonosis—good hand-cleaning hygiene usually sufficient to prevent infection of humans.
- Reduce fecal contamination in kennel situations—remove solid waste, disinfect runs and food and water bowls.

Abbreviations

FIP, feline infectious peritonitis; GI, gastrointestinal; IBD, inflammatory bowel disease.

Suggested Reading

Altekruse SF, Tollefson LK. Human campylobacteriosis: a challenge for the veterinary profession. *J Am Vet Med Assoc* 2003;223:445–452.

Brown C, Martin V, Chitwood S. An outbreak of enterocolitis due to *Campylobacter* spp. in a beagle colony. *J Vet Diagn Invest* 1999;11:374–376.

Fox JG. Enteric bacterial infections. In: Greene CE, ed. *Infectious Diseases of the Dog and Cat.* 2nd ed. Philadelphia: WB Saunders; 1998:226–229.

Author: Alfred M. Legendre
Consulting Editor: Stephen C. Barr

chapter 14

Candidiasis

DEFINITION/OVERVIEW

- Opportunistic yeast (part of the normal flora of the mouth, nose, ears, and gastrointestinal [GI] and genital tracts) that causes disease by colonizing damaged tissues of dogs and cats.

ETIOLOGY/PATHOPHYSIOLOGY

- *Candida albicans*—normal flora on mucous membranes of cats and dogs.
- Recovery of organisms from mucous membranes—does not imply disease.
- Opportunistic—colonizing damaged tissues or invading normal tissues of immunosuppressed animals.
- Pathogenic role—determined by identifying a fungemia, infiltration of organisms into the tissues, or signs of organisms in presumed sterile sites (e.g., urinary bladder).
- Conditions that suppress the immune system—increase the likelihood of isolation in asymptomatic animal.
- FIV—*C. albicans* has been isolated from throat cultures five times more often in FIV-infected cats than in asymptomatic, non–FIV-infected cats of a similar age and sex.
- Infection—rare.
- Infection—usually associated with neutropenia (secondary to parvovirus, retrovirus infection, bone marrow suppression), diabetes mellitus, retrovirus-induced immunosuppression, chronic glucocorticoid treatment, prolonged antibiotic treatment, and incomplete emptying of the bladder.

SIGNALMENT/HISTORY

- Cats—occurs less commonly than in dogs.
- Historically—skin damaged by burns, trauma, or necrotizing dermatitis predisposes to infection.
- Urinary tract—preferred site in diabetic cats, secondary to indwelling catheters, and cats that have urinary retention due to strictures secondary to urethrostomy.

CLINICAL FEATURES

- Urinary bladder involvement—cystitis (pollakiuria, hematuria, proteinuria, WBCs in urine).
- Ear infection—head shaking and scratching.
- Oral cavity involvement—drooling.
- Keratitis—rare, occasionally seen after extensive use of intraocular antibiotic-steroid treatment *(Fig. 14-1)*.

DIFFERENTIAL DIAGNOSIS

- Suspect candidiasis—when a primary infection (otitis, cystitis) does not respond to treatment, especially with antibiotics, but becomes worse.

DIAGNOSTICS

- Urinalysis—may show yeast form or clumps of mycelial elements (pseudohyphae) accompanied by an increase in inflammatory cells *(Fig. 14-2)*; normal fat globules in cat urine may adhere, giving the appearance of budding yeast.
- Pyuria without bacterial growth—culture for fungi and *Mycoplasma* organisms.
- Collect urine sample by cystocentesis—a culture of a large number of yeast colonies strongly supports a diagnosis.
- Neutropenic patients—inflammatory response may be absent.
- Biopsy sometimes needed to determine if *Candida* is truly a pathogen—requires demonstration of organisms penetrating the tissues.

■ **Fig. 14-1** Chronic keratitis in a cat caused by *C. albicans* (courtesy Dr. R. Riis, Cornell University).

■ **Fig. 14-2** Urinalysis from a dog with *C. albicans* infection of the urinary bladder showing the yeast form with some mycelial elements and increased numbers of inflammatory cells (courtesy Dr. T. Stokel, Cornell University).

- Otitis (dogs)—culture of *Candida* organisms or identification of yeast or mycelial elements on ear cytologic examination suggests the diagnosis.

 THERAPEUTICS

- Try to remove inciting factor:
  - Regulate diabetes mellitus.
  - Remove indwelling catheters.
  - Treat underlying cause of neutropenia.
  - Improve immune suppression, if possible (remove or modify chemotherapeutic drugs).

Drugs of Choice

Topical
- Treatment of infected mucous membranes.
- Nystatin (e.g., Nilstat cream).
- Clotrimazole (e.g., Lotrimin cream).
- Miconazole (e.g., Conofite cream).

Systemic
- Fluconazole (Diflucan [Pfizer, Exton, PA])—very effective; excreted unchanged in the urine, achieving a high concentration in commonly infected sites.
- Itraconazole (Sporanox [Janssen, Titusville, NJ])—effective but not as effective as fluconazole; use if the organism becomes resistant to fluconazole; not recommended for urinary tract infection (UTI) because it is not excreted in the urine.
- Clotrimazole (Lotrimin solution [Schering-Plough Animal Health, Union, NJ])—infused into the bladder if urinary tract *Candida* infection resistant to fluconazole (*Table 14-1*).

TABLE 14-1. Drug Therapy for Candidiasis in Dogs and Cats

Drug	Dose (mg/kg)	Route	Interval (Hours)	Duration (Weeks)
Nystatin cream (100,000 U/g)	—	Topical	8–12	2
Clotrimazole cream (1%)	—	Topical	6–8	1
Miconazole cream (2%)	—	Topical	12–24	3
Fluconazole	5	PO	12	4
Itraconazole	5–10	PO	12–24	4
Clotrimazole solution (1%)[a]	10–30 ml	Bladder infusion	48	—

[a] Infuse into the bladder every other day for 3 treatments.

Precautions/Interactions

- Fluconazole and itraconazole—hepatic toxicity; monitor serum ALT monthly and check if patient becomes anorexic; withdraw drug if ALT >200 U or with anorexia.
- After signs have resolved—obtain repeat culture of sites of infection; continue treatment for 2 weeks more; repeat culture examination 2 weeks after completion of treatment and again if signs recur.

 COMMENTS

- Prognosis—should resolve within 2 to 4 weeks of treatment.

Abbreviations

ALT, alanine aminotransferase; FIV, feline immunodeficiency virus; GI, gastrointestinal; UTI, urinary tract infection; WBC, white blood cell.

Suggested Reading

Forward ZA, Legendre AM, Khalsa HDS. Use of intermittent bladder infusion with clotrimazole for treatment of candiduria in a dog. *J Am Vet Med Assoc* 2002;220:1496–1498.

Greene CE, Chandler FW. Candidiasis, torulopsosis, rhodotorulosis. In: Greene CE, ed. *Infectious Diseases of the Dog and Cat*. Philadelphia: WB Saunders; 1998:414–417.

Lulich JP, Osborne CA. Fungal infections of the feline lower urinary tract. *Vet Clin North Am* 1996;26:309–315.

Author: Alfred M. Legendre
Consulting Editor: Stephen C. Barr

chapter 15

Canine Coronavirus Infection

DEFINITION/OVERVIEW

- A viral infection causing sporadic outbreaks of vomiting and diarrhea in dogs.

ETIOLOGY/PATHOPHYSIOLOGY

- Feces—primary source of infection.
- Infection—inapparent usually.
- Virus—restricted to upper two thirds of the small intestine and associated lymph nodes.
- Crypt cells spared—unlike in CPV.
- Mild to severe enteritis may occur—most dogs recover uneventfully.
- Death—reported in young pups.
- Virus shedding—in feces for about 2 weeks.
- Simultaneous infection with CPV—results in severe diarrhea; often fatal.
- Viremia or other manifestation of systemic disease—none.
- Distribution—worldwide, including wild canids.

SIGNALMENT/HISTORY

- Only wild and domestic dogs are known to be susceptible to disease.
- Cats can have inapparent infections.
- No age or breed predilection.
- Stress (e.g., intensive training, crowding) is greatest risk factor.
- Sporadic outbreaks occur in dogs attending shows and in kennels, where the introduction of new dogs is frequent.
- Crowding and unsanitary conditions—promote clinical illness.

CLINICAL FEATURES

- Adults—most infections inapparent.
- Puppies—may develop severe, fatal enteritis.
- Incubation period—short (1 to 3 days).

- Sudden onset of vomiting—usually only once.
- Vomiting—followed by diarrhea.
- Diarrhea—may be explosive; yellow-green or orange; loose or liquid; typically malodorous.
- Diarrhea—may persist for a few days up to 3 weeks; may recur later.
- Young pups—may suffer severe, protracted diarrhea and dehydration with anorexia and depression common.
- Fever rare—mild respiratory effects.

DIFFERENTIAL DIAGNOSIS

- Consider all causes of diarrhea—including systemic or metabolic disease as well as specific intestinal disorders.
- Other causes of acute enterocolitis in very young puppies—dietary indiscretion or intolerance; drugs (antibiotics); toxins (lead); parasites (cryptosporidiosis, giardiasis, hookworms, roundworms); infectious agents (parvovirus, salmonellosis, GI tract bacterial overgrowth, campylobacteriosis, clostridial enterotoxicosis); systemic organ dysfunction (renal, hepatic, pancreatic, cardiac); metabolic (hypoadrenocorticism, hypoglycemia); GI tract foreign body.

DIAGNOSTICS

- CBC and serum biochemical profile—usually normal unless severe dehydration.
- Serologic tests—available but not standardized.
- Antibody titers—generally low; may not indicate recent infection because of high rate of asymptomatic infection.
- Viral isolation—from feces in feline cell cultures at onset of diarrhea will identify virus; prolonged and often impractical.
- Immunofluorescent staining of frozen sections of the small intestine in fatal cases—may reveal viral antigen in cells lining the villous epithelium.
- Electron microscopy of feces—typical CCV particles (interpretation requires expertise).
- Because other enteric infections augment the disease—check feces for CPV and parasites.

THERAPEUTICS

- Most affected dogs recover without treatment.
- Hospitalization for supportive fluid and electrolyte treatment is indicated in severe infections with dehydration in very young puppies.

TABLE 15-1. Antibiotic Therapy to Consider for Use in Canine Coronaviral Enteritis

Drug	Dose (mg/kg)	Route	Interval (Hours)	Duration (Days)
Ampicillin	10–20	IV, IM, SC	6–8	5
Ceftiofur (Naxcel)	2–5	SC	12	5
Cefazolin (Ancef, Kefzol)	22	IV, IM	8	5
Gentamicin[a]	2–4	IM, SC	8	5

[a] Ensure animal is well hydrated before administration; check for nephrotoxicity by examining urine sediment. Can be given in combination with ampicillin.

Drugs of Choice

- Antibiotics—administer if enteritis is severe, or sepsis or respiratory illness are present.
- Use GI tract antibiotics—ampicillin, ceftiofur, cefazolin, gentamicin (*Table 15-1*).

Precautions/Interactions

- CCV—highly contagious and will spread rapidly.
- Strict isolation and sanitation—essential in the kennel.
- Infections by other enteric pathogens—believed to augment the disease.

 COMMENTS

- Vaccines—controversial.
- Inactivated and live viral vaccines available—appear to be safe but efficacy unknown, except for brief periods (2 to 4 weeks) after vaccination.
- Vaccination—not recommended.
- Diarrhea—may persist 10 to 12 days and may recur.
- Prognosis—normally good, except severe infections in young pups.
- Prognosis—majority recover after a few days of illness.
- Fluid or soft stools—may persist for several weeks.
- Virus—readily inactivated by disinfectants, drying, or steam cleaning.

Abbreviations

CBC, complete blood count; CCV, canine coronavirus; CPV, canine parvovirus; GI, gastrointestinal.

Suggested Reading

Hoskins JD. Canine viral enteritis. In: Greene, CE. *Infectious Diseases of the Dog and Cat*. Philadelphia: WB Saunders; 1998:45–47.

Author: Leland E. Carmichael
Consulting Editor: Stephen C. Barr

Canine Distemper

chapter 16

DEFINITION/OVERVIEW

- A viral infection of dogs causing acute to subacute febrile and often fatal disease with respiratory, GI, and CNS manifestations.

ETIOLOGY/PATHOPHYSIOLOGY

- Morbillivirus (in the Paramyxoviridae family)—affects many different species of the order Carnivora.
- Mortality rate—varies greatly among species.
- Natural route of infection—airborne and droplet exposure.
- Nasal cavity, pharynx, and lungs—macrophages carry the virus from these structures to local lymph nodes, where virus replication occurs.
- Within 1 week postinfection—virtually all lymphatic tissues become infected.
- Spreads via viremia—to surface epithelium of respiratory, GI, and urogenital tracts and to the CNS.
- Fever (for 1 to 2 days) and lymphopenia—may be the only findings during initial period.
- Further development of disease—depends on the virus strain and the immune response.
- Strong cellular and humoral immune response—may remain subclinical.
- Weak immune response—subacute infection; may survive longer.
- Failure of immune response—death within 2 to 4 weeks postinfection.
- Seizures and other CNS disturbances—frequent causes of death.
- Affects—all lymphatic tissues; surface epithelium in the respiratory, alimentary, and urogenital tracts; endocrine and exocrine glands; and nervous tissues.
- Domestic dogs—restricted to sporadic outbreaks.
- Wildlife (raccoons, skunks, fox)—fairly common.

SIGNALMENT/HISTORY

- Most carnivores are affected—Canidae, Hyaenidae, Mustelidae, Procyonidae, Viverridae; also felidae (large cats in zoos and wild).
- Young animals—more susceptible than are adults.

CLINICAL FEATURES

- Fever, first peak—3 to 6 days postinfection, may pass unnoticed.
- Fever, second peak—several days later (and intermittent thereafter); usually associated with nasal and ocular discharge, depression, and anorexia.
- Fever followed by GI and/or respiratory signs—often enhanced by secondary bacterial infection.
- CNS—many infected dogs; often, but not always, after systemic disease; depends on the virus strain.
- CNS presentation—either acute gray matter disease (seizures and myoclonus with depression) or subacute white matter disease (incoordination ataxia, paresis, paralysis, and muscle tremors).
- Meningeal signs of hyperesthesia and cervical rigidity—may be seen in both.
- Optic neuritis and retinal lesions—not uncommon; sometimes injected scleral blood vessels from anterior uveitis.
- Hardening of the footpads (hyperkeratosis) and nose—some virus strains; now much less common.
- Enamel hypoplasia of the teeth after neonatal infection—common.
- In utero infection of fetuses in antibody-negative bitches—rare.
- May lead to abortion or persistent infection—infected neonates may develop fatal disease by 4 to 6 weeks of age.

DIFFERENTIAL DIAGNOSIS

- Consider—in any young, unvaccinated dog with multifocal CNS disease and other organ involvement.
- Kennel cough—distemper can mimic the respiratory disease in young pups.
- Enteric signs—differentiate from CPV and CCV infections, parasitism (giardiasis, hookworms, roundworms), bacterial infections, gastroenteritis from toxin ingestion, or IBD.
- CNS form—differentiate from granulomatous meningoencephalomyelitis, protozoal encephalitis (toxoplasmosis, neosporosis), cryptococcosis or other infections (meningitis, ehrlichiosis, RMSF), pug dog encephalitis, and lead poisoning.

DIAGNOSTICS

- CBC—lymphopenia during early infection.

Diagnostic Feature

- **Blood cell inclusions—occasionally seen in circulating lymphocytes and, rarely, in monocytes, neutrophils, and RBCs *(Fig. 16-1)*.**

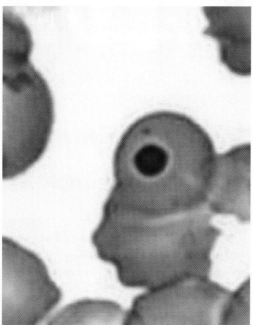

■ **Fig. 16-1** Inclusion bodies within the red blood cells of a dog infected with CDV. Distinguishable from Howell-Jolly bodies because CDV inclusions tend to be darker staining and larger. (**A,** Wright's stain. **B,** Giemsa stain, 1,400×.)

- Serology—limited value; positive antibody results do not differentiate between vaccination and exposure to virulent virus.
- Acute disease—patient may die from acute disease before neutralizing antibody can be produced.
- IgM responses—may be seen for up to 3 months after exposure to virulent virus and for up to 3 weeks after vaccination.
- CDV antibody in CSF—offers definitive evidence of distemper encephalitis because antibody is locally produced and not elevated even in vaccinated animals;

may see false positive titers if CSF is contaminated by blood during collection process or if a bleed into the CNS has occurred.

- To avoid false positive CSF antibody results—compare ratio of CDV antibody titer in CSF to serum; if .1 in association with consistent clinical signs, strongly indicative of distemper encephalitis.
- To increase predictive value of this ratio comparison even further—compare ratio to corresponding CSF/serum antibody ratio for another infectious agent against which the dog has been vaccinated (e.g., CPV or CAV); if CDV is greater, the only way elevation can occur is by the presence of distemper encephalitis.
- Vaccination or CDV infection without CNS involvement—will not increase CDV antibody titers in CSF.
- Viral antigen or viral inclusions—in buffy coat cells and conjunctival or vaginal imprints; negative results do not rule out the diagnosis.
- PCR on buffy coat and urine sediment cells—more sensitive.
- CSF—test for cell and protein content, CDV-specific antibody, interferon, and viral antigen early in disease course.
- Tissue immunofluorescence and/or immunocytochemistry, virus isolation, and/or PCR—preferred tissues from lungs, stomach, urinary bladder, lymph nodes, and brain.
- Virus may persist in skin for up to 60 days postinfection—PCR and immunocytochemistry may help in identifying CDV in skin biopsies; high false negative rate.

 THERAPEUTICS

- Inpatients and in isolation—to prevent infection of other dogs.
- Symptomatic nursing care—including intravenous fluids (with anorexia and diarrhea) or parenteral nutrition.
- Once fever and secondary bacterial infections are controlled—patients usually begin to eat again.

Drugs of Choice

- Antiviral drugs—none known to be effective.
- Antibiotics—to reduce secondary bacterial infection, because CDV is highly immunosuppressive.
- Anticonvulsant therapy—phenobarbital, potassium bromide; to control myoclonus and seizures.
- Vaccination—MLV-CD—prevents infection and disease.
- Two types of MLV-CD available:
  - Canine tissue culture–adapted vaccines (e.g., Rockborn strain)—induce complete immunity in virtually 100% of susceptible dogs; rarely, a postvaccinal fatal encephalitis develops 7 to 14 days after vaccination, especially in immunosuppressed animals.

- Chick embryo–adapted vaccines (e.g., Onderstepoort, Lederle strain)—safer; postvaccinal encephalitis does not occur; only about 80% of susceptible dogs seroconvert.
- Other species—chick embryo can safely be used in a variety of zoo and wildlife species (e.g., gray fox); Rockborn type is fatal in these animals.
- Killed vaccines—useful for species for which either type of MLV-CD is fatal (e.g., red panda, black-footed ferret).
- Canarypox recombinant CDV vaccine—recently available; being tested in other species.
- Because most pups lose protection from maternal antibody at 6 to 12 weeks of age—give 2 to 3 vaccinations during this period.
- Heterotypic (measles virus) vaccination—recommended for pups that have maternal antibody; induces protection from disease but not from infection.

Precautions/Interactions

- Corticosteroids—not to be used because they augment the immunosuppression and may enhance viral dissemination; may provide short-term control of signs.
- Tetracyclines—may produce renal tubular necrosis at high doses; produce yellow discoloration of teeth in young animals.
- Fluoroquinolones—may produce arthropathy in dogs up to 6 months of age; potentiate seizures in epileptic animals.

 COMMENTS

- Inform client—mortality rate is about 50% once the dog has contracted CDV.
- Death—typically occurs 2 weeks to 3 months postinfection.
- Dogs that appear to recover from early catarrhal signs—may later develop fatal CNS signs such as myoclonus (which may continue for several months).
- Owners can avoid infection of pups—by isolation to prevent infection from wildlife (e.g., raccoons, fox, skunks) or from CDV-infected dogs.
- Recovered dogs—are not carriers.
- Zoonotic risk—possible that humans may become subclinically infected with CDV.
- Immunization against measles virus—also protects humans against CDV infection.

Abbreviations

CAV, canine adenovirus; CBC, complete blood count; CCV, canine coronavirus; CDV, canine distemper virus; CNS, central nervous system; CSF, cerebrospinal fluid; CPV, canine parvovirus; GI, gastrointestinal; IBD, inflammatory bowel disease; MLV-CD, modified live virus of canine distemper; PCR, polymerase chain reaction; RBCs, red blood cells; RMSF, Rocky Mountain spotted fever.

Suggested Reading

Appel MJG, Summers BA. Pathogenicity of morbilliviruses for terrestrial carnivores. *Vet Microbiol* 1995;44:187–191.

Greene CE, Appel MJ. Canine distemper. In: Greene CE, ed. *Infectious Diseases of the Dog and Cat.* Philadelphia: WB Saunders; 1998:9–22.

Author: Max J. G. Appel
Consulting Editor: Stephen C. Barr

chapter 17

Canine Herpesvirus Infection

DEFINITION/OVERVIEW

- A rare systemic viral disease (although the virus is common in nature)—affects puppies <3 weeks of age, resulting in high mortality.
- Other canine species susceptible—wolves and coyotes.

ETIOLOGY/PATHOPHYSIOLOGY

- Canine herpesvirus—often found latent in several tissues, including the trigeminal nerve ganglia.
- Virus—may be excreted in nasal secretions in response to stress or corticosteroid use.
- Poor regulation of body temperature and immature immune response mechanisms—probably result in susceptibility of young puppies.
- Clinical disease very rare in pups >3 weeks of age—all organ systems involved.
- Pups—acquire infection as they pass through vagina during birth in an infected bitch.
- Mature nonpregnant dogs—often have subclinical infections (nasopharynx and external genitalia).
- Transplacental infections during last 3 to 4 weeks of gestation—can result in fetal deaths, often with mummification; abortions; birth of dead or dying pups.
- Localized genital infection—occurs in both sexes.

SIGNALMENT/HISTORY

- Puppy infections—sudden death usually occurs 9 to 14 days after birth.
- Sudden death—can occur as early as first day of life and as late as day 30 after birth.
- No breed predilection—most often reported in purebred dogs, however.

CLINICAL FEATURES

- Neonatal pups—4- to 6-days incubation period; sudden onset with death 12 to 36 hours later.

■ **Fig. 17-1** Vulval mucous membrane of a bitch. Note the lymphofollicular lesions and superficial excoriation on the vulva (*arrow*) (courtesy Dr. L. Carmichael, Cornell University).

- Some die with no signs; some develop mild signs—survive, but later develop ataxia, persistent vestibular signs, and blindness.
- Signs include:
  - Dyspnea.
  - Serous to mucopurulent nasal discharge.
  - Anorexia.
  - Yellow to green soft stool.
  - Crying.
  - CNS signs.
  - Petechial hemorrhages on mucous membranes.
  - Gasping before death.
- Surviving pups—may suffer deafness, blindness, encephalopathy, or renal damage.
- Mature females—lymphofollicular or hemorrhagic lesions on vaginal mucosa (*Fig. 17-1*).
- Mature dogs—conjunctivitis (very rare); keratitis reported.
- Infection of dams during last 3 weeks of gestation—fetal infection with death and mummification or ill pups that die shortly after birth.

DIFFERENTIAL DIAGNOSIS

- Other causes of sudden death in newborn pups—bacterial (brucellosis, coliform bacteria, streptococci, umbilical infections); toxoplasmosis; neosporosis; toxins; all fail to display the typical pathologic lesions of CHV.

- CPV type 1 (canine minute virus)—causes enteric and respiratory disease; distinguished from CHV by characteristic gross pathologic changes of CHV.
- Distemper and canine hepatitis (CAV type 1)—very rare and no characteristic renal gross pathologic changes.

DIAGNOSTICS

- CBC—thrombocytopenia occurs occasionally.
- Serology—of little value.

Diagnostic Feature
- **Diagnostic method of choice—gross and histopathology.**
- **Gross lesions—disseminated focal necrosis and hemorrhage in:**
    - Kidneys—diffuse hemorrhagic areas, necrotic foci, hemorrhagic infarcts (pathognomonic in young pups [Fig. 17-2]).
    - Lungs, liver, adrenal glands—diffuse foci of hemorrhage and necrosis.
    - Small intestine—variably affected.
    - Lymph nodes, spleen—generalized enlargement (consistent finding).
- Histopathologic examination—focal perivascular necrosis in kidneys, lung, liver, spleen, intestine, brain; necrotizing lesions in fetal placentas.
- Immunohistochemistry—viral antigens in most organs, especially in lesion areas.
- Viral isolation (on refrigerated samples, not frozen)—easily from lung or kidney.

■ **Fig. 17-2** Opened thorax and abdomen of a puppy that died of canine herpesvirus infection. Note the pathognomonic hemorrhagic infarcts over the kidney and liver surfaces (courtesy of Dr. L. Carmichael, Cornell University).

THERAPEUTICS

- Treatment—not recommended.
- Antiviral drug therapy—unsuccessful.
- Immune sera from a recovered bitch—may be beneficial in reducing pup deaths when given before onset of illness.

Drugs of Choice

- No vaccine available.

COMMENTS

- Normal litters can be expected from bitches that have previously suffered pup losses or abortion.
- Isolate pregnant dams (especially young bitches) when introduced into a kennel—adults commonly shed latent CHV in nasal secretions for 1 to 2 weeks after encountering newly introduced dogs.

Abbreviations

CAV, canine adenovirus; CBC, complete blood count; CHV, canine herpesvirus; CNS, central nervous system; CPV, canine parvovirus.

Suggested Reading

Carmichael LE, Greene CE. Canine herpesvirus infection. In: Greene CE, ed. *Infectious Diseases of the Dog and Cat.* Philadelphia: WB Saunders; 1998:28–32.

Author: Leland Carmichael
Consulting Editor: Stephen C. Barr

Canine Lungworm (*Crenosoma*)

chapter 18

DEFINITION/OVERVIEW

- A helminth parasite usually of foxes, wolves, and raccoons, but can invade the bronchial tree of domestic dogs to produce a persistent productive cough and a bronchointerstitial pattern on thoracic radiographs.

ETIOLOGY/PATHOPHYSIOLOGY

- *Crenosoma vulpis*—a metastrongyloidae parasite.
- Eggs and L1 larvae—are laid in the respiratory tree of infected dogs, ascend the trachea, and are swallowed back into the GI tract and passed in the feces.
- L1 larvae—infect snails and slugs, where they develop to L3 larvae.
- Dogs—become infected by eating infected mollusks or small amphibians and reptiles, which may serve as paratenic hosts.
- PPP = 19 days.

SIGNALMENT/HISTORY

- Affects dogs of all ages.
- Usually a history of unusual exposure to outdoors such as might occur with a suburban dog visiting a rural region for a period of time.
- Infected dogs usually present during mid to late summer.
- High prevalence amongst dogs on Prince Edward Island, Canada.

CLINICAL FEATURES

- Productive cough that is unresponsive to antibiotics.
- Cough develops approximately 2 to 3 weeks after likely exposure to parasite.
- Cough easily elicited on tracheal palpation (unlike cough caused by *Oslerus* [*Filaroides*] *osleri*).
- Dogs rarely debilitated by disease.

DIFFERENTIAL DIAGNOSIS

- A general differential diagnosis for cough includes such categories as:
  - Cardiovascular (pulmonary edema; enlarged heart, especially the left atrium; left-sided heart failure; pulmonary emboli).
  - Allergic (bronchial asthma, eosinophilic pneumonia or granulomatosis, pulmonary infiltrate with eosinophilia).
  - Trauma (foreign body, irritating gases, collapsing trachea, hypoplastic trachea).
  - Neoplasia (not only of the respiratory tree but also associated structures such as ribs, lymph nodes).
  - Inflammatory (pharyngitis, tonsillitis, kennel cough from such agents as *Bordetella bronchoseptica*, parainfluenza virus, infectious laryngotracheitis virus, and mycoplasma; bacterial bronchopneumonia; fungal pneumonia; aspiration pneumonia; chronic pulmonary fibrosis; pulmonary abscess or granuloma; chronic obstructive pulmonary disease).
  - Parasites (*Capillaria aerophila*, *Oslerus* [*Filaroides*] *osleri*, *Filaroides hirthi*, *F. milksi*, *Paragonimus kellicotti*, *Dirofilaria immitis*—heartworm disease).
- The L1 of all the canine lungworms (*F. hirthi*, *Oslerus* [*Filaroides*] *osleri*, *Crenosoma vulpis*, and *Filaroides milksi*) are very similar. *Oslerus* (*Filaroides*) *osleri* is best differentiated from the others by demonstrating nodules at the bifurcation of the trachea; the tail has a small kink making it similar to *F. milksi*. Thoracic radiographic changes for *F. hirthi*, *C. vulpis*, and *F. milksi* can be similar, but the L1 of *F. milksi* has a kinked tail; the other two do not. Differentiating *F. hirthi* and *C. vulpis* is difficult and requires comparing L1 larval differences: *F. hirthi* organisms have blunt, rounded oral ends, whereas *C. vulpis* organisms have bluntly conical oral ends and a straight-sided, more gradually tapering cone than that of *F. hirthi*. From a therapeutic perspective, differentiation of these latter two is unimportant because they are treated similarly.

 DIAGNOSTICS

Diagnostic Feature
- **L1 larvae can be identified in the feces using either ZSCT (specific gravity, 1.18), or Baermann's technique, which is usually more sensitive than finding parasites in a transtracheal wash *(Fig. 18-1)*.**
- Transtracheal wash usually contains L1 larvae (some L1 larvae are in eggs), eosinophils, some neutrophils.
- CBC occasionally demonstrates mild eosinophilia.
- Thoracic radiographs often show a diffuse bronchointerstitial pattern throughout the pulmonary parenchyma (*Fig. 18-2*).

■ **Fig. 18-1** L1 larvae of *C. vulpis* in an infected dog's feces. Note the nonkinked tail, which distinguishes this larva from *Oslerus (Filaroides) osleri*, and the relatively long esophagus that distinguishes this larva from those of Strongyloides and Ancylostoma.

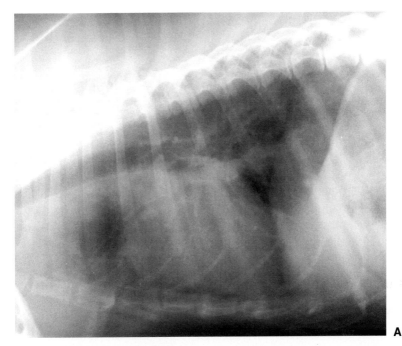

A

■ **Fig. 18-2** Lateral (**A**) and dorsoventral (**B**) thoracic radiographs of a dog with *C. vulpis* infestation. Note the diffuse bronchointerstitial lung pattern.

B

■ **Fig. 18-2** *Continued*

 THERAPEUTICS

- Response to drug therapy—usually rapid and complete with cessation of cough 3 days after beginning treatment with anthelmintic and prednisone.
- Radiographic changes—should be completely resolved by 6 weeks post-treatment.

Drugs of Choice

- Fenbendazole—not approved for use in dogs for this parasite.
- Levamisole—not approved for use in dogs and no current dog preparations.
- Prednisone—improves inflammation caused by the products of parasites killed off by anthelmintic therapy (*Table 18-1*).

Precautions/Interactions

- Levamisole—at high doses, may cause anxiety and neurologic signs.

TABLE 18-1. Drug Therapy for *Crenosoma vulpis* Infection in Dogs

Drug	Dose (mg/kg)	Route	Interval (Hours)	Duration (Days)
Fenbendazole (Panacur)	50	PO	24	3
Levamisole[a]	8	PO	Once	—
Prednisone	0.5	PO	12	5

[a] Multiple preparations of levamisole.

 ## COMMENTS

- The severity of the cough can be similar to that caused by kennel cough.
- Foxes do not acquire infections if raised on wire but do if raised on dirt; control of a dog's access to dirt and intermediate hosts should prevent infection.

Abbreviations

CBC, complete blood count; GI, gastrointestinal; PPP, prepatent period; ZSCT, zinc sulfate concentration technique.

Suggested Reading

Bihr T, Conboy GA. Lungworm (*Crenosoma vulpis*) infection in dogs on Prince Edward Island. *Can Vet J* 1999;40:555–559.

Peterson EN, Barr SC, Gould WJ, et al. Use of fenbendazole for treatment of *Crenosoma vulpis* in a dog. *J Am Vet Med Assoc* 1993;202:1483–1484.

Unterer S, Deplazes P, Arnold P, et al. Spontaneous *Crenosoma vulpis* infection in 10 dogs: laboratory radiographic and endoscopic findings. *Schweiz Arch Tierheilkd* 2002;144:174–179.

Author: Stephen C. Barr

Consulting Editor: Stephen C. Barr

chapter 19

Canine Lungworm
(Filaroides)

DEFINITION/OVERVIEW

- Adults of this helminth parasite live in the lung parenchyma of dogs, producing few clinical signs in most cases.
- May cause severe pneumonia (especially after treatment) in some cases.

ETIOLOGY/PATHOPHYSIOLOGY

- *Filaroides hirthi*—Metastrongyloidea nematode parasite.
- Adults—curl up in lung parenchyma; release thin-shelled eggs or L1 larvae into airways.
- L1 larvae—coughed up and swallowed, appearing in feces.
- L1 larvae—are infective, and horizontal transmission is common.
- PPP = 5 weeks.
- A second helminth, *Filaroides milksi*, has been very rarely demonstrated to cause verminous pneumonia in dogs in North America, Japan, and Belgium; details of life cycle, pathogenicity, and chemotherapy are unknown.

SIGNALMENT/HISTORY

- Although any dog can become infected, most infections are seen in dogs housed closely together (breeding facilities), where horizontal transmission and autoinfection are common.
- Transmission—by the fecal-oral route from a brood bitch to offspring is common.
- Small breeds—once treated specifically for infection or if immunosuppressed, can show severe signs of pneumonia.

CLINICAL FEATURES

- Most are asymptomatic.
- Those with clinical signs present with a mild cough on exercise.
- Dogs immunosuppressed with corticosteroids for long periods (weeks), suffering from Cushing's disease, or that have undergone prolonged nutritional stress may show severe and fatal signs of pneumonia.

- In dogs with severe pneumonia a cycle of autoinfection causing massive worm numbers to develop in the lungs usually precedes the fatal pneumonia.

 DIFFERENTIAL DIAGNOSIS

- A general differential diagnosis for cough includes such categories as:
  - Cardiovascular (pulmonary edema; enlarged heart, especially the left atrium; left-sided heart failure; pulmonary emboli).
  - Allergic (bronchial asthma, eosinophilic pneumonia or granulomatosis, pulmonary infiltrate with eosinophilia).
  - Trauma (foreign body, irritating gases, collapsing trachea, hypoplastic trachea).
  - Neoplasia (not only of the respiratory tree but also associated structures such as ribs, lymph nodes).
  - Inflammatory (pharyngitis; tonsillitis; kennel cough from such agents as *Bordetella bronchoseptica*, parainfluenza virus, infectious laryngotracheitis virus, and mycoplasma; bacterial bronchopneumonia; fugal pneumonia; aspiration pneumonia; chronic pulmonary fibrosis; pulmonary abscess or granuloma; chronic obstructive pulmonary disease).
  - Parasites (*Capillaria aerophila, Oslerus* [Filaroides] *osleri, Crenosoma vulpis, Paragonimus kellicotti, Dirofilaria immitis*—heartworm disease).
- The L1 of all the canine lungworms (*F. hirthi, Oslerus* [Filaroides] *osleri, Crenosoma vulpis,* and *Filaroides milksi*) are very similar. *Oslerus* (Filaroides) *osleri* is best differentiated from the others by demonstrating nodules at the bifurcation of the trachea; the tail has a small kink making it similar to *F. milksi*. Thoracic radiographic changes for *F. hirthi, C. vulpis,* and *F. milksi* can be similar, but the L1 of *F. milksi* has a kinked tail, whereas the other two do not. Differentiating *F. hirthi* and *C. vulpis* is difficult, requiring comparing L1 larval differences: *F. hirthi* organisms have blunt, rounded oral ends, whereas *C. vulpis* organisms have bluntly conical oral ends and a straight-sided, more gradually tapering cone than *F. hirthi*. From a therapeutic perspective, differentiation of these latter two is unimportant because they are treated similarly.

 DIAGNOSTICS

Diagnostic Feature
- **L1 larvae—best identified in feces using ZSCT (SpG; 1.18) instead of Baermann's technique; L1 larvae do not escape from the feces easily *(Fig. 19-1).***
- Transtracheal wash—can identify L1 larvae; mild eosinophil count also.
- Thoracic radiographs—lesions include linear and nodular interstitial infiltrates and occasional alveolar and peribronchial patterns.
- After anthelmintic treatment, pulmonary infiltrates often become more nodular and consolidated.

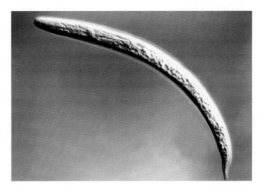

■ **Fig. 19-1** L1 larva of *Filaroides hirthi* in the feces of a dog. L1 of *F. hirthi* are very similar to although thicker than those of *Crenosoma vulpis* (no kinked tail and long esophagus), and thoracic radiographic changes can be similar. A careful history is required for the clinician to differentiate between the two. The L1 larvae of *F. hirthi* are best concentrated in the feces using ZSCT instead of Baermann's technique.

 THERAPEUTICS

- Patients can experience severe clinical signs 2 to 5 days after the onset of anthelmintic therapy.
- The author has found that treating for 5 days with anti-inflammatory levels of corticosteroids during the early stages of anthelmintic therapy decreases the severity and longevity of signs resulting from dying of parasites.

Drugs of Choice

- Fenbendazole
- Prednisone *(Table 19-1)*.

Precautions/Interactions

- Albendazole—effective therapy but possible side effects; can cause teratogenesis and myelosuppression in dogs and cats.
- Fenbendazole—can be used safely in pregnant and nursing bitches, stud male dogs, and puppies.

TABLE 19-1. Drug Therapy for *Filaroides hirthi* in Dogs

Drug	Dose (mg/kg)	Route	Interval (Hours)	Duration (Days)
Fenbendazole (Panacur)	50	PO	24	10–14
Albendazole (Valbazen)	25	PO	12	5[a]
Prednisone	0.5	PO	12	5

[a] Repeat in 2 weeks after end of first course.

COMMENTS

- If infected dogs are in contact with others—all dogs should be treated to attempt to break the horizontal transmission cycle.
- Feces from all dogs—should be screened using ZSCT; all dogs with positive test results should be isolated and treated.
- In a colony of experimental dogs—rigorous attempts must be made to clear the infection because lungworm lesions can lead to spurious results in drug toxicologic and carcinogenicity studies.

Abbreviations

PPP, prepatent period; ZSCT, zinc sulfate concentration technique.

Suggested Reading

Georgi JR. Parasites of the respiratory tract. In: Grieve RB, ed. *The Veterinary Clinics of North America: Parasitic Infections.* Philadelphia: WB Saunders; 1987:1430–1435.

Author: Stephen C. Barr
Consulting Editor: Stephen C. Barr

chapter 20

Canine Parvovirus Infection

DEFINITION/OVERVIEW

- Viral infection causing systemic illness with primarily GI and immunologic effects in young dogs (6 to 16 weeks of age) and occasionally cats.
- Clinically characterized by anorexia; vomiting; bloody, watery diarrhea; and sepsis as a result of absolute neutropenia.

ETIOLOGY/PATHOPHYSIOLOGY

- CPVs are small, nonenveloped single-stranded DNA viruses; two are pathogenic to dogs—CPV-1 (minute virus of canines) and CPV-2 (causing GI tract disease).
- CPV-1—uncertain pathogenicity; has been associated with "fading puppy syndrome"; causes lethargy, loose stools, respiratory distress, and sudden death in 1- to 3-day-old pups.
- CPV-2—first appeared in 1977; known simply as canine parvovirus and is closely related to feline panleukopenia virus and mink enteritis virus.
- Current isolates (CPV-2a appeared in 1980, and CPV-2b in 1984)—different antigenic structures, increased pathogenicity, and shorter incubation period (4 to 5 days versus 5 to 8 days) compared to CPV-2.
- CPV-2a and 2b—also replicate in cats.
- Vaccines made against the original CPV-2—protect against all 2a and 2b.
- Route of infection—fecal/oral followed by viral replication in tonsilar lymphoid tissue initially, with subsequent spread to other lymphoid tissue (bone marrow, mesenteric nodes, thymus).
- Viremia occurs by day 3 to 5 postinfection and precedes clinical signs—virus can be detected in intestinal epithelial cells by day 4 postinfection.
- Fecal shedding—occurs soon after viremia, with large amounts of virus excreted in feces in clinically affected dogs.
- Fecal shedding—usually lasts no longer than day 12 postinfection.
- CPV targets rapidly dividing cells in the intestine (crypt cells of distal duodenum and jejunum), bone marrow, and, under exceptional circumstances, myocardial tissue.

Enteritis

- Commonly seen in pups 6 to 16 weeks of age.
- Dividing crypt cells are killed; enteric cells moving up the villus to be lost into the intestinal lumen are not replaced by new cells; leads to denuded villus.
- Takes about 2 weeks for complete villus repair to occur.
- Virtually all clinical signs are as a consequence of crypt cell and lymphoid/bone marrow destruction.
- Severe cases develop sepsis and endotoxemia from gram-negative enteric bacteria (CPV infection alone in gnotobiotic dogs produces minimal signs).
- Sepsis causes circulatory collapse, multiple organ failure, and death.

Bone Marrow

- CPV causes necrolysis of both myeloid and erythroid stem cells in marrow—because RBCs have long half-lives (approximately 120 days), few effects are seen on the RBC indices, although anemia may occur as a result of blood loss from the bowel.
- Leukocyte counts reflect both peripheral consumption and myeloid destruction—with marked reduction beginning from day 3 to 5 postinfection.
- Myeloid destruction with profound reductions in WBC counts—occurs with, or just after, the onset of clinical signs (day 6 postinfection).
- In recovery—a left shift (appearance of band neutrophils) with rebound neutrophilia often predicts a successful treatment outcome.

Myocardial Disease

- Cardiac myocytes can only support CPV growth in first 2 weeks of puppies' life, so must be infected in utero or within first weeks of life—puppies with any degree of passive immunity from dam (today virtually 100%) are immune and will not become infected (syndrome rarely seen today, but was common in late 1970s).
- Although viral damage occurs in first 2 weeks—myocarditis not seen until pups are 6 to 8 weeks of age; causes acute death.

 ## SIGNALMENT/HISTORY

- Young dogs—usually between 6 and 16 weeks of age.
- Certain dog breeds—rottweilers, Doberman pinschers, pit bull terriers, German shepherds, English springer spaniels, Alaskan sled dogs, and perhaps Labrador retrievers seem more predisposed (more severe infection and can be infected as adults).
- Cats—can be infected with CPV 2a and 2b and show clinical signs similar to those seen in dogs, but this is rare.

 ## CLINICAL FEATURES

- Can be extremely variable depending on age, immunity, copathogens (parasites or enteric bacteria), and infective dose.
- Crowding and poor sanitation reduce the chances of successful response to immunization in kennels.

■ **Fig. 20-1** A diagnosis of parvovirus infection should be high on the list in a puppy between 6 and 16 weeks of age displaying clinical signs of depression, anorexia, vomiting, and bloody diarrhea. (Courtesy Dr. Leland Carmichael, Cornell University.)

- However, crowding and poor sanitation do not enhance severity of disease in individuals—not unusual to have some pups in a litter unaffected while others die acutely.
- Depression.
- Anorexia.
- Vomiting—with or without pyrexia.
- Pups vomit repeatedly—sometimes with roundworms in vomitus.
- Profuse mucoid then bloody diarrhea—with rapid severe weight loss (*Fig. 20-1*).
- Tachycardia—pale, tacky (5% to 8% dehydration) mucous membranes, abdominal pain or discomfort.
- Signs of cerebella hypoplasia—although occurs in dogs very rarely, more often found in feline panleukopenia infection.

 DIFFERENTIAL DIAGNOSIS

- All causes of diarrhea, including systemic or metabolic disease, as well as specific intestinal disorders, should be considered, although those affecting puppies should receive a higher priority.
- Other causes of acute enteritis: dietary indiscretion, foreign body, IBD, HGE, intussusception, drugs (antibiotics); toxins (lead), parasites (roundworms, cryptosporidiosis, giardiasis, coccidiosis, whipworms), infectious agents (salmonellosis, *Campylobacter* spp., GI tract bacterial overgrowth, clostridiosis, coronavirus), systemic organ dysfunction (renal, hepatic, pancreatic), metabolic (hypoadrenocorticism), and neoplasia (GI tract lymphoma or adenocarcinoma) in older dogs.

■ **Fig. 20-2** A blood smear showing a profound neutropenia in a puppy with depression, anorexia, vomiting, and bloody diarrhea is virtually diagnostic of parvovirus infection.

- Parvovirus may be distinguished from other causes of acute diarrhea by the presence of a profound neutropenia apparent even on a stained direct blood smear without cell counts (*Fig. 20-2*).

 DIAGNOSTICS

- CBC—profound neutropenia and lymphopenia.
- Neutrophils—often show toxic changes.
- Rebound leukocytosis with left shift—in recovery.
- Biochemical profile—reflects dehydration; electrolyte abnormalities (metabolic acidosis, hypokalemia) and hypoglycemia are common.
- Panhypoproteinemia initially as the signs progress—hypoalbuminemia may become progressively more severe with persistent diarrhea.
- Chemistry profile—may reflect multiorgan failure with sepsis.
- Imaging (radiology or abdominal ultrasonography)—perform to rule out foreign body, intussusception; shows fluid-filled bowel without gas.
- Fecal ELISA (Snap Parvo Antigen Test Kit [IDEXX Laboratories, Westbrook, ME])—for parvovirus antigen; false negative results may be seen due to relatively short time of viral shedding; false positive results may be seen with recent vaccination (prior 5 to 15 days); test is effective in detecting CPV in cat feces also.
- Less commonly used tests—viral isolation, fecal PCR, electron microscopy, fecal hemagglutionation assay, serum for hemagglutination inhibition.

THERAPEUTICS

- Intensive therapy with hospitalization—significantly improves survival.
- Isolate from other patients—affected patients excrete large amounts of virus.
- Puppies that are not vomiting and not significantly dehydrated—treat on an out-patient basis.
- Intravenous crystalloid fluid therapy is mainstay of therapy—account for dehydration and ongoing losses from vomiting and diarrhea.
- Avoid subcutaneous fluid administration in neutropenic patients to avoid abscess formation.
- Extreme care in catheter maintenance should be taken—a high proportion (up to 22%) of CPV patients develop bacterial colonization of IV catheters.
- Colloid therapy may be useful in patients with hypoalbuminemia—whole blood and plasma may also be used if blood loss in diarrhea is severe.
- Withhold water and food until vomiting has abated—initiate small amounts of water after 24 hours with no vomiting.
- Enteral nutrition via a nasogastric feeding tube soon after admission—improves morbidity, time to recovery, and survivability of CPV-affected dogs.
- Glutamine supplementation—improves enterocyte health.
- When ready to initiate food—use a bland diet (Hill's i/d, Purina EN), with gradual transition to normal diet.

Drugs of Choice

- Antiemetics—use if vomiting protracted. Metoclopramide or the serotonin receptor antagonist ondansetron are prefered. Phenothiazines (promethazine, chlorpromazine) may worsen lethargy and hypotension.
- H_2 blockers (famotidine)—may reduce nausea.
- Antibiotics—to prevent and treat sepsis; use broad-spectrum agents to include gram-negative organisms; ampicillin, cefazolin, ceftiofur, sometimes in combination with gentamicin (unless patient is very young or dehydrated).
- Anthelmintic therapy (fenbendazole)—for concurrent parasitism should be considered once vomiting has ceased.
- rIFNΣ—may improve survivability of CPV-affected dogs (*Table 20-1*).
- Equine endotoxin antiserum, granulocyte colony-stimulating factor, TNF, corticosteroids, and NSAIDs—do not seem to improve survivability or recovery time.
- Vaccination—MLV given at 6, 9, 12, and 16 weeks of age. High-risk breeds may require longer initial period, extending out to 22 weeks.
- Main reason for vaccine failure—interference from maternal antibody.
- Yearly booster vaccination—advised by most vaccine manufacturers, but dogs probably only require booster vaccination every 3 years.
- Dogs acquire natural boostering throughout their lives from exposure to wild-type CPV isolates in the environment—negates the need for regular booster vaccination.

TABLE 20-1. Drug Therapy for Canine Parvovirus Infections

Drug	Dose (mg/kg)	Route	Interval (Hours)	Duration (Days)
Metoclopramide	0.2–0.4	SC	6–8	5[a]
	1–2	IV–CRI	—	5[a]
Ondansetron	0.5–1	IV	12–24	5[a]
Famotidine	0.5–1	SC, IM	12–24	5
Ampicillin	10–20	SC, IM, IV	6–8	10[b]
Cefazolin	22	IM, IV	8	10[b]
Ceftiofur	2.2–4.4	SC	12	10[b]
Gentamicin	2–4	SC, IM	8	5[c]
Fenbendazole	50	PO	24	3[d]
rIFNΣ	2,500,000 U/kg	IV	24	3

[a] Or as long as needed.
[b] Or until oral medications can be taken.
[c] Not for use in dehydrated patient; monitor for nephrotoxicity.
[d] Use once vomiting has stopped.
CRI, constant rate infusion; rIFNΣ, recombinant feline interferon omega.

Precautions/Interactions

- Avoid fluoroquinolones in puppies because of risk of cartilage defects.
- Avoid use of gentamicin in dehydrated patients—monitor use of gentamicin by examining urine for appearance of casts to avoid nephrotoxicity.
- Avoid any surgical intervention while severe neutropenia is present.
- Extended antibiotic therapy may result in development of oral and intestinal candidiasis.

 COMMENTS

- Recovery—usually complete within 7 to 10 days, even in severely affected.
- Immunity after infection is long term—probably lifelong, negating the need for future parvoviral vaccination.
- Complications of infection—can include intussusception, DIC, endotoxic shock, or sepsis.
- CPV—ubiquitous in the environment and extremely resistant.
- CPV—can be killed using a 1:32 dilution of bleach.

Abbreviations

CBC, complete blood count; CPVs, canine parvoviruses; DIC, disseminated intravascular coagulation; DNA, deoxyribonucleic acid; ELISA, enzyme-linked immunosorbent assay; GI, gastrointestinal tract; HGE, hemorrhagic gastroenteritis; IBD, inflammatory bowel disease; MLV, modified live vaccine; NSAIDs, nonsteroidal anti-inflammatory drugs; PCR, polymerase chain reaction; RBCs, red blood cells; rIFNΣ, recombinant interferon omega; TNF, tumor necrosis factor; WBC, white blood cell.

Suggested Reading

Bohm M, Thompson H, Weir A, et al. Serum antibody titres to canine parvovirus, adenovirus and distemper virus in dogs in the UK which had not been vaccinated for at least three years. *Vet Rec* 2004:154;457–463.

De Mari K, Maynard L, Eun HM, et al. Treatment of canine parvoviral enteritis with interferon-omega in a placebo-controlled field trial. *Vet Rec* 2003:152;105–108.

Mohr AJ, Leisewitz AL, Jacobson LS, et al. Effect of early enteral nutrition on intestinal permeability, intestinal protein loss, and outcome in dogs with severe parvoviral enteritis. *J Vet Intern Med* 2003:17;791–798.

Mouzin DE, Lorenzen MJ, Haworth JD, et al. Duration of serologic response in five viral antigens in dogs. *J Am Vet Med Assoc* 2004:224;55–60.

Author: Jo Ann Morrison
Consulting Editor: Stephen C. Barr

chapter 21

Canine Tracheal Worm *(Oslerus)*

DEFINITION/OVERVIEW

- A helminth parasite that forms nodules within the mucosa at the bifurcation of the trachea of dogs.
- Causes cough, respiratory distress, and eventually tracheal obstruction.

ETIOLOGY/PATHOPHYSIOLOGY

- *Oslerus* (Filaroides) *osleri*—Metastrongyloidea parasite.
- Adult parasites—live in fibrous nodules within the tracheal bifurcation submucosa/mucosa; release eggs containing L1 larvae directly into the tracheal lumen.
- L1 larvae—are directly infective to other dogs (a unique feature of these parasites; other infective larvae require further development before becoming infective).
- Dogs—acquire infection directly from L1 in feces from infected dogs or when an infected dam regurgitates food.
- Regurgitated food—becomes contaminated with L1 larvae as the food passes over the oropharynx.
- Pups eating regurgitated food become infected—a feature more common of wild canids (wolves, coyotes, foxes, dingoes); may explain why infection is more common in wild canids than in domestic dogs.

SIGNALMENT/HISTORY

- Usually found in young dogs (4 to 6 months of age)—usually become infected months earlier because the nodules take months to develop after infection.
- Infected dogs—often have a history of contact with wild canids or at least frequent terrain where wild canids live; become infected by eating infected regurgitated food or feces.
- PPP = 10 to 14 weeks.

CLINICAL FEATURES

- First signs—harsh cough (often exercise induced or in cold weather).
- Tracheal pressure—usually does not elicit the cough, unlike other causes of tracheobronchitis in the dog.
- After coughing several times—dog often retches a brown phlegm, which is usually swallowed.
- Advanced and severe stages of disease—the trachea becomes so obstructed with nodules that harsh wheezes can be auscultated over the hilar region, especially on expiration (Fig. 21-1).
- Tachypnea.
- Increased inspiratory effort.
- Prolonged expiration.

DIFFERENTIAL DIAGNOSIS

- A general differential diagnosis for cough includes such categories as:
  - Cardiovascular (pulmonary edema; enlarged heart, especially the left atrium; left-sided heart failure; pulmonary emboli).
  - Allergic (bronchial asthma, eosinophilic pneumonia or granulomatosis, pulmonary infiltrate with eosinophilia).
  - Trauma (foreign body, irritating gases, collapsing trachea, hypoplastic trachea).
  - Neoplasia (not only of the respiratory tree but also associated structures such as ribs, lymph nodes).
  - Inflammatory (pharyngitis; tonsillitis; kennel cough from such agents as *Bordetella bronchoseptica*, parainfluenza virus, infectious laryngotracheitis virus, and mycoplasma; bacterial bronchopneumonia; fungal pneumonia; aspiration pneumonia; chronic pulmonary fibrosis; pulmonary abscess or granuloma; chronic obstructive pulmonary disease).
  - Parasites (*Capillaria aerophila, Filaroides hirthi, Crenosoma vulpis, Paragonimus kellicotti, Dirofilaria immitis*—heartworm disease).
- The L1 of all the canine lungworms (*Filaroides hirthi, Oslerus* [Filaroides] *osleri, Crenosoma vulpis,* and *F. milksi*) are very similar. *Oslerus.* (*Filaroides*) *osleri* is best differentiated from the others by demonstrating nodules at the bifurcation of the trachea; the tail has a small kink making it similar to *F. milksi*. Thoracic radiographic changes for *F. hirthi, C. vulpis,* and *F. milksi* can be similar, but the L1 of *F. milksi* has a kinked tail and the other two do not. Differentiating *F. hirthi* and *C. vulpis* is difficult, requiring comparing L1 larval differences: *F. hirthi* have blunt, rounded oral ends, whereas *C. vulpis* have bluntly conical oral ends and a straight-sided, more gradually tapering cone than *F. hirthi*. From a therapeutic perspective, differentiation of these latter two is unimportant because they are treated similarly.

■ **Fig. 21-1** Endoscopic view (**A**) and gross pathology specimen (**B**) of the tracheal bifurcation of a dog with *Oslerus* (*Filaroides*) *osleri* infestation. Note the nodes protruding into the tracheal lumen and, in the gross specimen, totally obliterating the lumen even down into bronchioles.

DIAGNOSTICS

Diagnostic Features

- **In large-breed dogs—bronchoscopy will reveal the nodules at the tracheal bifurcation and down into the mainstem bronchus.**
- Biopsies of nodules through the bronchoscope—reveal sections of adult parasites, eggs, and many L1 larvae *(Fig. 21-2).*
- In small-breed dogs (where bronchoscopy cannot be used)—transtracheal wash reveals L1 larvae and eggs.
- Fecal examinations for L1 larvae—often produce false negative results; may need multiple fecal examinations to find L1 larvae *(Fig. 21-3).*
- ZSCT (specific gravity, 1.18)—superior to Baermann's technique because of the lethargy of these larvae.

■ **Fig. 21-2** Histologic section of the trachea at the level of the bifurcation. Note the adult worm coiled within the nodule protruding from the mucosa.

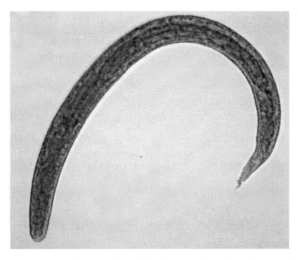

■ **Fig. 21-3** L1 larva of *Oslerus (Filaroides) osleri*. The kinked tail and relatively long esophagus distinguishes this L1 from those of *Strongyloides* and *Ancylostoma* spp.

- The larvae of *O.* (Filaroides) *osleri* are indistinguishable from those of *F. hirthi*—identifying the location of the lesion will help differentiate infestations by these parasites.
- Thoracic radiographs: trachea—may show soft tissue densities within the tracheal lumen at the bifurcation on severe infestations.
- Thoracic radiographs: diaphragm—may be flattened and lung volume increased on expiratory films in dogs with severe tracheal obstruction.

 THERAPEUTICS

- The author finds that physical removal of the nodules visualized during bronchoscopy using the biopsy forceps attachment of the endoscope (in medium and large-breed dogs) greatly improves respiratory signs such as cough and inspiratory difficulty.
- In severe cases—nodules may need to be removed during several procedures over days.
- During this procedure, the dog may require continuous ventilatory support with a high-frequency jet ventilator (using a rate of 100 breaths/min, a drive pressure of 20 psi, and an inspiratory fraction of 0.30).
- After nodule removal—tracheal mucosal inflammation and respiratory discomfort can be markedly reduced by administering prednisone.

Drugs of Choice

- Oxfendazole (Synanthic Bovine Dewormer Suspension 9.06%, Fort Dodge, Fort Dodge, IA)—not registered for use in the dog *(Table 21-1)*.
- Other anthelmintics (ivermectin, milbemycin, fenbendazole, levamisole, albendazole, and pyrantel pamoate) are ineffective.

TABLE 21-1. Drug Therapy for *Oslerus* (*Filaroides*) *osleri* Infection in Dogs				
Drug	Dose (mg/kg)	Route	Interval (Hours)	Duration (Days)
Oxfendazole (Synanthic Bovine Dewormer)	10	PO	24	28
Prednisone	0.2	PO	12	5

Precautions/Interactions

▪ Although not reported in dogs treated with oxfendazole, albendazole (a related benzimidazole) can cause myelosuppression in dogs. Given the few dogs ever treated with oxfendazole, it is advisable to perform a CBC at 2 and 4 weeks after starting oxfendazole treatment in dogs.

 COMMENTS

▪ Prevent dogs from frequenting terrain used by wild canids or from eating regurgitated food or feces of infected dogs (wild canids particularly).
▪ The feces of infected dogs, although of relatively low infectivity compared to regurgitated material, should be disposed of to prevent other in-contact dogs from becoming infected.

Abbreviations

CBC, complete blood count; PPP, prepatent period; ZSCT, zinc sulfate concentration technique.

Suggested Reading

Barr SC, Lavelle RB, Harrigan KE, et al. *Oslerus* (*Filaroides*) *osleri* in a dog. *Aust Vet J* 1986;63:334–336.

Bjorling DE, Lappin MR, Whitfield JB. High-frequency jet ventilation during bronchoscopy in a dog. *J Am Vet Med Assoc* 1985;187:1373–1375.

Kelly PJ, Mason PR. Successful treatment of *Filaroides osleri* infection with oxfendazole. *Vet Rec* 1985;116:445–446.

Author: Stephen C. Barr
Consulting Editor: Stephen C. Barr

Chagas' Disease (American Trypanosomiasis)

chapter 22

DEFINITION/OVERVIEW

- A systemic protozoal infection of dogs, initially causing acute myocarditis, that may progress to chronic dilated cardiomyopathy.
- Diffuse neurologic signs are occasionally seen.

ETIOLOGY/PATHOPHYSIOLOGY

- *Trypanosoma cruzi*—zoonotic hemoflagellated protozoan transmitted in the feces of vectors (*Triatominae protracta* and *T. sanguisuga* or "kissing bug").
- Infection in dogs—can occur by eating infected vectors or reservoir hosts (raccoons, skunks, opossums) or by organisms in the feces of the vector entering a bite wound or mucous membrane, by blood transfusion, or by the transmammary or transplacental route of transmission.
- After intracellular multiplication at site of entry, parasitemia develops (trypomastigotes)—followed by invasion of cardiac myocytes, where more cycles of multiplication/cell rupture/add to parasitemia occurs (coincides with acute myocarditis).
- Peak parasitemia—occurs 14 to 21 days postinfection.
- Parasitemia levels drop as antibody titer to protozoa rises.
- Subpatent infection—occurs 30 days postinfection.
- Dogs that survive acute myocarditis—enter protracted asymptomatic stage with insidious progression in some patients to end-stage dilated cardiomyopathy 1 to 5 years later.
- United States—occurs in dogs (and reservoir hosts and vectors) mostly in Texas, but also in other southern and southeastern coastal states (as far north as Virginia); reservoir hosts and vectors also reported in the west (California, New Mexico) and as far north as Maryland.

SIGNALMENT/HISTORY

- Acute myocarditis—dogs <2 years of age; chronic disease in older dogs.
- Dogs diagnosed at an older age (>5 years) tend to survive longer (2 to 5 years) than younger (<5 years) dogs (survive up to 5 months).
- Hunting breeds and male dogs overrepresented.
- Cats—infected in South America; not reported in North America.

CLINICAL FEATURES

Acute Myocarditis (Occasionally Encephalitis)

- Sudden death.
- Lethargy.
- Depression.
- Weakness.
- Exercise intolerance.
- Syncope.
- Generalized lymphadenopathy.
- Pale mucous membranes.
- Poor capillary refill.
- Both left- and right-sided heart failure—tachycardia with reduced QRS complexes and prolonged P-R interval (heart block).
- Neurologic weakness, ataxia, chorea, seizures.

Chronic Dilated Cardiomyopathy

- Weakness.
- Exercise intolerance.
- Syncope.
- Occasionally sudden death.
- Ventricular tachycardias.

DIFFERENTIAL DIAGNOSIS

- Cardiomyopathy, congenital cardiac disease, traumatic myocarditis.
- Distemper, *Neospora* spp., toxoplasma.

DIAGNOSTICS

Acute Stage

Diagnostic Features
- **Trypomastigotes on blood smear *(Fig. 22-1)* or on a buffy coat.**
- Visualized organisms (403 objective) above the buffy coat in a microhematocrit tube spun down for PCV.
- Antibody titer (ELISA or IFA)—may be negative in acute cases; repeat in 3 weeks.
- Blood culture—LIT medium (special laboratory—CDC).
- PCR—effective but offers little specificity or sensitivity over antibody titer (research laboratories only).

■ **Fig. 22-1** Trypomastigotes of *Trypanosoma cruzi* in the blood smear of a dog (Wright's-Giemsa stain, 1,000×).

- Thoracic radiologic examination—cardiomegaly and pulmonary edema, slight pleural effusion.
- ECG—AV block, depression of R wave and QRS amplitude, right bundle branch block (*Fig. 22-2*).
- Echocardiography—usually normal.

Chronic Stage

Diagnostic Feature
- Antibody titers are very sensitive and specific if they rule out *Leishmania* spp.; cross-reaction with *Leishmania* spp.

■ **Fig. 22-2** Electrocardiogram showing second-degree heart block and depressed QRS complexes typical of those found in acute Chagas' disease.

■ **Fig. 22-3** Electrocardiogram showing ventricular arrhythmias typical of those found in chronic Chagas' disease.

- Trypomastigotes—sometimes found in lymph nodes or effusions, but virtually impossible to find in blood; may culture in LIT if use a large blood volume (50 ml).
- Thoracic radiologic examination—enlarged cardiac silhouette, ascites, pleural effusion.
- ECG—low QRS amplitude, right bundle branch block, ventricular arrhythmias (initially VPC, then multiform, then degenerates into all types) *(Fig. 22-3)*.
- Echocardiography—reduced ejection fraction, fractional shortening, thinning of the right and left ventricular free wall; initially right, then bilateral, chamber dilation.

 THERAPEUTICS

- Medical treatment rarely produces a clinical cure.
- In severe cases of acute myocarditis coupled with high parasitemia, prognosis is poor and zoonotic risk higher (to those handling blood products), so consider euthanasia.
- If dogs survive acute disease, progression to chronic stage tends to occur more quickly (in about 1 to 2 years) in dogs diagnosed at a younger age (<2 years) than dogs diagnosed at an older age (>4 years), which survive longer (3 to 5 years).
- Treat cardiac failure and arrhythmias specifically.

Drugs of Choice

Acute Stage
- Benznidazole (Ragonil [Roche SA, Buenos Aires, Argentina])—preferred drug; produces cures in humans and dogs.

TABLE 22-1. Drug Therapy for Chagas' Disease (American Trypanosomiasis)					
Drug[a]	Table Size (mg)	Dose (mg/kg)	Route	Interval (Hours)	Duration (Months)
Benznidazole (Ragonil)	100	5–10	PO	24	2
Nifurtimox (Lampit)	120	2–7	PO	6	3–5

[a] Both drugs are available from the Centers for Disease Control and Prevention, Atlanta, Ga.

- Nifurtimox (Bayer 2502 or Lampit [Bayer Ag, Leverkusen–Bayerwerk, Germany])—combined with corticosteroids may remove parasitemia and improve mortality (*Table 22-1*).
- Both drugs—available in the United States only from the CDC.

Chronic Stage
- Neither nifurtimox nor benznidazole show efficacy during the chronic stage of disease.

Precautions/Interactions

- Neither drug is registered for use in dogs.
- Nifurtimox side effects are common and usually limit treatment to 3 to 4 weeks; side effects include anorexia, vomiting, weight loss, CNS signs, polyneuritis, pulmonary infiltrates, and skin eruptions.
- Benznidazole side effects are less common than those with nifurtimox; include vomiting.

COMMENTS

- Zoonosis—transmission to humans can occur by accidental injection of infected blood into a person.
- Warning—warn laboratory staff of potential infectivity of samples from a suspected patient.
- Risk of infection—from dog to human by vector is very low because of the absence of specific species of vectors (that do not occur in North America but do in South America).
- Kennel of dogs are infected—investigate mode of transmission so source of infection can be recognized and blocked.
- Chronic disease—organisms may be difficult to identify on histopathologic examination of the cardiac tissue (pseudocysts containing amastigotes; *Fig. 22-4*), necessitating the use of immunohistochemistry (*Fig. 22-5*).
- Serum antibody titer—usually still present in spite of drug treatment, although reported to drop in humans treated with benznidazole.

■ **Fig. 22-4** Pseudocyst of *Trypanosoma cruzi* within the myocardium of an infected dog (hematoxylin and eosin stain, 1,000×).

■ **Fig. 22-5** Pseudocyst of *Tryanosoma cruzi* within the myocardium of an infected dog (immunohistochemistry stain, 1,000×).

Abbreviations

AV, atrioventricular; CDC, Centers for Disease Control and Prevention; CNS, central nervous system; ECG, electrocardiogram; ELISA, enzyme-linked immunosorbent assay; IFA, immunofluorescence assay; LIT, liver infusion tryptose; PCR, polymerase chain reaction; PCV, packed cell volume; VPC, ventricular premature contraction.

Suggested Reading

Araujo FM, Bahia MT, Magalhaes NM, et al. Follow-up of experimental chronic Chagas' disease in dogs: use of polymerase chain reaction (PCR) compared with parasitological and serological methods. *Acta Trop* 2002;81:21–31.

Barr SC. American trypanosomiasis. In: Greene CW, ed. *Infectious Diseases of the Dog and Cat.* Philadelphia: WB Saunders; 1998;445–448.

Bradley KK, Bergman DK, Woods JP, et al. Prevalence of American trypanosomiasis (Chagas disease) among dogs in Oklahoma. *J Am Vet Med Assoc* 2000;217:1853–1857.

Yabsley MJ, Noblet GP. Seroprevalence of *Trypanosoma cruzi* in raccoons from South Carolina and Georgia. *J Wildl Dis* 2002;38:75–83.

Author: Stephen C. Barr
Consulting Editor: Stephen C. Barr

chapter 23

Cheyletiellosis

DEFINITION/OVERVIEW

- A highly contagious parasitic skin disease of dogs, cats, and rabbits, caused by infestation with *Cheyletiella* spp. mites.
- Signs of scaling and pruritus can mimic other more common diseases.
- Often referred to as "walking dandruff," because of the large mite size and excessive scaling.
- Prevalence varies by geographic region owing to mite susceptibility to common flea-control insecticides.
- Human (zoonotic) lesions can occur.

ETIOLOGY/PATHOPHYSIOLOGY

- *Cheyletiella yasguri*—dogs (Fig. 23-1).
- *C. blakei*—cats.
- *C. parasitivorax*—rabbits.

SIGNALMENT/HISTORY

- Dogs and cats.
- More common in young animals.
- Cocker spaniels, poodles, and long-haired cats are frequent asymptomatic carriers.
- Cats may exhibit bizarre behavioral signs or excessive grooming.
- Pruritus—none to severe, depending on the individual's response to infestation.
- Infestation may be suspected after lesions in humans have developed.
- Young animals and those in frequent contact with others are most at risk.
- Common sources of infestation—animal shelters, breeders, and grooming establishments.

CLINICAL FEATURES

- Scaling—most important clinical sign; diffuse or plaquelike; most severe in chronically infested and debilitated animals (*Fig. 23-2*).
- Lesions—dorsal orientation is commonly noted.

■ **Fig. 23-1** *Cheyletiella yasguri* (dog). (From Rhodes KH: *The 5-Minute Veterinary Consult Clinical Companion: Small Animal Dermatology*. Baltimore, Md: Lippincott Williams & Wilkins; 2002.)

■ **Fig. 23-2** Cheyletiellosis in a cat. Note the excessive scaling within the hair coat. (From Rhodes KH: *The 5-Minute Veterinary Consult Clinical Companion: Small Animal Dermatology*. Baltimore, Md: Lippincott Williams & Wilkins; 2002.)

- Underlying skin irritation—may be minimal.
- Cats—may exhibit bilaterally symmetrical alopecia.

 ## DIFFERENTIAL DIAGNOSIS

- Cheyletiellosis should be considered in every animal that has scaling, with or without pruritus.
- Also consider—seborrhea, flea-allergic dermatitis, *Sarcoptes* spp. mite infestation, atopy, food hypersensitivity, and idiopathic pruritus.

 ## DIAGNOSTICS

- Examination of epidermal debris—very effective in diagnosing infestation.
- Collection of debris—flea combing (most effective), skin scraping, and acetate tape preparation.
- *Cheyletiella* mites are large and can be visualized with a simple handheld magnifying lens; scales and hair may be examined under low magnification; staining is not necessary.
- Response to insecticide preparations may be required to definitively diagnose suspicious cases in which mites cannot be identified.

THERAPEUTICS

- Must treat all animals in the household.
- Clip long coats to facilitate treatment.
- Mainstay—6 to 8 weekly baths to remove scale, followed by rinses with an insecticide.
- Lime-sulfur and pyrethrin rinses—cats, kittens, puppies, and rabbits.
- Pyrethrin or organophosphates—dogs.
- Routine flea sprays and powders—not always effective.
- Environmental treatment with frequent cleanings and insecticide sprays—important for eliminating infestation.
- Combs, brushes, and grooming utensils—discard or thoroughly disinfect before reuse.
- Zoonotic lesions—self-limiting after eradication of the mites from household animals.
- Alternatives (or additions) to topical therapy—amitraz and ivermectin.
- Amitraz (Mitaban)—use on dogs (four rinses at 2-week intervals).
- Ivermectin—highly effective (300 μg/kg, SC, 3 times at 2-week intervals); dogs, cats, and rabbits >3 months old; pour-on forms have shown efficacy in cats (500 μg/kg 2 times at 2-week intervals).

COMMENTS

- Ivermectin—not FDA-approved for this use in dogs, cats, or rabbits; client disclosure and consent are paramount before administration; several dog breeds (e.g., collies, shelties, Australian shepherds) have shown increased sensitivity and should not be treated.
- Treatment failure—necessitates reevaluation for other causes of pruritus and scaling.
- Reinfestation—may indicate contact with an asymptomatic carrier or the presence of an unidentified source of mites (e.g., untreated bedding).
- Zoonotic potential—a pruritic papular rash may develop in areas of contact with the pet.

Suggested Reading

Moriello KA. Cheyletiellosis. In: Griffin CE, Kwochka KW, MacDonald JM, eds. *Current Veterinary Dermatology: The Science and Art of Therapy.* St. Louis: Mosby; 1993.

Author: Alexander H. Werner
Consulting Editor: Karen Helton Rhodes

chapter 24

Chlamydiosis: Cats

DEFINITION/OVERVIEW

- A chronic respiratory tract infection of cats caused by an intracellular bacterium, characterized by conjunctivitis, mild upper respiratory tract signs, and mild pneumonitis.

ETIOLOGY/PATHOPHYSIOLOGY

- *Chlamydia psittaci*—an obligate intracellular bacterium.
- Replicates on the mucosa of the upper and lower respiratory tract epithelium, producing a persistent commensal flora—causes a local irritation with resulting mild upper and lower respiratory signs.
- Ophthalmic—chronic conjunctivitis, often unilateral but may be bilateral.
- Colonization—can colonize the mucosa of the GI tract (with or without signs) and reproductive tract (without signs).
- Incidence of clinical disease—sporadic.
- May get outbreaks of respiratory disease—especially in multicat facilities.
- Overall incidence—5% to 10% chronically infected.
- Incubation period—7 to 10 days.

SIGNALMENT/HISTORY

- Kittens 2 to 6 months of age—usually clinically affected.
- Carriers—any age carriers.
- Historically—kittens show upper respiratory tract signs with sneezing, watery eyes, coughing, occasionally difficulty breathing with anorexia, especially if concurrent infections present.

CLINICAL FEATURES

- Conjunctivitis—often granular; initially unilateral, sometimes becoming bilateral (*Fig. 24-1*).
- Lacrimation.
- Photophobia.

■ **Fig. 24-1** Chemosis associated with conjunctivitis caused by *Chlamydia psittaci* (courtesy Dr. R. Riis, Cornell University).

- Blepharospasm.
- Rhinitis with nasal discharge—usually mild.
- Pneumonitis—with the inflammatory process in the alveoli.
- Airways—audible wheezes on auscultation.

 DIFFERENTIAL DIAGNOSIS

- Feline viral rhinotracheitis—short incubation period (4 to 5 days), rapid onset of bilateral conjunctivitis, severe sneezing, and ulcerative keratitis.
- Feline calicivirus infection—short incubation period (3 to 5 days); ulcerative stomatitis; and severe pneumonia.
- Feline reovirus infection—very mild upper respiratory tract infection; short incubation and duration.
- Bronchial pneumonia caused by bacteria such as *Bordetella bronchiseptica*—focal bronchoalveolar pattern on lung radiographs.

 DIAGNOSTICS

- CBC—neutrophilic leukocytosis.
- Thoracic radiographs of animals with pneumonitis—mild diffuse interstitial pattern.
- Conjunctival scrapings stained with Giemsa—intracytoplasmic inclusions.
- Isolation of organism—conjunctival swabs submitted to laboratory for cell culture.
- IFA—detects chlamydial antigen in conjunctival smear samples.

THERAPEUTICS

- Generally as outpatient.
- Inpatient only if complicated by concurrent infections causing anorexia or respiratory distress.
- Physically clean discharge away from nostrils and eyes.
- Quarantine affected cats from contacting other cats (do not let affected cats outside).
- Both inactivated and modified live vaccines are available to reduce the severity of infection.
- Vaccines do not prevent infection, but do reduce severity and duration of illness.
- Give a single vaccination on the initial visit; revaccinate 1 year later; then give annual revaccination.
- American Association of Feline Practitioners classifies vaccination as noncore.

Drugs of Choice

- Systemic antibiotics—doxycycline or tetracycline (*Table 24-1*).
- Ocular—ophthalmic ointments containing tetracycline (q8h).

Precautions/Interactions

- Tetracyclines—discolor growing teeth.
- Doxycycline—has been associated with esophagitis/strictures in cats; give with food.
- Adverse vaccine reactions—mild clinical disease; small percentage of vaccinated cats.

COMMENTS

- Colonies—the entire colony may have to be treated.
- Treatment—may have to be continued for as long as 6 weeks.
- Inform clients—of the causative organism, anticipated chronic course of disease, and need to vaccinate other cats before exposure.
- Prognosis—tends to be chronic, lasting for several weeks or months, unless successful antibiotic treatment is given.
- Zoonosis—*C. psittaci* can infect humans.
- Limited number of reports in humans—mild conjunctivitis transmitted from infected cats.
- Role of *C. psittaci* as a pathogen during pregnancy—unclear.

TABLE 24-1. Drug Therapy for Chlamydiosis in Cats				
Drug	Dose (mg/kg)	Route	Interval (Hours)	Duration (Weeks)
Doxycycline	5	PO	12	3–4
Tetracycline	22	PO	8	3–4

- Organism can colonize the reproductive mucosa—severe conjunctivitis neonatorum can occur in neonatal kittens infected at or shortly after birth.
- *C. psittaci* does not cause sexually transmitted disease in humans (caused by *C. trichomatosis*).

Abbreviations

CBC, complete blood count; GI, gastrointestinal; IFA, immunofluoresence assay.

Suggested Reading

Elston T, Rodan I, Flemming D, et al. 1998 report of the American Association of Feline Practitioners and Academy of Feline Medicine Advisory Panel on Feline Vaccines. *J Am Vet Med Assoc* 1998;212:227–241.

Greene CE. Chlamydial infections. In: Greene CE, ed. *Infectious Diseases of the Dog and Cat.* 2nd ed. Philadelphia: WB Saunders; 1998:172–174.

Author: Fred W. Scott
Consulting Editor: Stephen C. Barr

chapter 25

Clostridial Enterotoxicosis

DEFINITION/OVERVIEW

- A syndrome characterized by diarrhea in dogs and cats associated with the production of enterotoxin by normal bacterial flora in the GI tract.

ETIOLOGY/PATHOPHYSIOLOGY

- *Clostridium perfringens*—common enteric inhabitant generally found in the vegetative form living in a symbiotic relationship with the host.
- Certain strains of *C. perfringens* (generally type A based on PCR analysis)—produce enterotoxin that binds to the enteric mucosa, alters cell permeability, and results in cell damage with subsequent local enterocyte death, but no systemic illness.
- *C. perfringens* enterotoxin—probably associated with enteric sporulation.
- Enterotoxin production—a number of intrinsic host-related factors influence enterotoxin production and pathogenicity of *C. perfringens*.
- Pathogenicity of *C. perfringens*—may depend on the metabolic, mucosal, and immunologic integrity of the GI tract.
- IgA deficiency—possibly.
- Alkaline intestinal luminal environment—promotes *C. perfringens* sporulation and enterotoxin production.
- Incidence—unknown.
- Chronic large bowel diarrhea—suspected that up to 20% of cases of chronic large bowel diarrhea in dogs are *C. perfringens*–related.
- Cats—infection less common than in dogs.

SIGNALMENT/HISTORY

- Most animals tend to be middle-aged or older.
- No sex or breed predilections.
- Historically, large bowel diarrhea with mucus.
- Small amounts of fresh blood.
- Tenesmus with increased frequency commonly reported.
- Small bowel diarrhea signs (large volume of watery stool) also reported.
- Vomiting.

- Flatulence.
- Abdominal discomfort.
- Stress factors to the GI tract, dietary change, concurrent disease, or hospitalization may precipitate signs.

CLINICAL FEATURES

- Signs usually associated with either:
  - An acquired acute, self-limiting large bowel diarrhea lasting for 5 to 7 days
  - Chronic intermittent diarrhea.
  - Signs associated with other GI or non-GI tract disease.
- Chronic disease—often characterized by intermittent episodes occurring every 2 to 4 weeks that may persist for months to years.
- The syndrome may develop from a nosocomial (hospital-acquired) infection—with signs developing during or shortly following hospitalization or kennel boarding.
- *C. perfringens*—occasionally associated with cases of parvovirus and acute hemorrhagic gastroenteritis.

DIFFERENTIAL DIAGNOSIS

- All causes of diarrhea, including systemic or metabolic disease and specific intestinal disorders, should be considered.
- Other causes of acute enterocolitis are dietary indiscretion; IBD; neoplasia (especially GI tract lymphoma); drugs (antibiotics); toxins (lead); parasites (cryptosporidiosis, trichomoniassis, whipworms, giardiasis); infectious agents (parvovirus, FIP, salmonellosis, rickettsia, GI tract bacterial overgrowth, histoplasmosis, leishmaniasis, pythiosis); systemic organ dysfunction (renal, hepatic, pancreatic, cardiac); metabolic (hypoadrenocorticism, feline hyperthyroidism).

DIAGNOSTICS

- CBC and biochemical panel—usually normal except may reflect dehydration.
- Diagnostic confirmation of. *C. perfringens* enterotoxicosis—as yet controversial.
- Testing—no test appears to be completely accurate.
- Anaerobic fecal cultures—generally identify high concentrations of *C. perfringens* organisms but occasionally will be negative.
- Specific fecal spore cultures—will detect high concentrations of *C. perfringens* spores ($>10^6$ spores per gram of feces) in affected animals and correlate well with clinical disease but are rarely performed.
- Fecal enterotoxin assay by ELISA (Tech Labs, Blacksburg, VA)—positive result in conjunction with clinical signs, fecal culture, and response to antibiotic therapy support *C. perfringens* as a contributing pathogen.

- Assay—requires 1 g (pea-size sample) of feces, can be frozen.
- False positive and false negative results—can occur.
- PCR to identify *C. perfringens* enterotoxin—not commercially available but correlates well with clinical disease.
- Reverse passive latex agglutination assay for enterotoxin—considered inaccurate.

Diagnostic Features
- **Fecal cytology—high numbers of *C. perfringens* endospores in the feces does not always correlate with clinical disease or fecal enterotoxin assay**
- Cytologic examination—performed by making a thin fecal smear on a microscope slide, air-drying or heat-fixing, and staining with Diff-Quik or Wright's stain.
- *C. perfringens* spores—have a typical "safety-pin" appearance with an oval structure and a dense body at one end of the spore wall *(Fig. 25-1).*

 THERAPEUTICS

- Outpatient—most treated as outpatients.
- Hospitalize—when diarrhea or vomiting is severe, resulting in dehydration and electrolyte imbalance.
- Dietary manipulation—plays an important role in the treatment and management of cases with chronic recurring disease.
- High-fiber diets—either soluble (or fermentable) or insoluble fiber, often result in clinical improvement.
- High-fiber diets—reduce enteric clostridial numbers, acidify the distal intestine, thus limiting *C. perfringens* sporulation and enterotoxin production.

■ **Fig. 25-1** Clostridial spores *(one identified by arrow)* in the feces of a dog with clostridial enterotoxicosis.

TABLE 25-1. Drug Therapy for Clostridial Enterotoxicosis

Drug	Dose (mg/kg)	Route	Interval (Hours)	Duration (Days)
Metronidazole	10	PO	8–12	5–7
Tylosin (Tylan soluble powder)[a]	10–20	PO	12	5–7
Amoxicillin/clavulanic acid	22	PO	12	5–7
Ampicillin	22	PO	8–12	5–7
Clindamycin	10	PO	12	5–7

[a] Given with the food or formulated in capsules for long-term management (~3 g/tsp).

- Commercial high-fiber diets—can be supplemented with psyllium (½ to 2 tsp/day) as a source of soluble fiber.
- Diets low in fiber—supplement with either course bran (1 to 3 tbsp/day) as a source of insoluble fiber or psyllium added as a source of soluble fiber.

Drugs of Choice

- Acute self-limiting disease—5- to 7-day antibiotic course (e.g., oral ampicillin or amoxicillin, clindamycin, metronidazole, or tylosin) (*Table 25-1*).
- Acute cases—most patients respond well to appropriate antibiotic therapy.
- Chronic reoccurring cases—often require prolonged antibiotic therapy.
- Chronic cases—tylosin (Tylan Soluble powder [Elanco, Indianapolis, IN], 100-g container, ~3 g/tsp) best for long-term management.
- High doses of antibiotics—may not be necessary to prevent recurrence in chronic cases.
- Administration of oral antibiotics at submicrobial inhibitory concentrations—may be effective in chronic cases.
- Low antibiotic levels—may not actually reduce enteric *C. perfringens* numbers but may change the ecologic microenvironment, preventing sporulation and enterotoxin production.

 COMMENTS

- Inform owners—acute disease is often self-limiting.
- Inform owners—chronic cases may require prolonged therapy.
- Infection—associated with environmental contamination, and disinfection is difficult.
- Feeding high-fiber diets—may decrease the incidence of nosocomial diarrhea.
- Most animals respond well to therapy—although chronic cases may require lifelong therapy to control clinical signs.
- A failure in response—suggests concurrent disease (such as parvovirus, acute HGE, or IBD), and further diagnostic evaluation is indicated.

Abbreviations

CBC, complete blood count; ELISA, enzyme-linked immunosorbent assay; FIP, feline infectious peritonitis; HGE, hemorrhagic gastroenteritis; GI, gastrointestinal; IBD, inflammatory bowel disease; PCR, polymerase chain reaction.

Suggested Reading

Foley J, Hirsh DC, Pedersen NC. An outbreak of *Clostridium perfringens* enteritis in a cattery of Bengal cats and experimental transmission to specific pathogen free cats. *Feline Pract* 1996;24:31–35.

Kirth SA, Prescott JF, Welch MK, et al. Nosocomial diarrhea associated with enterotoxigenic *Clostridium perfringens* infection in dogs. *J Am Vet Med Assoc* 1989;195:331–334.

Marks SL, Kather EJ, Kass PH, et al. Genotypic and phenotypic characterization of *Clostridium perfringens* and *Clostridium difficile* in diarrheic and healthy dogs. *J Vet Intern Med* 2002;16:533–540.

Twedt DC. *Clostridium perfringens* associated enterotoxicosis in dogs. In: Kirk RW, Bonagura JD, eds. *Current Veterinary Therapy XI*. Philadelphia: WB Saunders; 1992:602–604.

Weese JS, Staempfli HR, Prescott JF, et al. The roles of *Clostridium difficile* and enterotoxigenic *Clostridium perfringens* in diarrhea in dogs. *J Vet Intern Med* 2001;15:374–378.

Author: David C. Twedt
Consulting Editor: Stephen C. Barr

chapter 26

Coccidioidomycosis

DEFINITION/OVERVIEW

- A systemic mycotic infection affecting dogs (usually <4 years old) and, rarely, cats.

ETIOLOGY/PATHOPHYSIOLOGY

- *Coccidioides immitis*—grows several inches deep in the soil, where it survives high ambient temperatures and low moisture.
- After a period of rainfall—organism returns to the soil surface, where it sporulates, releasing many arthroconidia that are disseminated by wind and dust storms.
- Infection—by inhalation of arthroconidia.
- Exposure to large doses of fungus in contaminated soil—associated with aggressive nosing about in soil and underbrush; dust storms after rainy season; earthquakes; land developments.
- After inhalation—fever, lethargy, inappetence, cough, and joint pain may be noticed before dissemination (10 days postinfection) to other organs.
- Asymptomatic infections—may occur.
- Immunity—some animals develop immunity without onset of clinical signs.
- Skin lesions—usually associated with dissemination; penetrating wounds have rarely been associated with skin lesions.
- Signs of dissemination—may not be evident for several months after the initial infection.
- Dissemination occurs—to long bones, joints, eyes, skin, liver, kidneys, CNS, cardiovascular system (pericardium and myocardium), and testes.

SIGNALMENT/HISTORY

- An uncommon disease, even in endemic areas.
- Endemic regions are southwestern United States in the geographic Lower Sonoran Life Zone: Southern California, Arizona, and southwest Texas; less prevalent in New Mexico, Nevada, and Utah.
- Historically—anorexia, cough, fever unresponsive to antibiotics, lameness, weakness with paraparesis, back and neck pain, seizures, visual changes, and weight loss.

CLINICAL FEATURES

Dogs

- Pulmonary signs—cough, dyspnea, fever.
- Disseminated disease—bone swelling, joint enlargement, lameness, cachexia, lethargy, and lymphadenopathy.
- Neurologic signs—both central and peripheral neurologic deficits may be present.
- Skin ulcers—with draining tracts.
- Ocular signs—uveitis, keratitis, iritis, and retinitis.

Cats

- Cachexia.
- Draining skin lesions.
- Dyspnea.
- Lameness caused by bone involvement.
- Uveitis.

DIFFERENTIAL DIAGNOSIS

- Pulmonary lesions—resemble those of other systemic mycoses (e.g., histoplasmosis, blastomycosis).
- Lymphadenopathy—lymphosarcoma, other systemic mycoses, and localized bacterial infections.
- Bone lesions—primary or metastatic bone tumors or bacterial osteomyelitis.
- Skin lesions—abscesses or other bacterial disease processes.

DIAGNOSTICS

- CBC—mild nonregenerative anemia, neutrophilic leukocytosis, monocytosis.
- Serum chemistry profile—hyperglobulinemia, hypoalbuminemia, azotemia with renal involvement.
- Urinalysis—low urine specific gravity; proteinuria with inflammatory glomerulonephritis.
- Serologic tests for antibody to *C. immitis*—several technologies available, including AGID, ELISA, and latex agglutination, as well as the two classical tests based on two types of antigen:
  - TP—detects mainly IgM response, so positive titers appear early in disease (by 14 days postexposure); titers increase with dissemination or reactivation; may become negative 4 to 6 weeks postinfection.

■ **Fig. 26-1** Radiograph of a toe of a dog with coccidioidomycosis showing a proliferative lesion containing both lysis and bone production and extending into the joint, atypical for bone neoplasia.

- CF—detects mainly IgG response; good test for quantitative titers; the higher the complement fixation titer, the more likely it is that the disease is disseminated; positive titer can just indicate past exposure or healing or localized lesion; often positive in chronic cases when TP has become negative; higher CF titers ≥1:64 most often seen with disseminated or severe pulmonary disease; remain elevated months after successful treatment, then slowly decrease; false negative result in immunosuppressed or anergic animals.
- Radiology—lung (interstitial infiltrates) and bone lesions (osteolysis; *Fig. 26-1*).

Diagnostic Feature
- **Definitive method of diagnosis—microscopic identification of the large spherule form of *C. immitis* in lesion or biopsy material, lymph node aspirates, impression smears of skin lesions or draining exudates *(Fig. 26-2)*.**
- Cultures—only performed by trained personnel in laboratories designed for the task.
- Mycelial form is highly contagious.

■ **Fig. 26-2** Impression smear from a draining tract of a dog with coccidioidomycosis showing a spherule (usually between 10 to 80 μm, double walled, containing endospores) surrounded by neutrophils and macrophages (Wright's stain, 1,000×).

■ **Fig. 26-3** Histopathology of *C. immitis* in a lung biopsy taken from a dog with coccidioidomycosis. Note the presence of the endospores, which differentiates the organism from blastomycosis organisms (PAS stain, 1,000×).

- Biopsy of infected tissue—often preferred to avoid false-negative results, but tissues involved (lung) may be impractical to obtain *(Fig. 26-3)*.
- Serologic testing—more logical approach in an animal with consistent clinical signs from an endemic region.

 THERAPEUTICS

- Generally treated as outpatients.
- Concurrent clinical symptoms (e.g., seizures, pain, coughing) should be treated appropriately.
- Animals with a CF titer >1:8 should be monitored; if a repeat titer shows a rise after 4 weeks, institute drug therapy.
- The necessity, expense, possible treatment failure, and possible side effects of the drugs used should be reviewed with the owner.
- Surgical removal of a focal granulomatous organ (lung lobe, eye, and kidney) may be indicated.

Drugs of Choice

- Fluconazole—drug of choice; crosses the blood/brain barrier; can be expensive in large-breed dogs.
- Veterinary compounding pharmacies in Arizona and California have made fluconazole available more cheaply—however, not all compounding pharmacies are reliable.

- Ketoconazole—not as effective as fluconazole; give with food to improve absorption; continue for at least 1 year; monitor for side effects.
- Itraconazole—produces no better clinical response than ketoconazole; fewer side effects but more expensive.
- Amphotericin B—rarely recommended because of the high risk of renal damage and lack of availability of an oral preparation of the drug (*Table 26-1*).

Cats

- As per dogs, the azoles are preferred.

Precautions/Interactions

- Monitor—liver enzyme levels (rises in ALT) monthly when using azoles, especially ketoconazole, for extended periods.
- Ketoconazole—teratogenic, so should be used in pregnant animals only if the potential benefit justifies the potential risk to offspring.
- Amphotericin B—monitor for renal damage by frequent examination of urine sediment; discontinue treatment if granular casts are noted in the urine; consider lipid-encapsulated amphotericin B to decrease side effects.
- Pulmonary disease resulting in severe coughing—may temporarily worsen after therapy is begun, owing to inflammation in the lungs associated with killing of organisms.
- Low-dose, short-term oral prednisone and cough suppressants—may be required to alleviate the respiratory signs.

  COMMENTS

- Coccidioidomycosis is considered one of the most severe and life-threatening of the systemic mycoses with treatment of disseminated disease.
- Often requires at least 1 year of aggressive antifungal therapy.

TABLE 26-1. Drug Therapy for Coccidioidomycosis in Cats and Dogs

Drug	Species	Dose	Route	Interval (Hours)	Duration (Months)
Fluconazole	D	5 mg/kg	PO	12	10–12[a]
	C	25–100/cat	PO	12–24	[a]
Ketoconazole	D	5–10 mg/kg	PO	12	[a]
	C	50 mg/cat	PO	12–24	[a]
Itraconazole	D	5 mg/kg	PO	12	[a]
	C	25–50/cat	PO	12–24	[a]
Amphotericin B	D	0.3–0.5 mg/kg	IV	48–2[b]	[c]

[a] Usually treat for 12 months or until clinical resolution and complement fixation titers,1:4.
[b] Give 3 days a week.
[c] Until a total cumulative dose of 8 to 11 mg/kg.
C, cats; D, dogs.

- Decision for termination of drug therapy is based on resolution of clinical disease, radiographic appearance of bone and lung lesions (progressive or not), and CF titers.
- Monitor CF titers 3 to 4 months, with animals being treated until their titers fall to less than 1:4.
- Animals displaying poor response to therapy should have a 2- to 4-hour postpill drug (fluconazole) level measured to ensure adequate absorption of the drug.
- Prognosis is guarded to grave.
- Many dogs improve after oral therapy, but relapses are common, especially if therapy is shortened.
- Overall recovery rate is approximately 60% (some report 90%) response to fluconazole therapy.
- In cats the prognosis is not well documented, but rapid dissemination requires long-term therapy.
- Spontaneous recovery from disseminated coccidioidomycosis without treatment is extremely rare.
- No vaccine is available for dogs or cats
- Caution should be used if culturing draining lesions suspected of being infected with *C. immitis*; although the spherule-form of the fungus found in animal tissues is not directly transmissible to humans or other animals, the mycelial form is highly contagious.

Abbreviations

AGID, agar gel immunodiffusion; ALT, alanine aminotransferase; CBC, complete blood count; CF, complement fixation; CNS, central nervous system; ELISA, enzyme-linked immunosorbent assay; TP, tube precipitin.

Suggested Reading

Gionfriddo JR. Feline systemic fungal infections. *Vet Clin North Am Small Anim Pract* 2000;30:1029–1050.

Greene RT. Coccidioidomycosis. In: Greene CE, ed. *Infectious Diseases of the Dog and Cat*. 2nd ed. Philadelphia: WB Saunders; 1998:391–398.

Kerl ME. Update on canine and feline fungal disease. *Vet Clin North Am Small Anim Pract* 2003;33:721–747.

Author: Nita Kay Gulbas
Consulting Editor: Stephen C. Barr

chapter 27

Coccidiosis

DEFINITION/OVERVIEW

- An enteric protozoan infection of dogs and cats traditionally confined to the GI tract and showing strict host specificity.
- Does not include *Toxoplasma*, *Cryptosporidium*, *Sarcocystis*, *Besnoitia*, or *Hammondia* spp. (see specific chapters).

ETIOLOGY/PATHOPHYSIOLOGY

- *Isospora canis* (dogs) and *I. felis* (cats)—obligate intracellular coccidian protozoa potentially able to infect and cause diarrhea in puppies and kittens.
- *Eimeria* spp.—not parasitic in dogs or cats; oocysts can appear in carnivore feces as a result of coprophagy or ingesting *Eimeria*-infected prey.
- *Isospora* spp.—host specific.
- Direct life cycles (fecal-oral transmission)—pass oocysts (relatively large at 32 to 53 μm, unsporulated) in feces.
- Damage to the host's small intestinal enterocytes—can cause watery diarrhea in the very young or immunosuppressed.
- Autoinfection—common, causing a continual recycling within the intestinal tract and loss of mucosal lining.
- The direct role of *Isospora* spp. in causing disease—still in question because there are few studies elaborating pathogenesis.
- Virtually every dog and cat becomes infected during its life (usually during the first month)—few show clinical disease.

SIGNALMENT/HISTORY

- Puppies and kittens.

CLINICAL FEATURES

- Diarrhea—watery.
- Diarrhea—can persist for weeks.
- Diarrhea—can occasionally contain mucus or blood.

DIFFERENTIAL DIAGNOSIS

- Other causes of diarrhea in young animals, including:
  - Dietary—indiscretion or poor nutrition.
  - Parasites—giardiasis, cryptosporidiosis, trichomoniasis.
  - Other infectious agents—parvovirus, FIP, FeLV, salmonellosis, rickettsia, *Campylobacter*, clostridia, or colibacillosis.
- Consider also—systemic organ dysfunction (renal, hepatic, pancreatic, cardiac, peritonitis); drugs (antibiotics); toxins (lead, organophosphates).

DIAGNOSTICS

- CBC and biochemical panel—may reflect fluid and electrolyte loss from diarrhea.
- Fecal examination—*Isospora* spp. oocysts, unsporulated and >30 μm long.
- Oocysts—should be differentiated from those of other species:
  - Cat—*Isospora revolta* (unsporulated, <30 μm), *Besnoitia* and *Toxoplasma gondii* (unsporolated, 10 to 14 μm).
  - Dog—*Hammondia* spp. (unsporulated).
  - Both cats and dogs—*Sarcocystis* spp. and *Cryptosporidia* (both sporulated, 9 to 16 μm and <5 μm, respectively) (*Figs. 27-1 and 27-2*).

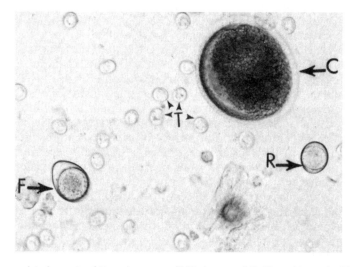

■ Fig. 27-1 Unsporulated oocysts of *Toxoplasma gondii* (*T*), *Isospora felis* (*F*), and *I. revolta* (*R*) with an egg of the helminth *T. cati* (*C*) in flotation of feline feces (unstained, 200×). (From Dubey JP: A review of *Sarcocystis* of domestic animals and of other coccidian of cats and dogs. *J Am Vet Med Assoc* 1976;169:1061–1078; with permission).

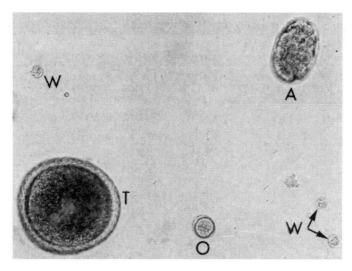

■ **Fig. 27-2** Unsporulated oocysts *of Isospora ohioensis* (*O*) and *Hammonida heydornia* (*H*) compared with eggs of the nematodes *Toxocara canis* (*C*) and *Ancylostoma caninum* (*A*) in a flotation of canine feces (unstained, 200×). (From Dubey JP: A review of *Sarcocystis* of domestic animals and of other coccidian of cats and dogs. *J Am Vet Med Assoc* 1976;169:1061–1078; with permission).

 THERAPEUTICS

- Most animals will respond to coccidiostat therapy alone—without parenteral support.
- Very young animals—may need fluid support if diarrhea is extreme.
- Coccidiosis is rarely the sole cause of diarrhea—every effort should be made to identify other concurrent factors or infections.
- Examine for host stress factors and factors within the kennel—concurrent parasitism, weaning, poor diet, poor environmental conditions, or immunosuppression.

Drugs of Choice

- Sulfadimethoxine (Albon [Pfizer Animal Health, Exton PA])—tables, 5% oral suspension.
- Trimethoprim-sulfadiazine (Tribrissen [Schering-Plough, Union, NJ])—tablets, injectable.
- Amprolium (Corid 9.6% oral solution [Merial, Iselin, NJ])—off-label use for prevention or treatment (*Table 27-1*).

Precautions/Interactions

- TMS—can produce keratoconjunctivitis sicca; should not be used in dogs with a reduced Schirmer tear test; may occur 1 week after beginning drug; monitor Schirmer tear test weekly.

TABLE 27-1. **Drug Therapy for Coccidiosis in Dogs and Cats**					
Drug	Species	Dose (mg/kg)	Route	Interval (Hours)	Duration (Days)
Sulfadimethoxine (Albon)	B	50–60[a]	PO	24	14–21
Trimethoprim-sulfadiazine (Tribrissen)	B	30–60[b]	PO, SC	24[c]	6
Amproline (Corid)	D	100–200	PO[d]	24	7
	C	20–40[e]	PO	24	10

[a] After first dose of 50 to 60 mg/kg, can halve dose until asymptomatic but not to exceed 3 weeks.
[b] If >4 kg body weight. Halve the dose if <4 kg body weight.
[c] Dose may be divided into two daily doses.
[d] Added to food or water.
[e] Can increase the dose to 300 mg/kg and give for 5 days.
B, both cats and dogs; C, cats; D, dogs.

- TMS—been associated with folate acid–deficient anemias, hepatotoxicity, immune-mediated polyarthritis, retinitis, glomerulitis, vasculitis, thrombocytopenia, toxic epidermal necrolysis, and cutaneous drug eruptions.
- Cats—TMS causes profound hypersalivation in cats; give as whole tablets, do not break; also, supplement cats with folic acid (2.5 mg/kg/day) to avoid development of megaloblastic anemia.

 # COMMENTS

- Coccidiosis outbreaks—can occur even in well-managed kennels or catteries, especially when young animals are present in large numbers.
- Eradication—not usually possible.
- Concentrate on controlling outbreaks by strict hygiene—live steam, ammonia or phenol-containing disinfectants.
- Dry, hot conditions—will kill cysts.
- Combination of sulfadimethoxine (55 mg/kg) and ormetoprim (11 mg/kg) daily for 23 days mixed with feed during pups' exposure to infective oocysts—shown to markedly reduce oocyst shedding and severity/incidence of diarrhea.

Abbreviations

CBC, complete blood count; FeLV, feline leukemia virus; FIP, feline infectious peritonitis; GI, gastrointestinal; TMS, trimethoprim-sulfadiazine.

Suggested Reading

Bowman DD, ed. *Georgi's Parasitology for Veterinarians.* 8th ed. Philadelphia: WB Saunders; 2003:92–95.

Author: Julie Ann Jarvinen
Consulting Editor: Stephen C. Barr

chapter 28

Colibacillosis

DEFINITION/OVERVIEW

- Bacterial infection of dogs and cats causing a range of conditions, including septicemia in the very young, sometimes complicating other causes of enteritis (parvovirus), UTI, and so on.
- Can be isolated as normal flora from the GI tract and prepuce and vagina of dogs and cats.

ETIOLOGY/PATHOPHYSIOLOGY

- *Escherichia coli*—gram-negative Enterobacteriaceae, normal inhabitant of the GI tract of most mammals.
- Under certain circumstances (immunosuppression; presence of other disease, such as GI disease or other pathogens)—can become systemic to affect other organs or contaminate other tissue/organ sites (urogenital system, skin, mammary gland).
- Virulence factors (various, depending on strains) exist—ability to cause septicemia probably due more to the immune status of host rather than virulence factors of bacterium.

SIGNALMENT/HISTORY

- Mainly affects neonatal puppies and kittens <1 week of age—especially if they have not received colostrum.
- Predisposition—overpopulated housing.
- Older dogs and cats—mainly diarrhea, urogenital (cystitis, endometritis, pyelonephritis, prostatitis, mastitis), otitis, pneumonia, hepatobiliary disease, endocarditis, and, rarely, meningoencephalomyelitis.

CLINICAL FEATURES

Neonates (First 2 Weeks of Life)

- Sudden onset.
- Vomiting.
- Weakness.

- Lethargy.
- Diarrhea—often watery.
- Hypothermia.
- Loss of sucking reflex.
- Cyanosis.
- Usually multiple animals in litter affected.
- Bitch/queen—may have poor health and nutritional status.
- Unable to provide good care and colostrum to offspring.
- Overcrowding and poor hygiene will precipitate fecal-oral spread of infection.

Puppies/Kittens and Adults

- Vomiting.
- Diarrhea.
- Rapid dehydration.
- Fever with some strains.
- Concurrent diseases (parvovirus, panleukopenia, parasitism) and use of antimicrobial agents that upset GI flora, or immunosuppression often precipitate disease.

DIFFERENTIAL DIAGNOSIS

- Dietary indiscretion, IBD; neoplasia (especially GI tract lymphoma); drugs (antibiotics); toxins (lead, organophosphates); parasites (giardiasis, cryptosporidiosis, trichomoniasis, whipworms); infectious agents (parvovirus, FIP, FeLV, salmonellosis, rickettsia, *Campylobacter*, clostridia, histoplasmosis, coronavirus); systemic organ dysfunction (renal, hepatic, pancreatic, cardiac, pyometra, peritonitis); metabolic (hypoadrenocorticism).

DIAGNOSTICS

- CBC and biochemical panel—usually neonates die very rapidly, not allowing too many changes.
- Hypoglycemia—usually present.
- Adults—may show consequences of electrolyte and fluid losses from diarrhea.
- Culture of *E. coli* from blood or other tissues (urine, aspirates) where not normally found—required to show that it is not a contaminant.

THERAPEUTICS

- Acutely ill neonates—must receive good nursing care in a heated environment.
- Parenteral fluids—containing glucose.

TABLE 28-1. Drug Therapy for *Escherichia coli* Infections in Dogs and Cats if Culture and Sensitivity Results Are Not Available

Drug	Dose (mg/kg)	Route	Interval (Hours)	Duration (Days)
Amoxicillin	10–20	PO, IV, SC	12	7
Trimethoprim-sulfa	30	PO	12	7–10
Enrofloxacin[a]	2.5–5	PO	12	7–10
Cefixime (Suprax)	5–10	PO	12	10
Cefaclor (Ceclor)	10	PO	8	7–10
Cefadroxil (Cefatabs)	22	PO	12	7

[a] For adult animals.

- When stronger and able to take food orally—tube feeding with balanced milk substitute is indicated.
- Attention must be paid to warmth, elimination, and hydration.

Drugs of Choice

- Antibiotic use—should be based on culture and sensitivity results, especially for UTI, and other non–life-threatening conditions (allowing time to get results back from lab).
- Empirically—use broad spectrum.
- Amoxicillin.
- TMS.
- Fluoroquinolones such as enrofloxacin (Baytril [Bayer, Bayer Co., Shawnee Mission, KS]) for adult animals.
- Cephalosporins such as cefixime (Suprax oral suspension [Lederle, Wayne, NJ]); cefaclor (Ceclor [Eli Lily, Indianapolis, IN]); cefadroxil (Cefa-tabs [Fort Dodge, Fort Dodge, IA]); third-generation injectable cephalosporins (*Table 28-1*).

Precautions/Interactions

- TMS can cause keratoconjunctivitis sicca—should not be used in dogs with a reduced Schirmer tear test.
- TMS—associated with folate acid–deficient anemias, hepatotoxicity, immune-mediated polyarthritis, retinitis, glomerulonephritis, vasculitis, thrombocytopenia, toxic epidermal necrolysis, and cutaneous drug eruptions.
- Do not use enrofloxacin in pregnant, growing, or neonatal animals.
- High doses of enrofloxacin—may cause blindness in cats, particularly with concurrent ocular diseases.

 COMMENTS

- Enterobacteriaceae can change resistance to antibiotics over time—ideally, important to base antibiotic use on culture and sensitivity results.

Abbreviations

CBC, complete blood count; FeLV, feline leukemia virus; FIP, feline infectious peritonitis; GI, gastrointestinal; IBD, inflammatory bowel disease; TMS, trimethoprim-sulfadiazine; UTI, urinary tract infection.

Suggested Reading

Kruth SA. Gram-negative bacterial infections. In: Greene CE, ed. *Infectious Diseases of the Dog and Cat.* Philadelphia: WB Saunders; 1998:217–222.

Author: Patrick L. McDonough and Kenneth W. Simpson
Consulting Editor: Stephen C. Barr

chapter 29

Cryptococcosis

DEFINITION/OVERVIEW

- A systemic or localized fungal infection causing granulomas, usually in the nose, sinuses, and eyes of cats and brain, nasal passages, and sinuses of dogs.

ETIOLOGY/PATHOPHYSIOLOGY

- *Cryptococcus neoformans*—an environmental yeastlike fungus able to form a heteropolysaccharide capsule in tissues.
- Environment—found mainly in bird droppings and decaying vegetation (where it can survive for 2 years).
- Infection—occurs by localization of the yeast in nasal passages after inhalation; some organisms may reach the terminal airways to establish lung infection (rare).
- Hematogenous dissemination—to brain, eyes, lymph nodes, and other tissues may occur; local spread to the skin of the nose, eyes, and lymph nodes can occur.

SIGNALMENT/HISTORY

- Most common at 2 to 7 years of age.
- Higher incidence in areas of southern California and Australia.

Dogs

- Rare in North America; prevalence ~0.00013%.
- Doberman pinschers, Labrador retrievers, and American cocker spaniels overrepresented.
- No sex predilection.

Cats

- About 10 times more common than in dogs.
- Siamese overrepresented.
- Occurs more commonly in males.
- Patients concurrently infected with FeLV or FIV are at higher risk and suffer more extensive disease.

CLINICAL FEATURES

- Lethargy.
- Fever.
- Signs vary depending on organ system affected.

Dogs

- Organs mainly affected—brain, nasal passages, sinuses; also draining lymph nodes, eyes, periorbital tissue; rarely lungs and abdominal organs.
- Usually neurologic signs—ataxia, seizures, paresis, blindness.
- Lymphadenopathy.
- Nasal discharge.
- Skin mass or ulceration.

Cats

- Organs mainly affected—nose, sinuses, facial skin, nasopharynx, brain, and eyes.
- Firm mass over the bridge of the nose.
- Masses—may ulcerate, develop weeping granulomatous tissue *(Fig. 29-1)*.
- Nasal discharge—occasional sneezing, snuffling.
- Lymphadenopathy—especially submandibular, prescapular.
- Nasopharyngeal mass lesions—snoring, stertor, inspiratory dyspnea.
- Lower respiratory tract signs—rare.
- CNS disease—cranial nerve involvement is common manifestation.
- Ocular signs—common with CNS disease.
- Blindness—due to exudative retinal detachment, granulomatous chorioretinitis *(Fig. 29-2)*, panophthalmitis, anterior uveitis.

■ **Fig. 29-1** Ulcerated mass lesion over the bridge of the nose of a cat with cryptococcosis.

■ **Fig. 29-2** Chorioretinitis and hemorrhage near the optic disc of a cat with cryptococcosis.

 ## DIFFERENTIAL DIAGNOSIS

Dogs

- Neurologic disease—both focal and diffuse; tumors, rickettsial diseases, other fungal diseases, granulomatous meningoencephalomyelitis, toxins such as lead, distemper, neosporosis, toxoplasmosis, idiopathic epilepsy.
- Nasal disease—immune mediated, especially when at the mucocutaneous junction; tumors, foreign body; other fungal infections; allergic rhinitis; and dental disease.
- Lymphadenopathy—lymphosarcoma; other infections, such as with *Leishmania* spp.
- Ocular disease—other fungal infections, distemper, neoplasia, toxoplasmosis, rickettsial diseases.

Cats

- Nasal disease—tumors, chronic rhinitis, sinusitis, or nasopharyngeal polyps.
- Ulcerative skin lesions—bacterial infection, cat bite abscess, tumor (squamous cell carcinoma).
- Ocular disease—neoplasia (lymphoma), toxoplasmosis, feline infectious peritonitis (FIP).

 ## DIAGNOSTICS

- CBC—anemia of chronic disease (normocytic, normochromic); eosinophilia occasionally seen in some cats.

- Serum biochemistry profile—usually normal; may show mild elevations in globulin proteins.
- Imaging (radiographs, CT, MRI) of nasopharynx—may show cryptococcal granuloma as a soft tissue density that can on occasion erode dorsal nasal bones/turbinates.
- Thoracic radiographs—diffuse mixed interstitial-alveolar pattern in animals with lung involvement.
- Latex agglutination or ELISA—detect cryptococcal capsular antigen in serum, CSF, urine, or even nasal discharge; are very sensitive and reasonably specific tests.
- Can get low false positive titers (1:4)—due to reaction with talc from latex gloves or latex from rubber stoppers of blood collection tubes contaminating the sample.
- Monitor capsular antigen titers—because magnitude correlates with extent of infection, these titers can be used to monitor treatment efficacy.
- Cultures—on Sabouraud's agar with antibiotics confirms diagnosis.
- NOTE:—unlike in-house cultures of *Blastomyces* and *Histoplasma* organisms, *Cryptococcus* spp. do not present a zoonotic risk to staff.

Diagnostic Feature
- **Definitive diagnosis—cytologic examination of aspirates of granulomas, nasal discharge material, lymph nodes, or CSF stained with Diff-Quik or Wright's stains (although New Methylene Blue and Gram's stain are the best) usually reveals pleomorphic yeast forms with clear mucopolysaccharide capsule (*Fig. 29-3*).**
- Biopsy—although definitive, is usually not required.

■ **Fig. 29-3** Lymph node aspirate cytologic specimen of a cat with cryptococcosis. Note the pleomorphic yeast-like organisms surrounded by a halo (Wright's stain, 1,000×).

THERAPEUTICS

- Surgically debulk mass lesions—especially if associated with respiratory distress (especially upper airway of cats), then administer systemic antifungal therapy.
- Nutritional support—especially cats after surgery (esophageal or PEG tube).
- Treat stable animals as outpatients—neurologic cases may need in-hospital supportive care initially.

Drugs of Choice

- Itraconazole (Sporanox [Janssen, Titusville, NJ])—first choice in cases without ocular or neurologic involvement because it does not penetrate into these tissues; less expensive than fluconazole; give with fatty food (such as canned) to improve absorption.
- Fluconazole (Diflucan [Pfizer, Exton, PA])—first choice in cases with ocular or neurologic involvement because it does penetrate into these tissues.
- Flucytosine (Ancobon [Roche, Nutley, NJ])—best if used with trizoles (itraconazole or fluconazole) or amphotericin B when infection not responding well to single agent.
- Amphotericin B deoxycholate (Fungizone [Squibb, New York, NY])—use if other therapies too expensive; often most successful when used with flucytosine; administer in conjunction with fluid therapy to protect against nephrotoxicity; using SC route in cats will reduce toxicity.
- Amphotericin B lipid complex (Abelcet [Liposome Co., Princeton, NJ])—use in place of deoxycholate because it is less toxic but more expensive.
- Terbinafine (Lamisil [Sandoz, Dayton, NJ])—effective in cats with infections resistant to the triazoles; expensive *(Table 29-1)*.

TABLE 29-1. Drug Therapy for Cryptococcosis

Drug	Species	Dose (mg/kg)	Route	Interval (Hours)	Duration (Months)
Itraconazole—100 mg capsules/ 100 mg/ml liquid	D	5.0	PO	12	6–10
	C	10–15	PO	24	6–10
Fluconazole—50, 100, 150, 200 mg tablets	B	5–15	PO	24	6–10
Flucytosine[a]—250, 500 mg capsules	B	30	PO	8	1–9
Amphotericin B (deoxycholate)—50 mg/vial powder for injection	C	0.1–0.5	IV	3 times/week	[b]
	C	0.5–0.8	SC	3 times/week	[c]
	D	0.25–0.5	IV	3 times/week	[b]
Amphotericin B (lipid)—100 mg/20 ml vial solution for injection	D	1.0	IV	3 times/week	[d]
Terbinafine—125, 250 mg tablets	B	5–10	PO	24	1–3

[a] Give with amphotericin B.

[b] Give to a total cumulative dose of 4 to 10 mg/kg.

[c] Add each dose to 400 ml of 0.45% saline/2.5% dextrose, to a total cumulative dose of 8 to 26 mg/kg.

[d] Can be given to a total cumulative dose of up to 12 mg/kg.

B, both cats and dogs; C, cats; D, dogs.

Precautions/Interactions

- Triazoles (itraconazole and fluconazole)—hepatotoxic (monitor for liver enzyme elevations monthly); can cause GI tract signs.
- Itraconazole—ulcerative dermatitis (usually develops toward treatment end but needs to be differentiated from cryptococcal lesions); do not give with the antihistamines terfenadine and astemizole, or with cisapride (fatal cardiac arrhythmias may occur).
- Fluconazole—water soluble, so excreted via kidneys; reduce dose in animals with renal insufficiency.
- Flucytosine—can cause drug eruptions (depigmentation of lips or nose, ulceration, exudation, and crusting of skin), myelosuppression; avoid in neonates, pregnant animals or in animals with renal insufficiency.
- Amphoteracin B deoxycholate—nephrotoxic (monitoring urine for casts is the most sensitive method for detecting nephrotoxicity; creatine and BUN elevations are not as sensitive or specific but have been used to monitor nephrotoxicity).
- Amphotericin B lipid complex—much less toxic than deoxycholate but more expensive.
- Terbinafine—reduce dosage by at least half in animals with reduced renal and hepatic function; may show GI tract signs.

 COMMENTS

- Owner needs to be aware that triazole therapy is expensive and disease requires months of therapy—usual duration is 3 to 12 months.
- Drug choice—generally, itraconazole is used in nonocular or non-neurologic disease, fluconazole when ocular and neurologic disease is present, and amphotericin B in patients in situations in which financial restraints are present; the latter can be used inexpensively with SC administration on an outpatient basis.
- Assure owner—that infection is not zoonotic.
- Inform owner—that organism is acquired from the environment and that animal could be at increased risk, especially if immunosuppressed.
- Monitor liver enzymes—monthly in patients receiving triazole antifungals.
- Use clinical signs and capsular antigen titers to monitor efficacy of therapy—check titers first, 2 months after onset of therapy (should be markedly reduced); generally, titers decline by 2- to 4-fold/month during successful treatment; if not responding to treatment, try another triazole or add flucytosine; stop treatment after capsular antigen titers become negative or reduced by 32-fold from beginning titer.
- Cats with FIV or FeLV—have a poorer prognosis.

Abbreviations

BUN, blood urea nitrogen; CBC, complete blood count; CNS, central nervous system; CSF, cerebrospinal fluid; CT, computed tomography; ELISA, enzyme-linked immunosorbent assay; FeLV, feline leukemia virus; FIP, feline infectious peritonitis; FIV, feline immunodeficiency virus; GI, gastrointestinal; MRI, magnetic resonance imaging; PEG, percutaneous endoscopic gastrostomy.

Suggested Reading

Berthelin CF, Bailey CS, Kass PH, et al. Cryptococcosis of the nervous system in dogs, Part 1: epidemiologic, clinical and neuropathologic features. *Prog Vet Neurol* 1994;5:88–97.

Berthelin CF, Legendre AM, Bailey CS, et al. Cryptococcosis of the nervous system in dogs, Part 2: diagnosis, treatment, monitoring and prognosis. *Prog Vet Neurol* 1994;5:136–146.

Jacobs GJ, Medleau L, Clavert C, et al. Cryptococcal infection in cats: factors influencing treatment outcome, and results of sequential serum antigen titers in 35 cats. *J Vet Int Med* 1997;11:1–4.

Malik R, Craig AJ, Wigney DI, et al. Combination chemotherapy of canine and feline cryptococcosis using subcutaneously administered amphotericin B. *Aust Vet J* 1996;73:124–128.

Medleau L, Jacobs GJ, Marks A. Itraconazole for the treatment of cryptococcosis in cats. *J Vet Intern Med* 1995;9:39–42.

Author: Alfred M. Legendre
Consulting Editor: Stephen C. Barr

chapter 30

Cryptosporidiosis

DEFINITION/OVERVIEW

- A coccidian protozoa causing diarrhea in dogs and cats; also infects humans and many other mammals, including calves, foals, rodents.

ETIOLOGY/PATHOPHYSIOLOGY

- Multiple species occur—including *Cryptosporidium canis* and *C. felis*.
- Morphologically—species very similar.
- Some species are host specific—others (e.g., *C. parvum*) infect multiple species.
- *C. parvum*—main species to infect small animals.
- Infection—occurs by ingestion of sporulated oocysts; sporozoites are released from oocysts to infect intestinal epithelial cells; multiply (asexually); merozoites released to infect other cells.
- PPP = 5 to 10 days in cats.
- Immunocompetent animals—develop intestinal infection, which is usually asymptomatic; excrete oocysts in feces for about 2 weeks, then stop shedding.
- Immunocompromised animals—usually have signs of enteritis, but can develop infections of respiratory tract, liver, biliary tree, and pancreas.

SIGNALMENT/HISTORY

- No sex or breed predilection in either cats or dogs.

Dogs

- Virtually all clinical cases occur in dogs <6 months of age.
- Older dogs can excrete cysts but not show signs unless complicated by intestinal disease (IBD or neoplasia such as GI tract lymphoma).

Cats

- Serologic examination results suggest approximately 15% exposure rate in cats in the United States.
- Virtually all clinical cases reported in immunocompromized cats.
- More common in young and newborn kittens <6 months of age.

CLINICAL FEATURES

- Most commonly, asymptomatic oocyst shedding.
- Small bowel diarrhea, although large bowel diarrhea reported.

DIFFERENTIAL DIAGNOSIS

- Anything that causes acute small bowel diarrhea, including dietary indiscretion; IBD; neoplasia (especially GI tract lymphoma); drugs (antibiotics); toxins (lead); parasites (giardiasis, trichomoniasis, whipworms); infectious agents (parvovirus, FIP, salmonellosis, rickettsia, GI bacterial overgrowth, clostridia, histoplasmosis, leishmaniasis); systemic organ dysfunction (renal, hepatic, pancreatic, cardiac); metabolic (hypoadrenocorticism, hyperthyroidism of cats).
- NOTE: Patients with diarrhea and *Cryptosporidia* cysts in their feces invariably have an underlying disease process that could include a systemic cause for immunosuppression (neoplasia, FIP, FeLV, FIV, distemper, chronic corticosteroid use) or underlying intestinal tract disease (IBD, intestinal lymphoma, chronic antibiotic use).

DIAGNOSTICS

- CBC, biochemical panel, urinalysis, imaging—are usually normal unless altered by underlying disease process.
- Identify oocysts in feces—sugar and zinc sulfate flotation (specific gravity = 1.18).
- Because the organism is so small—identification of the oocysts is often difficult and best accomplished by experienced laboratory staff.
- Routine salt flotation—often fails because oocysts are very small (4 to 8 μm). (*Fig. 30-1*).
- Preferred stain—modified acid-fast; oocysts stain orange-red (*Fig. 30-2*).
- Crystal violet will stain fecal material but not oocysts—making visualization clearer (negative staining).
- NOTE: When submitting feces to a laboratory—mix 1 part 100% formalin with 9 parts feces to inactivate oocysts and decrease health risk to laboratory staff.
- Direct fluorescent antibody kits (Merifluor, [Meridian Diagnostics, Cincinnati, OH]) are effective in cats and dogs but often only available in diagnostic laboratories.
- Antigen detection methods (ProSpecT, *Cryptosporidium* Mitrotiter Assay [Alexon, Sunnyvale, CA]; Color-Vue *Cryptosporidium* [Seradyn, Indianapolis, IN])—are available but unknown if detect *C. felis* and *C. canis*.
- PCR techniques—available in specific research laboratories; not generally for diagnostic use.
- PCR—approximately 10 to 100 times more sensitive for the diagnosis of cryptosporidiosis in cats than other techniques.
- Intestinal biopsy or cytology—may reveal organisms in epithelial cells but can produce false-negatives results.

■ **Fig. 30-1** *Cryptosporidium* cysts in a fecal smear from a dog.

■ **Fig. 30-2** *Cryptosporidium* cysts in the feces of a cat (modified acid fast stain, 1,200×).

 THERAPEUTICS

- In immunocompetent animals—the diarrhea is usually very mild and self-limiting.
- Wait 2 weeks—then check for oocyst shedding again (unless public health/zoonosis issues of primary concern).

- Underlying diseases—treat aggressively.
- Mild diarrhea—treat on outpatient basis; withhold food for 24 to 48 hours; supplement with oral glucose-electrolyte solutions (Entrolyte, [Pfizer, Exton, PA]).
- Severe diarrhea—NPO, parental fluids (isotonic with potassium added at least to 30 mEq/liter).

Drugs of Choice

- None of these drugs are registered for this use in small animals.

Paromomycin (Humatin [ParkDavis, Morris Plans, NJ])
- Stops oocyst shedding in both cats and dogs.
- Not absorbed from GI tract if intact.
- If the drug is absorbed from the GI tract (possible in animals with hemorrhagic diarrhea, very young animals), it can cause renal failure and deafness (similar to other aminoglycosides).
- Toxicity responds to diuresis; monitor renal toxicity by monitoring urine for casts.

Tylosin (Tylan [Elanco, Indianapolis, IN])
- Has been used successfully in cats, but long treatment course required.

Nitazoxanide (Alinia [Romark Labs, Tampa, FL])
- Registered for the treatment of cryptosporidiosis and giardiasis in humans.
- Stops oocyst shedding in cats.
- Dosing usually associated with vomiting, which can be ameliorated by antiemetics (chlorpromazine) (*Table 30-1*).

Precautions/Interactions

- Paromomycin—will be absorbed across the blood-GI tract barrier in very young animals and animals with hemorrhagic diarrhea; because it is an aminoglycoside, its side effects of renal failure and deafness will be exacerbated in animals receiving parenteral aminoglycosides (gentamicin).
- Nitazoxanide—has only been used in a limited number of cats with cryptosporidiosis and needs further evaluation; few side effects other than vomiting.

TABLE 30-1. Drug Therapy for Cryptosporidiosis in Small Animals					
Drug	Species	Dose (mg/kg)	Route	Interval (Hours)	Duration (Days)
Paromomycin[a]—250 mg capsules	B	125–165	PO	12	5
Tylosin—100 g containers (~3 g/tsp)	C	11	PO	12	28
Nitazoxanide—100 mg/5ml suspension	C	25	PO	24	7–28

[a] Monitor closely for renal toxicity
B, cats and dogs; C, cats.

COMMENTS

- Zoonosis.
- Although some studies suggest that the incidence of cryptosporidiosis in HIV-positive people who own dogs is not increased, it would be prudent to make such owners are aware of the infectivity of the organism.

Disinfection

- Resistant to commercial bleach (5.25% sodium hypochlorite) and chlorination of drinking water.
- A 10% formaldehyde solution and 5% ammonia solution will kill oocysts, but requires 18 hours of exposure.
- Higher concentrations of ammonia (50%) will kill oocysts in 30 min.
- Moist heat (steam or pasteurization [>55°C]), freezing and thawing, or thorough drying are also effective.

Abbreviations

CBC, complete blood count; FeLV, feline leukemia virus; FIV, feline immunodeficiency virus; FIP, feline infectious peritonitis; GI, gastrointestinal; IBD, inflammatory bowel disease; HIV, human immunodeficiency virus; NPO, nothing per os; PCR, polymerase chain reaction; PPP, prepatent period.

Suggested Reading

Gookin JL, Nordone SK, Argenzio RA. Host responses to *Cryptosporidium* infection. *J Vet Intern Med* 2002;16:12–21.
Lappin MR. Diagnosis and management of cryptosporidiosis in dogs and cats. *Proc Am Col Vet Intern Med* 2002;20:654–656.

Author: Stephen C. Barr
Consulting Editor: Stephen C. Barr

chapter 31

Cuterebriasis

DEFINITION/OVERVIEW

- A disease caused by the migration through tissues of the larvae of flies (genus *Cuterebra*) in dogs and cats.

ETIOLOGY/PATHOPHYSIOLOGY

- *Cuterebra* spp. are obligatory parasites of rodents and lagomorphs (rabbits).
- The fly lays eggs on blades of grass or in the host's nest; the eggs hatch, and larvae crawl onto the skin of a passing host.
- The small maggot enters a body orifice, migrates through various internal tissues, and, eventually, migrates to the skin where it makes a warble.
- These small maggots (3 to 5 mm in length) are sometimes the parasite found to cause clinical disease.
- Once matured, the maggot (now up to 1 inch long) drops out of the host to pupate in the soil (*Fig. 31-1*).
- Cats and dogs infected in same way as other hosts.
- Signs are associated with either the warble in the skin or migration of the larvae through tissues (nares, upper respiratory tract, skin of the face, ocular tissue, brain).

SIGNALMENT/HISTORY

- All ages and breeds of outdoor dogs and cats may be affected.
- Disease mainly seen during mid to late summer (northern states) or nearly year round (southern states) when flies are most active.

CLINICAL FEATURES

Skin Warble

- More common in dogs but also cats.
- Appears as a single draining 2- to 5-mm cutaneous fistula (*Fig. 31-2*).
- Sometimes, a bot with protruding spiracles can be seen within the fistula.
- Before the bot penetrates the skin, the early developing warble can appear as a tender 1-cm swelling of the subcutis.

■ **Fig. 31-1** Second-instar larva of *Cuterebra* removed from the skin lesion of a cat.

Tissue Migration

- Neurologic disease—most common form in cats.
- Larvae—migrate through the cribriform plate into the brain, causing acute onset of ataxia, circling, paralysis, blindness and recumbency *(Fig. 31-3)*.
- Nasal irritation—migration may be preceded by 4 to 14 days of signs of nasal irritation.
- Respiratory—serous nasal discharge with sneezing as larvae migrate through nares; usually cats affected.
- Swelling—can see unilateral facing swelling.
- Larvae migration to nasopharynx and larynx—may see respiratory distress and stridor.

■ **Fig. 31-2** A draining fistula or warble in the neck of a cat after a *Cuterebra* larva has been removed.

■ **Fig. 31-3** A *Cuterebra* larva (*arrow*) on the frontal lobe of a cat's brain, where it was found at necropsy. Note the area of necrosis anterior to the larvae (courtesy Dr. A. Delahunta, Cornell University).

- Migration into lungs—can cause eosinophilic respiratory disease.
- Ophthalmic lesions—larvae migrate into globe or conjunctiva.

 DIFFERENTIAL DIAGNOSIS

Skin Warble

- Mature warble is unmistakable because larvae with characteristic spiracles can be seen on the bot within the wound.
- Immature warble (before breaking through the skin) needs to be differentiated from subcutaneous foreign body, aggressive neoplasia, focal infectious lesion due to bacterial abscess, nocardia, fungal (blastomycosis).

Tissue Migration

- Neurologic—rabies, distemper, brain neoplasia, trauma, inflammatory neurologic disease, *Angiostrongylus* infection, toxoplasmosis, neosporosis, fungal diseases.
- Respiratory.
  - Cats—causes of acute respiratory distress are feline asthma; lungworms; cardiomyopathy; upper respiratory tract viruses (herpes virus, calicivirus); nasopharyngeal foreign body or abscess; pleural effusion; pneumonia; diaphragmatic hernia; pulmonary edema (electric shock).
  - Dogs—causes of acute respiratory distress are allergic bronchitis; pneumonia; cardiac disease; parasitic disease.
- Ophthalmic—foreign body; larval hypoderma.

 DIAGNOSTICS

- CBC—usually normal but may show mild neutrophilia and eosinophilia.

- Aspirate cytologic examination of immature warble—neutrophils and eosinophils on proteinacious background.
- CSF tap—usually normal but may show increased protein and mild increase in cell content.
- MRI—demonstrates larval migration tract through brain; CT scan not as sensitive.

Diagnostic Feature
- **Identification of larvae in a cutaneous fistula.**

THERAPEUTICS

- Remove maggot from subcutaneous lesion—increase size of hole through skin using a scalpel, grasp maggot with forceps and remove intact.
- Shaving hair around fistula tract—improves rate of healing.
- Breaking maggot—may result in severe foreign body reaction but rarely occurs and may be alleviated by pretreatment with chlorpheniramine.
- Manifestations of respiratory tract and neurologic disease—may be alleviated with the use of corticosteroids.
- Neurologic disease—requires hospitalization and fluid and nutritional support during first week of recovery period.

Drugs of Choice

- Ivermectin—thought to kill migrating larvae.
- Prednisone—improves neurologic disease and reduces inflammation associated with larval migration through soft tissues, especially respiratory tract (nasopharynx).
- Chlorpheniramine—antihistamines proposed to alleviate anaphylactic reaction if parasite is ruptured during removal or during kill off by ivermectin (Table 31-1).

Precautions/Interactions

- Check dogs for heartworm microfilaria before using ivermectin.
- Do not use these doses of ivermectin in ivermectin-sensitive collies or collie-cross dogs.

TABLE 31-1. Drug Therapy for Cuterebriasis				
Drug	Dose (mg/kg)	Route	Interval (Hours)	Duration (Days)
Ivermectin	0.2	SC, PO	24	3
Prednisone	1–2	PO	12	3–5
Chlorpheniramine	2–12	PO	8	5

COMMENTS

- Once larvae are removed from warble, fistula track heals quickly.
- Larval migration seems to induce poor immunity because cats can become infected often in same year and subsequent years.
- Application of monthly heartworm preventives (avermectin-containing products), flea development control products (lufenuron-containing products), or topical flea and tick treatments may prevent the maggots from either developing in the dog or cat or may kill them before they have time to gain access to an orifice for entry.
- Most cats with neurologic cuterebriasis have improved function after treatment, but prognosis has to be guarded.

Abbreviations

CBC, complete blood count; CSF, cerebrospinal fluid; CT, computed tomography; MRI, magnetic resonance imaging.

Suggested Reading

Bowman DD. In: *Georgis' Parasitology for Veterinarians.* 8th ed. Philadelphia: WB Saunders; 2003: 95–97.

Bowman DD, Hendrix CM, Lindsay DS, et al. In: *Feline Clinical Parasitology,* Ames: Iowa State University Press; 2002:430–431.

Dvorak LD, Bay JD, Crouch DT, et al. Successful treatment of intratracheal cuterebrosis in two cats. *J Am Anim Hosp Assoc* 2000;36:304–308.

Glass EN, Cornetta AM, deLahunta A, et al. Clinical and clinicopathologic features in 11 cats with cuterebra larvae myiasis of the central nervous system. *J Vet Intern Med* 1998;12:365–368.

Author: Stephen C. Barr
Consulting Editor: Stephen C. Barr

chapter 32

Cytauxzoonosis

DEFINITION/OVERVIEW

- Fatal tick-borne protozoal disease of domestic and feral cats (especially bobcats) affecting the vascular system of the lungs, liver, spleen, kidneys, and brain, with development stages in the RBCs.

ETIOLOGY/PATHOPHYSIOLOGY

- *Cytauxzoon felis*—distributed in the south central and southeastern United States (Kansas and Oklahoma).
- Large schizonts (tissue phase)—develop in macrophages, causing them to line the lumen of veins of almost every organ, leading to occlusion of the vessels (especially in lungs).
- DIC—often the final outcome.
- Merozoites bud from the schizonts in macrophages—rupture cell to infect other macrophages and RBCs (1 to 3 days before death).
- Vector—*Dermacentor variabilis*, but probably others also involved.

SIGNALMENT/HISTORY

- No sex, age, or breed predisposition.

CLINICAL FEATURES

- Usually severe debilitation at presentation.
- Anemia (beginning 5 to 6 days postinfection).
- Depression.
- Anorexia.
- Dehydration.
- High fever.
- Icterus.
- Splenomegaly.
- Hepatomegaly.

DIFFERENTIAL DIAGNOSIS

- Other causes of regenerative anemia—immune-mediated hemolytic anemia, Heinz body anemia, *Haemobartonella* spp., *Babesia* spp., blood loss or hemorrhage (GI tract neoplasia, intercavity hemorrhage, GI tract parasitism).

DIAGNOSTICS

- CBC—regenerative anemia due to hemolysis and hemorrhage.
- Parasitemia phase—leukopenia, left shift and toxic neutrophils, thrombocytopenia, normocytic, normochromic nonregenerative anemia may be present.
- *Cytauxzoon* RBC forms—usually indicates late stage of disease *(Fig. 32-1)*.
- Splenic and bone marrow aspirates—extraerythrocytic form.
- Biochemical profile and urinalysis—reflect DIC and changes due to severe anemia (organ hypoxia).
- In cats that die—histopathologic examination demonstrates marginalization of mononuclear cells in veins within most organs, but particularly lungs *(Fig. 32-2)*.

■ **Fig. 32-1** Feline RBCs infected with *Cytauxzoon felis* piroplasms. Note the Howell-Jolly body for comparison in the RBC in the bottom right (Giemsa stain, 1,000×).

■ **Fig. 32-2** Infected monocytes lining the walls of veins within a lung from a *Cytauxzoon felis*–infected cat (Hematoxylin and eosin stain, 1,000×).

  THERAPEUTICS

- Antibiotics—indicated if sepsis present (due to leukopenia).
- DIC—aggressive treatment, including:
  - IV isotonic fluids.
  - Heparin (150 IU/kg, SC, q8h).
  - Plasma, and whole blood if anemia particularly severe.

Drugs of Choice

- Imidocarb dipropionate (Imizol [Schering-Plough, Union, NJ]; Forray-65 [Hoechst Marion Roussel, Kansas City, MO]).
- Diminazene acetate (Berenil [Bayer, Shawnee Mission, KS], not available in United States) (*Table 32-1*).

Precautions/Interactions

- Imidocarb dipropionate—administer preanesthetic doses of atropine or glycopyrrolate.

TABLE 32-1. Drug Therapy for *Cytauxzoon felis* in Cats

Drug	Dose (mg/kg)	Route	Interval (Hours)	Repeat Dose (Days)
Imidocarb dipropionate (Imazol)	2	IM	Once	3–7
Diminazene acetate[a] (Berenil)	2	IM	Once	3–7

[a] Not available in the United States.

- Imidocarb dipropionate—produces pain and swelling at the injection site as well as postinjection vomiting; other side effects can include periorbital edema, hypersalivation, diarrhea, signs similar to organophosphate toxicity.
- Cats—may become anorectic, febrile, and depressed after initial treatment with diminazene acetate.

 COMMENTS

- The majority of cats will die if aggressive treatment is not begun immediately.
- Prevent tick transmission of disease by using products containing pyrethrin (collars, sprays) or fipronil (Frontline [Merial, Iselin, NJ]).

Abbreviations

CBC, complete blood count; DIC, disseminated intravascular coagulation; GI, gastrointestinal; RBCs, red blood cells.

Suggested Reading

Green CE, Latimer K, Hopper E, et al. Administration of diminazene or immidocarb dipropionate for treatment of cytauxzoonosis in cats. *J Am Vet Med Assoc* 1999;215:497–500.

Meinkoth J, Kocan AA, Whitworth L, et al. Cats surviving natural infection with *Cytauxzoon felis*: 18 cases (1997–1998). *J Vet Intern Med* 2000;14:521–525.

Author: Johnny D. Hoskins
Consulting Editor: Stephen C. Barr

chapter 33

Demodicosis

DEFINITION/OVERVIEW

- An inflammatory parasitic disease of dogs and, rarely, cats that is characterized by an increased number of mites in the hair follicles, which often leads to furunculosis and secondary bacterial infection.
- May be localized or generalized in dogs.

ETIOLOGY/PATHOPHYSIOLOGY

Dogs

- *Demodex canis*—a mite; part of the normal fauna of the skin; typically present in small numbers; resides in the hair follicles and sebaceous glands of the skin (*Fig. 33-1*).
- Pathology—develops when number of mites exceed that tolerated by the immune system.
- Initial proliferation of mites—may be the result of a genetic or an immunologic disorder.

Cats

- Poorly understood disorder.
- Mites have been identified on the skin and within the otic canal.
- Two species: *D. cati* and an unnamed species.

Dog/Cat

- Dead and degenerate *D. canis* mites may be found in noncutaneous sites (e.g., lymph node, intestinal wall, spleen, liver, kidney, urinary bladder, lung, thyroid gland, blood, urine, and feces) and are considered to represent drainage to these areas by blood and/or lymph.

SIGNALMENT/HISTORY

- Dogs and rarely cats.
- Potential increased incidence—Siamese and Burmese cat breeds.
- Localized—usually in young dogs; median age 3 to 6 months.
- Generalized—both young and old animals.

■ **Fig. 33-1** *Demodex canis* mites in skin scraping. Note the different stages of the mite, including an egg. (From Rhodes KH: *The 5-Minute Veterinary Consult Clinical Companion: Small Animal Dermatology.* Baltimore, Md: Lippincott Williams & Wilkins; 2002.)

Dogs

- Exact immunopathologic mechanism unknown.
- Studies indicate that dogs with generalized demodicosis have a subnormal percentage of IL-2 receptors on their lymphocytes and subnormal IL-2 production.
- Genetic factors, immunosuppression, and/or metabolic diseases may predispose animal.

Cats

- Association—often with metabolic diseases (e.g., FIV, SLE, diabetes mellitus).
- Unnamed species—short and blunted; rarely a marker for metabolic disease; individual reports indicate that it may be transferable from cat to cat within the same household.

 CLINICAL FEATURES

Dogs

Localized
- Lesions—usually mild; consist of erythema and a light scale.
- Patches—several may be noted; most common site is the face, especially around the perioral and periocular areas; may also be seen on the trunk and legs.

Generalized
- Can be widespread from the onset, with multiple poorly circumscribed patches of erythema, alopecia, and scale (*Fig. 33-2*).

■ **Fig. 33-2** Patch of alopecia with erythema and scaling secondary to demodicosis. (From Rhodes KH: *The 5-Minute Veterinary Consult Clinical Companion: Small Animal Dermatology*. Baltimore, Md: Lippincott Williams & Wilkins; 2002.)

- As hair follicles become distended with large numbers of mites, secondary bacterial infections are common, often with resultant rupturing of the follicle (furunculosis) (*Fig. 33-3*).
- With progression, the skin can become severely inflamed, exudative, and granulomatous (*Fig. 33-4*).

■ **Fig. 33-3** Swelling of the digits caused by demodicosis and secondary furunculosis. (From Rhodes KH: *The 5-Minute Veterinary Consult Clinical Companion: Small Animal Dermatology*. Baltimore, Md: Lippincott Williams & Wilkins; 2002.)

■ **Fig. 33-4** Demodicosis with severe secondary bacterial infection of the facial and periauricular region. (From Rhodes KH: *The 5-Minute Veterinary Consult Clinical Companion*: *Small Animal Dermatology*. Baltimore, Md: Lippincott Williams & Wilkins; 2002.)

Cats

- Often characterized by partial to complete multifocal alopecia of the eyelids, periocular region, head, and neck.
- Lesions are variably pruritic with erythema, scale, and crust; those caused by the unnamed species often quite pruritic.
- Ceruminous otitis externa has been reported.

 DIFFERENTIAL DIAGNOSIS

Dogs

- Bacterial folliculitis/furunculosis.
- Dermatophytosis.
- Contact dermatitis.
- Pemphigus complex.
- Dermatomyositis.
- SLE.

Cats

- Allergic dermatitis
- Scabies.

DIAGNOSTICS

- May be useful—for identifying underlying metabolic diseases in cats.
- FeLV and FIV serologic examination—identify underlying metabolic diseases in cats.
- Skin scrapings—diagnostic for finding large numbers of mites in the majority of cases.
- Cutaneous biopsy—may be needed when lesions are chronic, granulomatous, and fibrotic (especially on the paw).

THERAPEUTICS

- Localized—conservative; most cases (90%) resolve spontaneously with no treatment.
- Evaluate—general health status of dogs with either the localized or the generalized form.
- Generalized (adult dog)—frequent management problem; expense and frustration with the chronicity of the problem are issues; many cases are medically controlled, not cured.

Drugs

Amitraz (Mitaban; Taktic-EC)
- A formamidine, which inhibits monoamine oxidase and prostaglandin synthesis; an α_2-adrenergic agonist.
- Use weekly (the label states every other week) at ½ vial (5 ml) per gallon of water until resolution of clinical signs and no mites are found on skin scrapings; do not rinse off; let air dry.
- Treat for 1 month after negative skin scrape.
- Apply a benzoyl peroxide shampoo before application of the dip as a bactericidal therapy and to increase exposure of the mites to the miticide through follicular flushing activity.
- The efficacy is proportional to the frequency of administration and the concentration of the dip.
- May be mixed with mineral oil (3 ml amitraz to 30 ml mineral oil) for application to focal areas, such as pododemodicosis.
- Success with the 9% amitraz collar has not been established, although there are positive anecdotal reports.
- Between 11% and 30% of cases will not be cured; may need to try an alternative therapy or control with maintenance dips every 2 to 8 weeks.

Ivermectin (Ivomec; Eqvalan Liquid)
- A macrocyclic lactone with GABA agonist activity.
- Daily oral administration of 0.3 to 0.6 mg/kg very effective, even when amitraz fails.
- Treat for 60 days beyond negative skin scrapings (average 3 to 8 months).

- Ivermectin is contraindicated in collies, Shetland sheepdogs, old English sheepdogs, other herding breeds, and crosses with these breeds; sensitive breeds appear to tolerate the acaricidal dosages of milbemycin (see below).

Milbemycin (Interceptor)
- A macrocylic lactone with GABA agonist activity.
- Dosage of 1 mg/kg, PO, q24h cures 50% of cases; 2 mg/kg, PO, q24h cures 85% of cases.
- Treat for 60 days beyond multiple negative skin scrapings.

Cats
- Exact protocols are not defined.
- Topical lime-sulfur dips or amitraz solutions applied weekly for four treatments often lead to good resolution of clinical signs.

 # COMMENTS

Amitraz

- Most common side effects—somnolence, lethargy, depression, anorexia seen in 30% of patients for 12 to 36 hours after treatment.
- Other side effects—vomiting, diarrhea, pruritus, polyuria, mydriasis, bradycardia, hypoventilation, hypotension, hypothermia, ataxia, ileus, bloat, hyperglycemia, convulsions, and death.
- The incidence and severity of side effects do not appear to be proportional to the dose or frequency of use.
- Humans—can develop dermatitis, headaches, and respiratory difficulty after exposure.
- Antidote—yohimbine 0.11 mg/kg, IV.

Ivermectin and Milbemycin

- Signs of toxicity—salivation, vomiting, mydriasis, confusion, ataxia, hypersensitivity to sound, weakness, recumbency, coma, and death.

Possible Interactions

- Amitraz—may interact with heterocyclic antidepressants, xylazine, benzodiazepines, and macrocyclic lactones.
- Ivermectin and milbemycin—cause elevated levels of monoamine neurotransmitter metabolites, which could result in adverse drug interactions with amitraz and benzodiazepines.
- Multiple skin scrapings and evidence of clinical resolution are used to monitor progress.
- Avoid breeding animals with generalized form.

Expected Course and Prognosis

- Prognosis (dogs)—depends heavily on genetic, immunologic, and underlying diseases.

- Localized—most cases (90%) resolve spontaneously with no treatment; <10% progress to the generalized form.
- Adult onset (dogs)—often severe and refractory to treatment.
- Adult onset—sudden occurrence is often associated with internal disease, malignant neoplasia, and/or immunosuppressive disease; approximately 25% of cases are idiopathic over a follow-up period of 1 to 2 years.

Abbreviations

FeLV, feline leukemia virus; FIV, feline immunodeficiency virus; GABA, gamma-aminobutyric acid; IL, interleukin; SLE, systemic lupus erythematosus.

Suggested Reading

Scott DW, Miller WH, Griffin CE, eds. *Muller & Kirk's Small Animal Dermatology*. 5th ed. Philadelphia: WB Saunders; 1995:417–432.

Author: Karen Helton Rhodes
Consulting Editor: Karen Helton Rhodes

chapter 34

Dermatophilosis

DEFINITION/OVERVIEW

- A crusting skin disease in dogs and a nodular subcutaneous and oral disease in cats.
- Reported infrequently.

ETIOLOGY/PATHOPHYSIOLOGY

- *Dermatophilus congolensis*—causative agent; gram-positive, branching filamentous bacterium classified as an Actinomycete; common cause of crusting dermatoses in hoofed animals, which causes crusted skin lesions of affected large animals and persists in their environment within crusts and other debris shed from infected hoof stock.
- Dogs, cats, and humans can rarely be secondarily infected.

SIGNALMENT/HISTORY

- Association—with farm animals or free-roaming lifestyle often reported.
- Cats—episode of trauma; existence of a foreign body; lesions generally chronic; no systemic clinical signs, except when internal organs or large oral lesions develop.
- Dogs, cats, and humans—can be exposed directly from lesions on large animals or from environmental exposure.
- Infectious stage—requires wetting for activation; probably cannot penetrate intact epithelium; thus antecedent minor trauma or mechanical transmission by biting ectoparasites required.
- Deeper infections—presumably acquired by traumatic inoculation of infectious material.

CLINICAL FEATURES

- Dogs—lesions: papular; crusted; mainly on the skin of the trunk or head; circular to coalescent; similar to those in superficial pyoderma caused by *Staphylococcus intermedius*; resemble dermatophilosis in horses (adherent thick, gray-yellow crusts that incorporate hair and leave a circular, glistening shallow erosion when removed); pruritus variable.

- Cats—subcutaneous, oral, or internal ulcerated and fistulated nodules or abscesses similar to lesions caused by other actinomycetes in this species.

 DIFFERENTIAL DIAGNOSIS

Dogs

- Staphylococcal pyoderma.
- Acute moist dermatitis.
- Dermatophytosis.
- Pemphigus foliaceus.
- Keratinization disorder.

Cats

- Actinomycosis and nocardiosis.
- Atypical mycobacterial granuloma.
- Sporotrichosis.
- Other subcutaneous fungal infection.
- Deep mycotic infection, especially.

Cryptococcosis

- Foreign body.
- Chronic bite/wound abscess.
- Bacterial L-form infection.
- *Rhodococcus equi* infection.
- Cutaneous or mucosal neoplasm, especially squamous cell carcinoma.

 DIAGNOSTICS

Dogs

- Cytologic examination of crusts—most important procedure; differentiates from more typical bacterial pyodermas.
- Organism—distinctive morphology in cytologic and histologic preparations; resembles railroad tracks as the bacterium forms chains of small diplococci; chains often branching.
- Cytologic diagnosis—from impression smears made of exudate from under crusts or by preparation of minced crusts; mince crusts finely in a drop of water and allow to macerate several minutes; then dry the preparation and stain with any Wright-Giemsa stain.
- Histopathologic specimens—from crusts.

Cats

- Histopathologic examination—biopsy of ulcerated nodules; procedure of choice.
- Cytologic examination—exudate obtained from aspiration or swabbing of a draining tract.
- Culture of biopsy specimens—may yield the organism; facilitated if the laboratory is alerted to the possible presence of *Dermatophilus* (aerobic, relatively slow growing, and easily obscured by contamination).
- Culture from crusts—requires the use of special selective medium; generally used to corroborate cytologic findings.

Pathologic Findings

- Dogs—crusting and superficial pustular dermatitis; palisading of the crusts with orthokeratotic and parakeratotic hyperkeratosis; organism visualized within the crusts, generally without the use of special bacterial stains.
- Cats—pyogranulomatous inflammation; central necrosis; fistulous tract formation; organism visualized near the necrotic center of granulomas, especially with Gram stain.

 THERAPEUTICS

- Dogs—antibacterial shampoo and gentle removal (and disposal) of crusts; shampoo may contain benzoyl peroxide, ethyl lactate, chlorhexidine, or selenium disulfide; one or two applications suffice in most cases.
- Cats—for pyogranulomas and abscesses: surgical débridement; exploration for foreign body; establishment of drainage for exudate; maintain effective drainage and postoperative wound care.

Drugs

- Penicillin V—10 mg/kg, PO, q12h for 10 to 20 days; drug of choice.
- Ampicillin—10–20 mg/kg, PO, q12h for 10 to 20 days.
- Amoxicillin—10–20 mg/kg, PO, q12h for 10 to 20 days.
- Tetracycline, doxycycline, or minocycline—standard dosage.

 COMMENTS

- Dogs—reexamine after 2 weeks of treatment to ensure complete resolution of symptoms; give an additional 7 days of systemic therapy.
- Cats—monitor biweekly for 1 month after apparent resolution of lesions, depending on their location.
- Dogs—excellent prognosis.
- Cats—prognosis varies with the location of lesions and extent of surgical débridement; complete resolution can be achieved with timely diagnosis and appropriate surgical and medical therapy.

- Veterinarians and animal care workers—very seldom infected, even after traumatic exposure when working with farm animals known to be infected.
- Dogs and cats—very unlikely to serve as a source for human infection; caution is warranted for exposure of immunocompromised individuals.

Suggested Reading

Greene CE. Dermatophilosis. In: Greene CE, ed. *Infectious Diseases of the Dog and Cat*. Philadelphia: WB Saunders; 1998:326–327.

Author: Carol S. Foil

Consulting Editor: Karen Helton Rhodes

Dermatophytosis: Keratinophilic Mycosis

DEFINITION/OVERVIEW

- A cutaneous fungal infection affecting the cornified regions of hair, nails, and occasionally the superficial layers of the skin.
- Most commonly isolated organisms are *Microsporum canis*, *Trichophyton mentagrophytes*, and *M. gypseum*.

ETIOLOGY/PATHOPHYSIOLOGY

- Exposure to or contact with a dermatophyte—does not necessarily result in an infection.
- Infection may not result in clinical signs.
- Dermatophytes grow in the keratinized layers of hair, nail, and skin; do not thrive in living tissue or persist in the presence of severe inflammation—incubation period: 1 to 4 weeks.
- Affected animal that does not show signs may remain in this inapparent carrier state for a prolonged period of time—some animals never become symptomatic.
- Corticosteroids—can modulate inflammation and prolong the infection.
- Cats—*M. canis* is by far the most common agent.
- Dogs—*M. canis*, *M. gypseum*, and *T. mentagrophytes*; incidence of each agent varies geographically.
- Reliance on clinical signs and incorrectly interpreted Wood's lamp examination results in overdiagnosis.

SIGNALMENT

- Cats—more common in long-haired breeds (*Fig. 35-1*).
- Clinical signs—more common in young animals.
- Incidence—although infection is ubiquitous, the incidence is higher in hot and humid regions.
- Lesions—may begin as alopecia or a poor hair coat.
- History of previously confirmed infection or exposure to an infected animal or environment (e.g., a cattery)—a useful but not consistent finding.

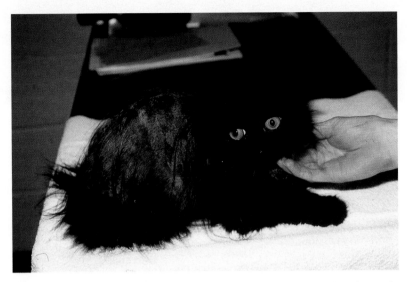

■ **Fig. 35-1** Persian cat with *Microsporum canis* infection. This breed is considered predisposed to dermatophytosis (courtesy Dr. Carol Foil).

Risk Factors

- Immunocompromising disease or immunosuppressive medication.
- High population density.
- Poor nutrition.
- Poor management practices.
- Lack of an adequate quarantine period.
- Vary from an inapparent carrier state to a patchy or circular alopecia.
- Classic circular alopecia common in cats; often misinterpreted in dogs (*Fig. 35-2*).
- Scales, erythema, hyperpigmentation, and pruritus are variable (*Fig. 35-3*).
- Paronychosis, granulomatous lesions, or kerions may occur.

■ **Fig. 35-2** Dermatophytosis (*Microsporum canis*) in a dog. Circular patches of alopecia and scale are more characteristic in humans and cats (courtesy Dr. Carol Foil).

■ **Fig. 35-3** Disseminated dermatophytosis caused by *Trichophyton mentagrophytes* (courtesy Dr. Carol Foil).

DIFFERENTIAL DIAGNOSIS

- Cats—miliary dermatitis and almost any other dermatitis.
- Dogs—folliculitis, furunculosis, and most cases of alopecia.
- Demodicosis and bacterial skin infection—epidermal collarettes more typical of a bacterial infection; grossly enlarged follicular ostia with furunculosis suggest demodicosis; these characteristics are not consistent; concurrent bacterial or mite infections can be seen with dermatophytosis; all three diseases can cause focal hyperpigmentation.
- Immune-mediated skin diseases—severe inflammation associated with dermatophytosis affecting the face or feet.

DIAGNOSTICS

- Reliance on clinical signs and incorrectly interpreted Wood's lamp examination results in overdiagnosis.

Fungal Culture with Macroconidia Identification

- Best means of confirming diagnosis.
- Hairs that exhibit a positive apple-green fluorescence under Wood's lamp examination are considered ideal candidates for culture.
- Pluck hairs from the periphery of an alopecic area; do not use a random pattern.
- Use a sterile toothbrush to brush the hair coat of an asymptomatic animal to yield better results.
- Test media change to red when they become alkaline; dermatophytes typically produce this color during the early growing phase of their culture; saprophytes, which also produce this color, do so in the late growing phase; thus, it is important to examine the media daily.

- Microscopic examination of the macroconidia necessary to confirm pathogenic dermatophyte and to identify genus and species; helps identify source of infection.
- Positive culture indicates existence of a dermatophyte; however, it may have been there only transiently, as commonly occurs when the culture is obtained from the feet, which are likely to come in contact with a geophilic dermatophyte.

Microscopic Examination of Hair

- Examination after using a clearing solution can help provide a rapid diagnosis.
- Time-consuming and often produces false negative results.
- Use hairs that fluoresce under Wood's lamp illumination to increase the likelihood of identifying the fungal hyphae associated with the hair shaft.
- Wood's lamp examination is not a very useful screening tool; many pathogenic dermatophytes do not fluoresce; false fluorescence is common; lamp should warm up for a minimum of 5 minutes and then be exposed to suspicious lesions for up to 5 minutes; a true positive reaction associated with *M. canis* consists of apple-green fluorescence of the hair shaft; keratin associated with epidermal scales and sebum will often produce a false-positive fluorescence.

Skin Biopsy

- Not usually needed.
- Can be helpful in confirming true invasion and infection.

Pathologic Findings

- Folliculitis, perifolliculitis, or furunculosis.
- Hyperkeratosis.
- Intraepidermal pustules.
- Pyogranulomatous reaction pattern.
- Fungal hyphae may be observed in H&E–stained sections; special stains allow easier visualization of the organism.

 THERAPEUTICS

- Zoonosis—consider quarantine owing to the infective and zoonotic nature of the disease.
- Griseofulvin—most widely prescribed systemic drug; microsized formulation: 25 to 60 mg/kg, PO, q12h for 4 to 6 weeks; ultramicrosized formulation: 2.5 to 5.0 mg/kg, PO, q12–24h; pediatric suspension: 10–25 mg/kg, PO, q12h; GI upset is the most common side effect; alleviate by reducing the dose or dividing the dose for more frequent administration.
- Griseofulvin—fatty meal improves absorption.
- Ketoconazole—not labeled for use in dogs or cats in the United States; dose: 10 mg/kg, PO, q24h or divided twice per day for 3 to 4 weeks; anorexia is the most common side effect.
- Ketoconazole—acid meal (add tomato juice) enhances absorption.

Griseofulvin Precautions

- Bone marrow suppression (anemia, pancytopenia, and neutropenia)—can occur as an idiosyncratic reaction or with prolonged therapy.
- Neutropenia—most common fatal reaction in cats; can persist after discontinuation of drug; weekly or biweekly CBC is recommended; can be life-threatening in cats with FIV infection.
- Side effects—neurologic.
- Do not use during the first two trimesters of pregnancy—it is teratogenic.

Ketoconazole Precautions

- Hepatopathy has been reported and can be quite severe.
- Inhibits endogenous production of steroidal hormones in dogs.

Miscellaneous

- Vaccination—product literature claims are based on clinical signs and Wood's lamp findings; may be useful as an adjuvant to systemic therapy; may be valuable for treating asymptomatic carriers, which can be frustrating to the client and veterinarian and can complicate the diagnosis and management; studies involving dermatophyte cultures as a measure of achieving a cure or prevention are necessary to ensure true efficacy.
- Topical therapy and clipping—once strongly advocated; may help prevent environmental contamination; often associated with an initial exacerbation of signs after the procedures are initiated; lime sulfur (1:16), enilconazole (bottle dilution), and miconazole shampoo are the most effective agents; lime sulfur is odiferous and can stain; enilconazole is not available in the United States.

Alternative Drugs

- Itraconazole—similar to ketoconazole but with fewer side effects; probably more effective; expensive; supplied as 100-mg capsules; dose: 10 mg/kg, PO, q24h or 5 mg/kg, PO, q12h.

 COMMENTS

- Dermatophyte culture is the only means of truly monitoring response to therapy; many animals will clinically improve but remain culture positive.
- Repeat fungal cultures toward the end of the treatment regimen and continue treatment until at least one culture result is negative.
- In resistant cases, the culture may be repeated weekly, using the toothbrush technique; continue treatment until 2 to 3 consecutive culture results are negative.
- Initiate a quarantine period and obtain dermatophyte cultures of all animals entering the household to prevent reinfection from other animals.
- Consider the possibility of rodents aiding in the spread of the disease.
- Avoid infective soil, if a geophilic dermatophyte is involved.
- Consider using griseofulvin for 10 to 14 days as a prophylactic treatment of exposed animals.

- Many animals will self-clear a dermatophyte infection over a period of a few months.
- Treatment for the disease hastens clinical cure and helps reduce environmental contamination.
- Some infections, particularly in long-haired cats or multianimal situations, can be very persistent.

Client Education

- Inform owner—that many short-haired cats in a single-cat environment and many dogs will undergo spontaneous remission.
- Advise owner—that treatment can be both frustrating and expensive, especially in multianimal households or recurrent cases.
- Inform owner—that environmental treatment, including fomites, is important, especially in recurrent cases; dilute bleach (1:10) is a practical and relatively effective means of providing environmental decontamination; concentrated bleach and formalin (1%) are more effective at killing spores, but their use is not as practical in many situations; chlorhexidine was ineffective in pilot studies.
- Inform owner—that in a multianimal environment or cattery situation, treatment and control can be very complicated; referral to a veterinarian with expertise in this type of situation should be considered.

Abbreviations

CBC, complete blood count; GI, gastrointestinal; H&E, hematoxylin and eosin.

Suggested Reading

Moriello KA, DeBoer DJ. Dermatophytosis. In: August JR, ed. *Consultations in Feline Internal Medicine 2.* Philadelphia: WB Saunders; 1994:219–225.
Scott DW, Miller WH, Griffin CE, eds. *Muller & Kirk's Small Animal Dermatology.* 5th ed. Philadelphia: WB Saunders; 1995:332–350.

Author: W. Dunbar Gram
Consulting Editor: Karen Helton Rhodes

chapter 36

Ear Mites

DEFINITION/OVERVIEW

- *Otodectes cynotis* mites cause a hypersensitivity reaction that results in intense irritation of the external ear of dogs and cats (*Fig. 36-1*).

SIGNALMENT/HISTORY

- Common in young dogs and cats, although it may occur at any age.
- No breed or sex predilection.

CLINICAL FEATURES

- Pruritus—primarily located around the ears, head, and neck; occasionally generalized.
- Thick, red-brown or black crusts—usually seen in the outer ear.
- Crusting and scales—may occur on the neck, rump, and tail.
- Excoriations—often occur on the convex surface of the pinnae, owing to the intense pruritus.

DIFFERENTIAL DIAGNOSIS

- Flea bite hypersensitivity.
- Pediculosis.
- Pelodera dermatitis.
- Sarcoptic mange.
- Chiggers.
- Allergic dermatitis.

DIAGNOSTICS

- Skin scrapings—identify mites, if signs are generalized.
- Ear swabs placed in mineral oil—usually a very effective means of identification.

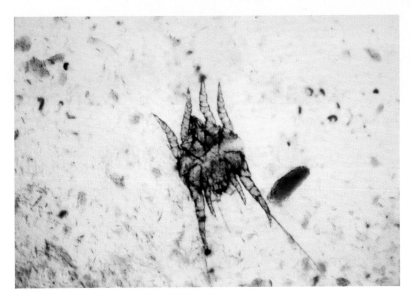

■ **Fig. 36-1** *Otodectes* mite from an ear swab. (From Rhodes KH: *The 5-Minute Veterinary Consult Clinical Companion: Small Animal Dermatology.* Baltimore, Md: Lippincott Williams & Wilkins; 2002.)

THERAPEUTICS

- Very contagious—important to treat all in-contact animals.
- Environment—thoroughly clean and treat.
- Cleanse the ears thoroughly—with mineral oil or a commercial ear cleaner to remove debris.
- Rotenone-based products—treat ears twice per week initially; then decrease to weekly; continue for 2 weeks after clinical cure.
- Ivermectin—as an alternative; use systemically or topically; systemic: (bovine 1%) 300 μg/kg, SC every 1 to 2 weeks for approximately four treatments was found to be effective; topical: place 500 μg directly in the ears every 1 to 2 weeks for approximately 5 weeks (associated with a higher incidence of recurrence); topical dosage not approved for use in dogs or cats in the United States; dogs with heartworm may exhibit a shocklike reaction, probably owing to dying microfilaria.
- Acarexx (Blue Ridge Pharmaceuticals, Greensboro, NC)—0.01% ivermectin otic suspension.
- Revolution (Pfizer, Exton, PA)—topical treatment placed on base of neck.
- Amitraz—topical; place 1 ml in 33 ml mineral oil directly into the ear; not approved for this use.
- Pyrethrin-based flea spray—treat entire animal weekly for 4 to 6 weeks if not using systemic ivermectin.

COMMENTS

- Environment—treat with a flea-type preparation 2 times, 2 to 4 weeks apart.
- Ivermectin—do not use in collies, shelties, their crosses, or other herding breeds; use only if absolutely necessary in animals <6 months of age; an increasing number of

toxic reactions have been reported in kittens.

- Amitraz—reported to cause adverse reactions in cats when used topically for generalized infestations; thus, use with caution.
- Ear swab and physical examination—should be done 1 month after therapy commences.
- Prognosis—is good for most patients.
- Allergy—rarely, the infestation will be cleared only to find an underlying allergy that keeps the otitis externa active.
- Humans—the mites will also bite humans (rare).

Suggested Reading

Scott DW, Miller WH, Griffin CE. *Muller & Kirk's Small Animal Dermatology.* 5th ed. Philadelphia: WB Saunders; 1995.

Author: Karen A. Kuhl and Jean S. Greek

chapter 37

Ehrlichiosis

DEFINITION/OVERVIEW

- A tick-borne disease of dogs and cats causing vasculitis, thrombocytopenia, hyperglobulinemia, and multisystem dysfunction.

ETIOLOGY/PATHOPHYSIOLOGY

Dogs

- Recently reclassified—moved from the family *Rickettsiaceae* into the family *Anaplasmataceae*.
- Within the family *Anaplasmataceae*—three pathogenic genera: *Ehrlichia*, *Anaplasma*, and *Neorickettsia*.
- *Ehrlichia* spp.—divided into three groups:
  - *E. canis*—ehrlichiosis found intracytoplasmically in circulating leukocytes.
  - *E. ewingii*—canine granulocytic ehrlichiosis; like *A. phagocytophila*, infects granulocytic cells in dogs, but differs in geographic distribution (mainly found in southeastern and south-central United States.)
  - *E. chaffeensis*—like *E. canis*, tropism for mononuclear cells; mainly a human pathogen but causes disease in dog.
- *Anaplasma* spp.—two organisms of importance:
  - *A. phagocytophila*—previously *E. equi*, *E. phagocytophila*, and HGE agent; infects mainly horses but also the granulocytic cells of dogs; serologically indistinguishable from *E. canis* infection; mainly found in northeastern and upper Midwestern states and California.
  - *A. platys*—previously *E. platys*; tropism for platelets; does not share serologic cross reactivity with *E. canis*.
- *Neorickettsia* spp.—two organisms of importance:
  - *N. risticii*—previously *E. risticii*; causes Potomac horse fever in horses but also infects dogs and cats; like other *Neorickettsia*, this organism is not transmitted by ticks; infections acquired by ingesting infected snails, free nematode life stages, or aquatic insects with encysted metacercaria; grazing or drinking from standing water explains why horses become infected more often than dogs; infected dogs have negative *E. canis* titers.
  - *N. helminthoeca*—causes salmon poisoning disease in dogs (see Chapter 92).

- Pathophysiology for *E. canis*—*Rhipicephalus sanguineus* (brown dog tick) transmits disease to dogs in saliva (*Dermacentor variabilis* also).
- Incubation period—1 to 3 weeks.
- Three stages of disease:
  - Acute—spreads from bite site to the spleen, liver, and lymph nodes (causes organomegaly), then subclinical, with mild thrombocytopenia; mainly endothelial cells affected; vasculitis; antiplatelet antibodies may exacerbate thrombocytopenia; variable leukopenia; mild anemia; severity depends on organism.
  - Subclinical—organism persists; antibody response increases (hyperglobulinemia); thrombocytopenia persists.
  - Chronic—impaired bone marrow production (platelets, erythroid suppression); marrow hypercellular with plasma cells.
- Multisystemic disease—including bleeding tendencies (thrombocytopenia and vasculitis), lymphadenopathy, splenomegaly, CNS, ocular (anterior uveitis), and lung (rarely affected by vasculitis).
- *E. chaffeensis*—vomiting, epistaxis, lymphadenopathy and anterior uveitis reported in naturally infected dogs; experimental infections demonstrate mild to inapparent signs.
- Only PCR will differentiate *E. chaffeensis* infection from that of *E. canis*.
- *E. ewingii*—serologic cross reactivity with *E. canis*; main clinical manifestation is polyarthritis with fever; splenomegaly, hepatomegaly, mild to moderate thrombocytopenia and meningitis also noted.
- Fatal infections due to *E. ewingii* are rare—quick recovery with appropriate therapy.
- *A. phagocytophila*—mild illness typified by fever, lethargy, and thrombocytopenia; polyarthritis occurs but is rare in comparison to infection with *E. ewingii*; most dogs present in autumn and are females; *E. canis* titers are usually negative.
- *A. platys*—moderate to severe cyclic thrombocytopenia but bleeding rare; co-infections with *E. canis* occur.
- *N. risticii*—lethargy, vomiting, bleeding disorders, and arthralgia are common signs.

Cats

- Extremely rare.
- *N. risticii* and *A. phagocytophila*.
- Serologic evidence suggests a species that cross reacts with *E. canis* can cause illness.

   SIGNALMENT/HISTORY

Dogs

- Worldwide distribution.
- North America—mainly Gulf Coast and eastern seaboard; also Midwest and California.
- Occurs throughout the year—insidious.
- Breed predilection—chronic (*E. canis*) disease may be more severe in Doberman pinschers and German shepherd dogs.

■ **Fig. 37-1** Conjunctival petechiation and fibrin within the anterior chamber of a dog with acute *E. canis* (courtesy Dr. R. Riis, Cornell University).

- Average age—5.22 years (range: 2 months to 14 years).
- Historically—may show lethargy, depression, anorexia and weight loss, fever, spontaneous bleeding, epistaxis, respiratory distress, ataxia, head tilt, and ocular pain (uveitis).

 CLINICAL FEATURES

Dogs

- Duration of clinical signs from initial acute illness to presentation—usually >2 months.

Acute

- Bleeding diatheses—petechiation of mucous membranes such as conjunctiva (*Fig. 37-1*) or retinal hemorrhage (*Fig. 37-2*) as a result of thrombocytopenia.
- Fever—with depression, anorexia, weight loss.
- Lymphadenopathy—generalized.

■ **Fig. 37-2** Retinal hemorrhage in a dog with thrombocytopenia infected with *E. canis* (courtesy Dr. R. Riis, Cornell University).

- Ticks—found in 40% of cases.
- Respiratory signs—dyspnea (even cyanosis) and increased bronchovesicular sounds.
- Diffuse CNS disease—meningitis.
- Ataxia—with upper motor neuron dysfunction.
- CNS—vestibular dysfunction.
- Hyperesthesia—generalized or local.
- Most dogs recover without treatment—then enter a subclinical state.

Chronic
- In nonendemic areas.
- Spontaneous bleeding.
- Anemia.
- Generalized lymphadenopathy.
- Polyarthritis.
- Scrotal and limb edema.
- Splenomegaly.
- Hepatomegaly.
- Uveitis.
- Hyphema.
- Retinal hemorrhages and detachment with blindness.
- Corneal edema.
- Seizures—rare.

Cats

- Fever—with anorexia, lethargy, and weight loss.
- Hyperesthesia—joint pain and irritability.
- Polyarthritis—some cases.
- Bone marrow hypoplasia or dysplasia—with pancytopenia and thrombocytopenia.
- Splenomegaly, lymphadenopathy, dyspnea, pale mucous membranes.

 DIFFERENTIAL DIAGNOSIS

Dogs

- RMSF (*Rickettsia rickettsii*)—usually seasonal between March and October; serologic testing for diagnosis; responds to same treatment as ehrlichiosis.
- Immune-mediated thrombocytopenia—not usually associated with fever or lymphadenopathy; serologic testing best distinguishes; may treat for both until results are known.
- SLE—ANA test usually negative with ehrlichiosis; serologic testing for diagnosis.
- Multiple myeloma—serologic testing to differentiate and determine cause of hyperglobulinemia; bone marrow cytology and punched-out bone lesions on radiology.

- Chronic lymphocytic leukemia—differentiate by lymphocytosis and cytology of bone marrow.
- Brucellosis—serologic testing for diagnosis and to determine cause of scrotal edema.

Cats

- Other causes of polyarthritis—feline syncytium-forming virus infection that may reflect coinfection with FIV (screen with antibody test; screen also for FeLV); septic joint disease (rare); immune-mediated polyarthritis.
- Bone marrow dyscrasias with thrombocytopenia, pancytopenia—consider FeLV (panleukopenia syndrome, lymphoma); feline panleukemia; immune-mediated, drug-induced bone marrow suppression (estradiol cypionate, chloramphenicol, albendazole).

 DIAGNOSTICS

Dogs

Acute

- CBC—thrombocytopenia (before onset of clinical signs), anemia, leukopenia (due to lymphopenia and eosinopenia), leukocytosis and monocytosis (as disease becomes more chronic).
- Morulae—intracytoplasmic inclusions in leukocytes rare (*Fig. 37-3*).

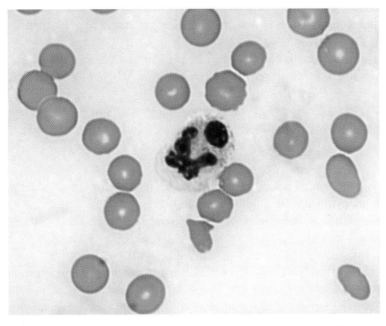

■ **Fig. 37-3** A canine neutrophil containing a morula in a dog with acute ehrlichiosis (Wright's-Giemsa stain, 1,000×).

- Nonspecific changes—mild increases in ALT, ALP, BUN, creatinine, and total bilirubin (rare).
- Hyperglobulinemia—progressively increases 1 to 3 weeks post-infection.
- Hypoalbuminemia—usually from renal loss.
- Proteinuria—with or without azotemia.

Chronic

- CBC—pancytopenia typical; monocytosis and lymphocytosis may be present.
- Serum biochemistry profile—hyperglobulinemia; magnitude of globulin increase correlates with duration of infection; usually polyclonal gammopathy, but monoclonal (IgG) gammopathies occur.
- Hypoalbuminemia.
- High BUN and creatinine—from primary renal disease, owing to glomerulonephritis and renal interstitial plasmacytosis.

Serologic Testing

- IFA—most clinically useful and reliable method.
- Highly sensitive—poor specificity with cross-reactivity between *E. canis* and *A. phagocytophila*, but not between *E. canis* and *A. platys*.
- Titers—reliable 3 weeks after infection; >1:10 diagnostic; paired titers recommended because single titer can reflect past infection; high seroprevalence compared to disease prevalence.
- Canine Snap 3Dx Diagnostic Test (IDEXX Laboratories, Westbrook, ME)—an in-house snap test that tests for antibodies against Lyme disease and *E. canis*, and heartworm antigen; detects positive titers to *E. canis* at an equivalent IFA titer of >1:100; sensitivity of 95%; specificity of 100% (according to manufacturer); however, as with any serologic test, predictive value also depends not only on sensitivity and specificity but also prevalence; in low-prevalence areas, likely to get a high false positive rate.
- Coombs'-positive anemia (rare)—may be present and confuse the diagnosis.
- PCR—proving to be more sensitive than IFA; tests whole blood samples; should be used in conjunction with serololgic testing.
- Test for other accompanying pathogens—*Babesiosis* spp., *Hemobartonellosis* spp. (erythrocytic mycoplasmal infections), *A. platys*, and *Hepatozoon canis*.

Cats

- CBC—nonregenerative anemia (not in all cats), leukopenia (in about a third of cats), and thrombocytopenia (in a quarter of cats).
- Morulae—found in about half of cases (none of the *E. canis*–infected cats had morulae).
- Isolation into monocyte culture—usually successful.
- Serum biochemical profile—hyperglobulinemia with polyclonal gammopathy in some.
- Serologic examination—all cats infected with *E. canis*–like organisms have positive ANA titer (highest reported at 1:640) and had negative results on conventional IFA serologic testing (some infected with other *Ehrlichia* spp. were positive).
- Cats infected with *E. canis*–like organisms—positive results on PCR of blood.

THERAPEUTICS

- Inpatient—initial medical stabilization for anemia and/or hemorrhagic tendency resulting from thrombocytopenia (balanced electrolyte solution or blood transfusion if indicated).
- Outpatient—stable patients; monitor CBC and response to medication frequently.

Drugs of Choice

- Doxycycline—see rapid (within 72 hours of onset of treatment) improvement of platelet count in acute cases.
- Imidocarb dipropionate (Imazol [Schering-Plough Animal Health, Union, NJ])— effective against both E. *canis* and babesiosis; reasonable alternative to doxycycline; pretreatment with atropine may lessen anticholinergic adverse effects (salivation, serous nasal discharge, diarrhea).
- Glucocorticoids (dogs only; cats treated with steroids do not eliminate infection when treated with doxycycline)—may be indicated when thrombocytopenia is life-threatening (thought to be a result of immune-mediated mechanisms); because immune-mediated thrombocytopenia is a principal differential diagnosis, may be indicated until results of serologic tests are available, and will not affect the outcome if final diagnosis is ehrlichiosis.
- Androgenic steroids (oxymetholone or nandrolone decanoate)—to stimulate bone marrow production in chronically affected dogs with hypoplastic marrows; oxymetholone or nandrolone decanoate *(Table 37-1)*.

Precautions/Interactions

- Tetracycline (and derivatives)—do not use in dogs <6 months old (permanent yellowing of teeth occurs); do not use with renal insufficiency (try doxycycline because it can be excreted via the gastrointestinal tract).
- Enrofloxacin—not effective against E. *canis*.
- Glucocorticoids—prolonged use at immunosuppressive levels may interfere with the clearance and elimination of E. *canis* after use of tetracycline.

TABLE 37-1. Drug Therapy for Ehrlichiosis in Dogs and Cats					
Drug	Species	Dose (mg/kg)	Route	Interval (Hours)	Duration (Days)
Doxycycline	B	10	PO	24	28
Imidocarb	B	5	IM	Once[a]	—
Prednisone	D	1–2	PO	12	14[b]
Oxymetholone	D	2	PO	24	Until response
Nandrolone	D	1.5	IM	Weekly	Until response

[a] Repeat 2 weeks later; pretreat with atropine.

[b] Gradually decrease dose as thrombocytopenia improves; taper in 50% decrements every 2 weeks.

B, cats and dogs; D, dogs.

COMMENTS

- Concurrent infection with *Babesia* spp., *Haemobartonella* spp., *A. platys,* and *Hepatozoon canis*—worsens clinical syndrome.
- Acute—prognosis excellent with appropriate therapy.
- Chronic—response may take 1 month; prognosis poor if the bone marrow is severely hypoplastic.
- Progression from acute to chronic—can be easily prevented by early, effective treatment; but many dogs remain seropositive and may relapse (even years later).
- German shepherd dogs and Doberman pinschers—more chronic and severe form of disease.
- Inform owner on how to control tick infestation—dips or sprays containing dichlorvos, chlorfenvinphos, dioxathion, propoxur, or carbaryl; flea and tick collars may reduce reinfestation but reliability unproven; selamectin topically (Revolution [Pfizer, Exton, PA]) monthly; avoid tick-infested areas.
- Removing ticks by hand—use gloves; ensure mouth parts are removed to avoid a foreign body reaction.
- Zoonotic potential—serologic evidence indicates that *E. canis* (or possibly a related species) occurs in humans; probably not directly infected from dogs; tick exposure thought to be necessary; *R. sanguineus* probably not the vector in humans.

Abbreviations

ALP, alkaline phosphatase; ALT, alanine aminotransferase; ANA, antinuclear antibody; BUN, blood urea nitrogen; CBC, complete blood count; CNS, central nervous system; FeLV, feline leukemia virus; FIV, feline immunodeficiency virus; HGE, human granulocytic ehrlichial agent; IFA, indirect fluorescent antibody; PCR, polymerase chain reaction; RMSF, Rocky Mountain spotted fever; SLE, systemic lupus erythematosus.

Suggested Reading

Breitschwerdt EB, Abrams-Ogg AC, Lappin MR, et al. Molecular evidence supporting *E. canis*-like infections in cats. *J Vet Int Med* 2002;16:642–649.

Cohn LA. Ehrlichiosis and related infections. *Vet Clin Small Anim* 2003;33:863–884.

Frank JR, Breitschwerdt EB. A retrospective study of ehrlichiosis in 62 dogs from North Carolina and Virginia. *J Vet Intern Med* 1999;13:194–201.

Greig B. Granulocytic ehrlichiosis. In: Bonagura JD, Kirk RW, eds. *Current Veterinary Therapy XIII.* Philadelphia: WB Saunders; 2000:298–300.

Neer TM, Breitschwerdt EB, Greene RT, et al. Consensus statement on ehrlichial disease of small animals for the infectious disease study group of the ACVIM. *J Vet Intern Med* 2002;16:309–315.

Author: Stephen C. Barr
Consulting Editor: Stephen C. Barr

chapter 38

Encephalitozoonosis

DEFINITION/OVERVIEW

- Uncommon protozoal disease of dogs and cats with a wide host range (including humans, rabbits, mice, foxes) in the United States.
- Causes lung, heart, kidney, and brain involvement.

ETIOLOGY/PATHOPHYSIOLOGY

- *Encephalitozoon cuniculi*—obligate intracellular protozoan (phylum Microspora).
- Mature spores—possess a polar filament and extrusion apparatus that distinguishes microsporidia from other protozoa.
- Infection—ingestion or inhalation of spores from urine or feces shed by infected host.
- Inoculation—transplacental and traumatic inoculation reported.
- Once internalized—spores invade host cells, multiply by schizogony, rupture cells to invade others or are shed in urine or feces.
- Localized infections—occur in kidney, liver, and brain of cats.
- Natural infections—rare in cats and dogs (no prevalence data reported).
- Kennels of dogs—whole kennel can be infected at once.

SIGNALMENT/HISTORY

- No sex, or breed predilection.
- Young animals (kittens) show more signs than older cats.

CLINICAL FEATURES

Neonates

- Signs—develop a few weeks postpartum.
- Growth—stunted.
- Unthriftiness—progresses to renal failure.
- Neurologic abnormalities—possible.

Adults

- Can include similar signs as neonates but usually not as severe.
- Aggressive behavior.
- Seizures.
- Blindness.

DIFFERENTIAL DIAGNOSIS

- Other infectious diseases causing neurologic signs—rabies, distemper, toxoplasmosis, *Neospora* infections, FeLV, cuterebriasis, systemic mycoses, GME, toxins (lead), hepatic encephalopathy.

DIAGNOSTICS

- CBC—mild normocytic, normochromic anemia, lymphocytosis, monocytosis.
- Biochemistry profile—elevated serum ALT and ALP.
- Serologic examination—IFA on CSF or blood (commercially available).
- IFA serum titer >1:20 considered positive—suggests previous exposure and not necessarily active infection.
- IFA—send refrigerated serum or CSF to Texas Veterinary Medical Diagnostic Laboratory, College Station, TX.
- Detect spores in urine, feces, or tissues—using Gram's or Ziehl-Neelson stains to identify organisms in renal epithelial cells.
- Modified trichrome stains—excellent for tissue spores (stain bright pink with pink band and clear posterior vacuole; *Fig. 38-1*).

Diagnostic Feature
- **Electronmicroscopy—still considered the definitive diagnostic technique of choice.**

THERAPEUTICS

- None reported to be effective.
- Euthanasia is indicated when severe neurologic signs develop.

Drugs of Choice

- Albendazole (Valbazen® [Pfizer, Exton, PA]).
- Fenbendazole (Panacur® [Intervet, Millsboro, DE] *(Table 38-1)*.

Precautions/Interactions

- Albendazole—reported to cause myelosuppression in cats and dogs.

■ **Fig. 38-1** Kidney aspirate from a dog infected with *Encephalitozoon cuniculi*. Note the bright pink organisms (modified trichrome stain, 1,000×).

 COMMENTS

- Currently—no effective drugs have been described in dogs and cats.
- Fenbendazole—although not reported for the treatment of *E. cuniculi* infections in cats and dogs, would probably be worth trying.
- Zoonosis—especially a risk to immunosuppressed humans.
- Sanitation—70% ethanol.

Abbreviations

ALP, alkaline phosphatase; ALT, alanine aminotransferase; CBC, complete blood count; CSF, cerebrospinal fluid; FeLV, feline leukemia virus; GME, granulomatous meningoencephalitis; IFA, indirect fluorescent antibody.

TABLE 38-1. Suggested Drug Therapy for Encephalitozoonosis in Dogs and Cats				
Drug	Dose (mg/kg)	Route	Interval (Hours)	Duration (Days)
Fenbendazole (Panacur)	50	PO	24	14[a]
Albendazole (Valbazen)	50	PO	8	7[b]

[a] Proposed by consulting editor. A dose of 20mg/kg, PO, q24h for 7 days treats rabbits, or medicated in feed for 4 weeks prevents infection in rabbits.

[b] This dose is effective in mice and humans; may cause myelosuppression in dogs and cats—monitor CBC.

Suggested Reading

Didier PJ, Didier ES, Snowden K, et al. Encephalitozoonosis. In: Greene CE, ed. *Infectious Diseases of the Dog and Cat*. 2nd ed. Philadelphia: WB Saunders; 1998:465–470.

Suter C, Muller-Doblies UU, Hatt JM, et al. Prevention and treatment of *Encephalitozoon cuniculi* infection in rabbits with fenbendazole. *Vet Rec* 2001;148:478–480.

Author: Johnny D. Hoskins
Consulting Editor: Stephen C. Barr

Feline Calicivirus Infection

DEFINITION/OVERVIEW

- A common viral respiratory disease of cats characterized by upper respiratory tract signs; ulceration on the tongue, hard palate, lips, or tip of nose or around claws; pneumonia; and occasionally arthritis.

ETIOLOGY/PATHOPHYSIOLOGY

- A small, nonenveloped single-stranded RNA virus.
- Numerous strains occur in nature—varying degrees of cross-reactivity.
- More than one serotype—most produce similar diseases.
- A very virulent hemorrhagic strain (FCV-ari) described first in California in 1998 but has caused several outbreaks since—causes a hemorrhagic disease syndrome developing 1 to 5 days after exposure; extremely infectious.
- Relatively stable—resistant to many disinfectants.
- Transmission—cats may become infected from FCV carriers (some carries shed virus virtually continuously and thus are always infectious to other cats); directly from other cats with acute disease; fomites within the environment (cages, bowls, etc.).
- Routes of infection—nasal, oral, and conjunctival.
- Once invades cells—rapid cytolysis with tissue damage and ulceration on mucosal surfaces.
- Clinical disease—common in multicat facilities and breeding catteries.
- Incubation period—clinical disease usually appears 3 to 4 days after exposure.
- Neutralizing antibodies—appear about 7 days after exposure, resulting in rapid recovery.
- Persistent infections (carrier states) are common—virus persists in tonsillar and oropharyngeal tissues, in some cats for life.
- FCV carriers—tend to be low, medium, or high shedders in that they shed fairly constant amounts of virus; high shedders are very infectious to other cats.
- Up to 25% of healthy cats may be shedding FCV at any one time—vaccinated cats can still be FCV shedders.
- Routine vaccination—has reduced incidence of clinical disease but has not decreased the prevalence of the virus.

SIGNALMENT/HISTORY

- Mainly affects young kittens >6 weeks of age.
- Cats of any age may show clinical disease.
- Historically, present with a sudden onset of anorexia.
- Owner may report dyspnea, open-mouth breathing.
- Acute onset of lameness due to arthritis.

CLINICAL FEATURES

- Patients are generally alert and in good body condition.
- Fever, especially in those cats with secondary bacterial infections.
- Ocular or nasal discharge with little or no sneezing may result in crusting around the face in young kittens (*Fig. 39-1*).
- Ulcers appear on the tongue and hard palate (*Fig. 39-2*), lips, or tip of nose (*Fig. 39-3*) or around claws.
- Ulcers may occur without any other signs; tongue ulcers are common; occasionally ulcers form on the hard palate and lips; rarely, ulcers can occur around nail beds, leading to pododermatitis and secondary bacterial infection.
- Intestinal ulceration usually does not cause clinical disease.
- Ophthalmic signs are acute serous conjunctivitis with matting of the hair below the eyes, usually without keratitis or corneal ulceration (*Fig. 39-4*).

■ **Fig. 39-1** Severe bilateral conjunctivitis resulting in a serous ocular discharge that has dried into crusts around the eyes and mouth of this young kitten with calicivirus infection (courtesy Dr. R. Riis, Cornell University).

■ **Fig. 39-2** Ulceration of the tongue and hard palate of a cat, caused by calicivirus infection (courtesy Dr. J. Richards, Feline Health Center, Cornell University).

■ **Fig. 39-3** Ulceration of the tip of the nose of a cat, caused by calicivirus infection (courtesy Dr. J. Richards, Feline Health Center, Cornell University).

■ **Fig. 39-4** Ocular discharge from conjunctivitis can become severe enough to cause the fur to matt below the eye and cause hair loss and irritation of the skin (courtesy Dr. R. Riis, Cornell University).

- Lameness, usually shifting, may or may not be associated with oral or respiratory signs; fever; dull and anorexia; full recovery after 24 to 48 hours; can occur secondary to FCV vaccination.
- Infections may be complicated by secondary bacterial invasion, resulting in pneumonia.
- Hemorrhagic syndrome may occur; as well as the typical signs (oral ulceration, nasal and ocular discharge), which are often severe; cats develop a fever; cutaneous edema usually over the head and limbs; alopecia, crusting, and ulceration on the nose, pinnae, occasionally distal limbs; pulmonary edema and pleural effusion develop in some cats; vomiting, diarrhea, and icterus if GI and liver involvement occur; DIC terminally.

DIFFERENTIAL DIAGNOSIS

- Feline viral rhinotracheitis—short incubation period (4 to 5 days); rapid bilateral conjunctivitis; severe sneezing; and ulcerative keratitis.
- Chlamydiosis—tends to have a longer incubation period (7 to 10 days); not characterized by ulcerative stomatitis or pneumonia (although can produce a mild pneumonitis); conjunctivitis mild.
- Feline reovirus infection—very mild upper respiratory tract infection; short incubation period and duration of infection.
- Bronchopneumonia caused by bacteria such as *Bordetella bronchiseptica*—occasionally, localized areas of density within the lungs on radiographs.

DIAGNOSTICS

- Diagnosis usually made based on history and clinical signs.
- CBC, serum biochemical profile, urinalysis—normal; except in hemorrhagic syndrome, in which changes include hyperbilirubinemia, hypoalbuminemia, hyperglycemia, elevated CK, AST, and ALT.
- Thoracic radiology—alveolar-interstitial lung pattern in cats with pneumonia.
- Serologic titers on paired serum samples demonstrate a rise in neutralizing antibody titers against the virus—rarely performed.
- Viral isolation—cultures of swabs from ocular and nasal discharge.
- PCR—not commercially available.

THERAPEUTICS

- Unless severe pneumonia is present, treat as an outpatient to decrease the risk of contamination of the hospital.
- Recommend that owners isolate cats from others to prevent transmission.
- Careful cleaning of ocular nasal discharges and enticing with highly palatable foods will encourage cats to start eating again; feed soft food if oral ulcers present.

■ Place a feeding tube until ulcers are healed sufficiently to allow cat to start eating.

■ Acute arthritis rarely requires treatment except for pain medication.

Vaccination

■ MLV or inactivated vaccines should be given when vaccinated against FHV (8 to 10 weeks of age) and booster 3 to 4 weeks later.

■ In breeding colonies with a severe problem, vaccinate kittens at an earlier age (4 to 5 weeks) or with intranasal administration at 10 to 14 days of age; follow-up vaccinations at 6, 10, and 14 weeks of age.

■ Annual booster vaccines recommended, although immunity undoubtedly lasts >1 year.

■ American Association of Feline Practitioners recommends vaccination of all cats with core vaccines (against FHV, FPV, and calicivirus) on initial visit, after 12 weeks of age, and then 1 year later; booster for FCV should then be given every 3 years.

■ Administer parenteral MLV vaccine carefully—vaccine virus may induce clinical signs if it reaches the oral-respiratory mucosa (if cat licks injection sites, or if an aerosol is produced with the syringe).

■ Intranasal MLV vaccination—induces quicker onset and better protection than parenteral MLV vaccination; however, intranasal vaccination may induce slight side effects including sneezing and ocular and nasal discharge; the best protection is achieved when both intranasal and parenteral vaccinations are given.

■ Inactivated adjuvant vaccines—not as effective as MLV vaccines but have a place in virus-free catteries because there is no risk of spread or revision to virulence; some are licensed for use in pregnant queens.

■ Vaccination—will not eliminate infection in a subsequent exposure but will prevent clinical disease caused by most strains of the virus; vaccination will not prevent shedding.

■ Hemorrhagic syndrome—isolation; aggressive fluid therapy including colloid-containing fluids (hetastarch); treat for DIC with heparin and plasma.

Drugs of Choice

■ Specific antiviral drugs are not available.

■ Broad-spectrum antibiotics—usually indicated to prevent secondary bacterial infections; Antibiotics—amoxicillin (22 mg/kg, PO, q12h) or doxycycline (10 mg/kg, PO, q24h).

■ Antibiotic eye ointment—reduce chance of secondary bacterial infections of the conjunctiva.

■ Human rα-interferon (Roferon [Roche, Nutley, NJ])—may improve cats but findings subjective (30 U/cat, PO, q24h for 7 days, repeated every other week).

Precautions/Interactions

■ Proper vaccination protocol should be explained to clients, especially those owning catteries, where kittens require vaccination before becoming infected (often at 6 to 8 weeks of age) from an infected queen.

■ MLV vaccines—not to be used in pregnant queens.

COMMENTS

- Monitor patients carefully—susceptible to developing interstitial pneumonia or secondary bacterial infections.
- Prognosis—clinical course is usually only 3 to 5 days in uncomplicated cases; rapid recovery usually occurs once neutralizing antibodies appear (~7 days after exposure).
- Prognosis excellent—unless severe pneumonia develops.
- Recovered cats—persistently infected for long periods; many will continuously shed small quantities of virus in oral secretions.

Abbreviations

ALT, alanine aminotransferase; AST, aspartate aminotransferase; CBC, complete blood count; CK, creatine kinase; DIC, disseminated intravascular coagulation; FCV, feline calicivirus; FHV, feline herpes virus; FPV, feline parvovirus; GI, gastrointestinal; MLV, modified live vaccine; PCR, polymerase chain reaction; RNA, ribonucleic acid.

Suggested Reading

Gaskell R, Dawson S. Feline respiratory disease. In: Green CE, ed. *Infectious diseases of the dog and cat.* Philadelphia: WB Saunders; 1998:97–106.
Hurley KF, Sykes JE. Update on feline calicivirus: new trends. *Vet Clin North Am Small Anim Pract* 2003;33:759–772.

Author: Fred W. Scott
Consulting Editor: Stephen C. Barr

chapter 40

Feline Immunodeficiency Virus

DEFINITION/OVERVIEW

- A viral infection causing immunodeficiency in domestic cats.

ETIOLOGY/PATHOPHYSIOLOGY

- Retrovirus (lentivirus)—same genus as HIV, the causative agent of AIDS in humans.
- Infection disrupts immune system function—feline lymphocytes and macrophages serve as the main target cells for virus replication.
- Acute infection—virus spreads from the site of entry (usually a cat bite) to the lymph tissues and thymus, first infecting T lymphocytes then macrophages.
- CD4+ and CD8+ cells—virus selectively and progressively decreases CD4+ (T helper) cells.
- CD4+:CD8+ ratio becomes inverted (from ~2:1 to <1:1)—develops slowly over time.
- An absolute decrease of CD4+ T cells—seen after several months of infection.
- Patients—remain clinically asymptomatic until cell-mediated immunity is disrupted.
- Humoral immune function—altered in advanced stages of infection.
- Macrophages—main reservoir of virus in affected cats; transport virus to tissues throughout the body; defects in function (e.g., increased production of TNF).
- Other cells infected—astrocyte and microglial cells in the brain, megakaryocytes and mononuclear bone marrow cells.
- Coinfection with FeLV—may increase the expression of FIV in many tissues, including kidney, brain, and liver.
- Distribution—worldwide.
- North America—incidence is 1.5% to 3% in the healthy cat population, 9% to 15% in cats with clinical illness.

SIGNALMENT/HISTORY

- Prevalence of infection—increases with age; mean age 5 years at time of diagnosis.
- Males mainly—more aggressive, roaming behavior increases likelihood of being bitten by another cat.

- Diverse historical findings—owing to immunosuppressive nature of infection.
- Associated disease—cannot be clinically distinguished from FeLV-associated immunodeficiencies.
- Recurrent minor illnesses—especially with upper respiratory and GI signs.

CLINICAL FEATURES

- Depend on occurrence of opportunistic infections.
- Lymphadenomegaly—mild to moderate.
- Gingivitis.
- Stomatitis.
- Periodontitis—25% to 50% of cases.
- Upper respiratory tract—rhinitis; conjunctivitis; keratitis (~30% of cases); often associated with feline herpesvirus and calicivirus infections.
- Chronic renal failure.
- Persistent diarrhea—10% to 20% of cases; bacterial or fungal overgrowth, parasite-induced inflammation; direct effect of FIV infection on the GI tract epithelium.
- Chronic, nonresponsive, or recurrent infections of the external ear and skin—from bacterial infections or dermatophytosis.
- Fever and wasting—especially in later stage; possibly from high levels of TNF.
- Ocular disease—anterior uveitis, pars planitis, glaucoma.
- Neoplasia—lymphosarcoma or other neoplasia.
- Neurologic abnormalities—disruption of normal sleep patterns, behavioral changes (pacing and aggression), peripheral neuropathies.

DIFFERENTIAL DIAGNOSIS

- Primary bacterial, parasitic, viral, or fungal infections.
- Toxoplasmosis—neurologic and ocular manifestations may be the result of *Toxoplasma* infection, FIV infection, or both.
- Nonviral neoplastic diseases.

DIAGNOSTICS

- CBC—usually normal, but may show anemia, lymphopenia, neutropenia.
- Neutrophilia—in response to secondary infections.
- Serum biochemistry profile—occasionally hypergammaglobulinemia; variety of other abnormalities depending on organ system involved.
- ELISA—routine screening test detects antibodies to FIV.
- Confirm positive ELISA results—additional testing, especially in healthy, low-risk cats or when diagnosis would result in euthanasia.
- Western blot (immunoblot)—confirmatory testing of ELISA-positive samples.

- Kittens—when <6 months old may have positive test result owing to passive transfer of antibodies from an FIV-positive queen.
- Kittens—a positive test does not indicate infection; retest at 8 to 12 months to determine infection.
- PCR—useful in vaccinated cats or kittens with maternal antibody; currently not commercially available.
- CD4+:CD8+ evaluation—helps determine extent of immunosuppression.
- Virus isolation or detection—experimental only.

 THERAPEUTICS

- Outpatient sufficient for most patients.
- Inpatient—with severe secondary infections until condition is stable; parenteral fluid and nutritional support.
- Manage secondary and opportunistic infections.
- Periodontitis—frequent dental cleaning, tooth extraction, gingival biopsy may be required.

Drugs of Choice

- AZT or zidovudine (Retrovir or Retrovis [Glaxo SmithKline, Philadelphia, PA])—direct antiviral agent; most effective against acute infection; neurologic FIV-related disease may show improvement; monitor for bone marrow toxicity (dose: 5 to 15 mg/kg PO, q12h).
- Immunomodulatory drugs—alleviate some clinical signs:
  - Human recombinant α-interferon (Roferon [Roche, Nutley, NJ])—may increase survival rates and improve clinical status.
  - *Propionibacterium acnes* (ImmunoRegulin [Neogen, Lexington, KY]).
  - Acemannan (Carrisyn [Carrington Labs, Irving, TX])—freeze-dried extract from aloe vera plant.
  - *Staphylococcus* protein A (Prozyme [Pharmacia Biotech, Piscataway, NJ]).
- Gingivitis and stomatitis—may be refractory to treatment.
- Antibacterial or antimycotic drugs—useful for overgrowth of bacteria or fungi; prolonged therapy or high dosages may be required; for anaerobic bacterial infections use metronidazole (Flagyl [Pfizer, Exton, PA]) or clindamycin (Antirobe Pharmacia and Upjohn Co, Kalamazoo, MI).
- Corticosteroids or gold salts—judicious but aggressive use may help control immune-mediated inflammation.
- Anorexia—appetite stimulation:
  - Short term—diazepam (Valium [Roche, Nutley, NJ]); oxazepam (Serax [Wyeth-Ayerst Collegeville, PA]); midazolam (Versed, [Roche], Nutley, NJ); cyproheptadine (Periactin [Merck, Whitehouse Station, NJ]) *(Table 40-1)*.
  - Long term—anabolic steroids or megestrol acetate; efficacy in FIV-positive cats unknown.
- Topical corticosteroids—for anterior uveitis; long-term response may be incomplete or poor; pars planitis often regresses spontaneously and may recur.

TABLE 40-1. Drugs Used to Manage Cats with Feline Immunodeficiency Virus Infections

Drug	Dose (mg/kg)	Route	Interval (Hours)	Duration (Days)
AZT (Retrovir)	5–15	PO	12	a
Human rα-interferon (Roferon)	30[b]	PO	24	7[c]
Propionibacterium acnes (Immunoregulin)	0.5[d]	IV	Once or twice	Weekly
Acemannan (Carrisyn)	100[e]	PO	24	28
Staphylococcus protein-A	0.01	IP	Twice, 1st week	f
Metronidazole (Flagyl)	7–15	PO	12	14
Clindamycin (Antirobe)	11	PO	12	14
Diazepam (Valium®)	0.2	IV	Once or twice	—
Oxazepam (Serax)	2.5[e]	PO	Once or twice	2
Midazolam (Versed)	0.02–0.05	IV	As needed	—
Cyproheptadine (Periactin)	2[e]	PO	12	As needed

a Until a response is seen.
b International unit total dose per cat.
c Repeat every other week.
d Milliliter total dose per cat.
e Milligram total dose per cat.
f After first week, treat once monthly.

- Glaucoma—standard treatment.
- Yearly vaccination for respiratory and enteric viruses with inactivated vaccines is recommended.

Precautions/Interactions

- Griseofulvin—avoid or use with extreme caution in FIV-positive cats; may induce severe neutropenia; neutropenia is reversible if the drug is withdrawn early enough but secondary infections associated with the condition can be life-threatening.
- MLV vaccines—may cause disease in immunosuppressed cats.
- Systemic corticosteroids—use with caution especially at high doses as may lead to further immunosuppression.
- Long-term use of megestrol acetate—may lead to development of diabetes mellitus.

 COMMENTS

- Inform client—infection is slowly progressive and healthy antibody-positive cats may remain healthy for years.
- Advise client that cats with clinical signs—will have recurrent or chronic health problems that require medical attention.

- Discuss the importance of keeping cats indoors—to protect them from exposure to secondary pathogens and to prevent spread of FIV.
- Quarantine and test incoming cats—before introducing into multicat households.
- Zoonosis—no known zoonotic potential.
- FIV-positive queens—reported abortions and stillbirths; transmission to kittens is infrequent if the queen is antibody-positive before conception.
- Prognosis—within the first 2 years after diagnosis or 4.5 to 6 years after the estimated time of infection, about 20% of cats die but >50% remain asymptomatic.
- In late stages of disease (wasting and frequent or severe opportunistic infections)—life expectancy is ≤1 year.
- Vaccination—dual subtype (A&D), inactivated whole virus vaccine (Fel-O-Vax FIV [Fort Dodge Animal Health, Fort Dodge, IA]).

  - Efficacy of 60% to 80% after three doses.
  - Cannot distinguish between vaccinated and FIV-infected cats with antibody assays.

- Yearly vaccination for respiratory and enteric viruses—inactivated vaccines are recommended.

Abbreviations

AIDS, acquired immunodeficiency syndrome; AZT, azidothymidine; CBC, complete blood count; ELISA, enzyme-linked immunosorbent assay; FeLV, feline leukemia virus; FIV, feline immunodeficiency virus; GI, gastrointestinal; HIV, human immunodeficiency virus; MLV, modified live virus; PCR, polymerase chain reaction; TNF, tumor necrosis factor.

Suggested Reading

Barr MC, Phillips TR. FIV and FIV-related diseases. In: Ettinger SJ, Feldman EC, eds. *Textbook of Veterinary Internal Medicine.* 5th ed. Philadelphia: WB Saunders; 2000:433–438.

Levy JK. CVT update: feline immunodeficiency virus. In: Bonagura JD, ed. *Kirk's Current Veterinary Therapy XIII: Small Animal Practice.* Philadelphia: WB Saunders; 2000:284–288.

Author: Margaret C. Barr
Consulting Editor: Stephen C. Barr

chapter 41

Feline Infectious Peritonitis

DEFINITION/OVERVIEW

- A viral disease of cats characterized by insidious onset, persistent nonresponsive fever, pyogranulomatous tissue reaction, accumulation of exudative effusions in body cavities, and high mortality.

ETIOLOGY/PATHOPHYSIOLOGY

- Two genomic types of FCoV: FCoV-1 (causes perhaps 85% of infections) and FCoV-2.
- Distinguishing between forms—there has been great effort to distinguish between the low-virulent or avirulent enteric strains (FECV) and the virulent strains.
- FECV and FIP virus—occur in both type 1 and type 2 forms.
- Spectrum of disease within each type—avirulent viruses (producing asymptomatic infections) to fatal FIP.
- Fecal shedding of virus—important in transmission.
- FIP virus—replicates locally in epithelial cells of the upper respiratory tract or oropharynx.
- Antiviral antibodies are produced—virus is taken up by macrophages.
- The virus is transported within monocytes/macrophages throughout the body—localizes at various vein walls and perivascular sites.
- Local perivascular viral replication and subsequent pyogranulomatous tissue reaction—produce the classic lesion.
- Multisystemic—pyogranulomatous or granulomatous lesions in the omentum, on the serosal surface of abdominal organs (e.g., liver, kidney, and intestines), within abdominal lymph nodes, and in the submucosa of the intestinal tract.
- Respiratory—lesions on lung surfaces.
- Pleural effusion—in the wet form.
- Nervous—vascular lesions can occur throughout the CNS, especially in the meninges.
- Ophthalmic—lesions may include uveitis and chorioretinitis.
- FIP virus can infect fetuses—resulting in fetal death or neonatal disease.
- Distribution—worldwide.

- Prevalence of antibodies against FCoV—high in most populations, especially in multicat facilities.
- Incidence of clinical disease—low in most populations, especially in single-cat households.
- Because of the difficulty in diagnosis, control, and prevention—outbreaks within breeding catteries may be catastrophic.
- In endemic catteries—risk of an FCoV antibody–positive cat eventually developing FIP is usually <10%.

SIGNALMENT/HISTORY

- Susceptibility—some families or lines of cats appear more susceptible.
- Highest incidence in kittens—3 months to 3 years of age.
- Incidence decreases—sharply after cats reach 3 years of age.
- Incidence increases—again in cats >10 years of age.
- Onset—insidious onset.
- Weight loss and decrease in appetite—gradual.
- Growth—stunting in kittens.
- Gradual increase in the size of the abdomen—giving a potbellied appearance.
- Persistent fever—fluctuating and unresponsive to antibiotics.

CLINICAL FEATURES

- Vary widely.
- Depend on—virulence of the strain, effectiveness of the host immune response, organ system affected.
- Two classic forms:
  - Wet or effusive form—targets the body cavities.
  - Dry or noneffusive form—targets a variety of organs.
- Depression.
- Poor condition.
- Stunted growth.
- Weight loss.
- Dull, rough hair coat.
- Icterus.
- Abdominal and/or pleural effusion (Fig. 41-1).
- Palpation of the abdomen—abdominal masses (granulomas or pyogranulomas) within the omentum, on the surface of viscera (especially the kidney), and within the intestinal wall.
- Mesenteric lymph nodes—may be enlarged.
- Ocular—anterior uveitis, keratic precipitates, fibrin in the anterior chamber, cataract formation, color change to the iris, and irregularly shaped pupil can all be presentations (Fig. 41-2, Fig. 41-3, Fig. 41-4).
- Neurologic—brain stem, cerebrocortical, or spinal cord.

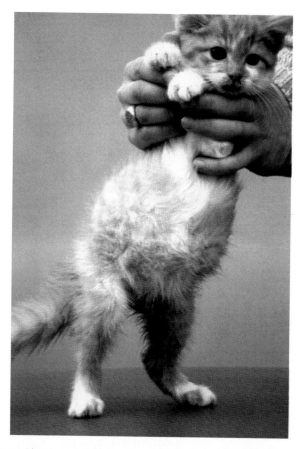

■ **Fig. 41-1** Young kitten with enlarged abdomen from ascitic fluid typical of feline infectious peritonitis infection (courtesy Dr. Fred Scott, Professor Emeritus, Cornell University).

■ **Fig. 41-2** Acute fibrin accumulation within the anterior chamber of a cat with acute-onset feline infectious peritonitis (courtesy Dr. Ron Riis, Cornell University).

■ **Fig. 41-3** Anterior uveitis with fibrin and keratic precipitate accumulation within the anterior chamber of a cat with feline infectious peritonitis (courtesy Dr. Ron Riis, Cornell University).

DIFFERENTIAL DIAGNOSIS

- Fever of unknown origin—when other causes of fever are ruled out.
- Cardiac disease causing pleural effusion—typically has low specific gravity and cell count.
- Lesions of lymphoma, especially in the kidney, on palpation.
- CNS tumors—most cats will have positive test for FeLV.
- FeLV-negative cats—biopsy the lesion (if accessible) for histopathology and immunohistochemistry for diagnosis of FCoV.
- Respiratory disease—FCV, FHV, chlamydiosis, or various bacteria.

■ **Fig. 41-4** Cataract formation with anterior uveitis in a cat with feline infectious peritonitis (courtesy of Dr. Ron Riis, Cornell University).

- Pansteatitis (yellow fat disease)—classic feel and appearance of fat within the abdominal cavity; pain on abdominal palpation; often a fish-only diet.
- Panleukopenia producing enteritis—leukopenia; positive fecal canine parvovirus antigen assay.
- Hepatic involvement—cholangiohepatitis, lymphoma (and other neoplasia), infectious.

 ## DIAGNOSTICS

- CBC.
    - Leukopenia—common early in the infection.
    - Later leukocytosis with neutrophilia and lymphopenia.
    - Mild to moderate anemia may occur.
- Serum biochemical profile—variety of abnormalities possible depending on organ involvement.
- High total plasma globulin—common.
- Hyperbilirubinemia and hyperbilirubinuria—often.
- Serum antibody tests—immunoassays, viral neutralization assays.
- Detect antibodies against FCoV—positive tests not diagnostic, indicate only previous infection or vaccination; correlation between height of titer and eventual confirmation of infection not high.
- PCR assays—detect viral antigen; accuracy of positive tests correlating with clinical disease is still being evaluated.
- RT-PCR assay of effusions and tissue—better positive predictive value for identifying cats with FIP.
- Both PCR reactions—available at commercial laboratories.
- Immunohistochemistry (immunoperoxidase) assays—detect FCoV within specific cells of biopsy samples or histopathologic sections of tissues from cats with fatal diseases.
- Immunohistochemistry—excellent for confirming cause of specific lesions, especially inflammatory abdominal disease, which often is not diagnosed as FIP.
- Fluid obtained via thoracocentesis and abdominocentesis—pale to straw colored, viscous, flecks of white fibrin often seen, will clot upon standing, specific gravity usually high (1.030–1.040), high protein concentrations (>3.5 g/dl).
- Laparoscopy or exploratory laparotomy—to observe specific lesions of the peritoneal cavity; to obtain a biopsy sample for histopathologic or immunohistochemistry confirmation.

Diagnostic Feature
- **The triad of hyperglobulinemia, FCoV serum antibody titer >160, and lymphopenia—very high predictive value for diagnosing FIP in a patient with consistent clinical signs.**

 ## THERAPEUTICS

- Inpatient or outpatient—depends on stage and severity of disease, and owner's willingness and ability to provide good supportive care.

- Therapeutic paracentesis—may relieve pressure on respiration from excessive ascites or pleural effusions.
- Diet—important to encourage the affected cat to eat.

Drugs of Choice

- Treatment—no treatment routinely effective.
- Patients with generalized and typical signs—almost invariably die.
- Most FCoV-positive cats—have subclinical infection or mild, localized granulomatous disease that is not diagnosed as FIP.
- Immunosuppressive drugs (e.g., prednisolone and cyclophosphamide)—limited success.
- Corticosteroids (subconjunctival injection)—may help ocular involvement.
- Interferon—effective in vitro; limited success in vivo; a recombinant interferon reported to have some success in Japan.
- Antibiotics—ineffective because generally not associated with secondary bacterial infections.
- Antiviral drugs—none proven to be efficacious.
- MLV intranasal vaccine—available against FIP virus; efficacy low; cannot rely on vaccination alone for control; may produce antibody-positive cats, complicating monitoring in catteries or colonies; should only be considered for seronegative cats that are at extremely high risk of exposure to FCoV.

Precautions/Interactions

- NA

 COMMENTS

- Inform client—of all the various aspects of disease, including the grave prognosis.
- Inform client—of the high prevalence of FCoV infection but low incidence of actual clinical disease.
- Less than 10% of FCoV antibody–positive cats <3 years of age eventually develop clinical disease.
- In mother/offspring—main method of transmission appears to be from asymptomatic carrier queens to their kittens at 5 to 7 weeks of age, after maternally derived immunity wanes.
- Break cycle of transmission—early weaning at 4 to 5 weeks of age kittens and isolating litter from direct contact with other cats, including the queen.
- Routine disinfection of premises, cages, and water/food dishes—readily inactivates virus and reduces transmission.
- Introduce only FCoV antibody–negative cats to catteries or colonies that are free of virus.
- Restrict household cats to indoor environments.
- Clinical course—lasts a few days to several months.
- Prognosis is grave once typical signs occur—mortality nearly 100%.

Abbreviations

CBC, complete blood count; CNS, central nervous system; FCoV, feline coronavirus; FCV, feline calicivirus; FECV, feline enteric coronavirus; FeLV, feline leukemia virus; FHV, feline herpes virus; FIP, feline infectious peritonitis; MLV, modified live virus; PCR, polymerase chain reaction; RT-PCR, reverse transcriptase polymerase chain reaction.

Suggested Reading

Barr MC, Olsen CW, Scott FW. Feline viral diseases. In: Ettinger SJ, Feldman EC, eds. *Veterinary Internal Medicine*. 4th ed. Philadelphia: WB Saunders; 1995:409–439.

Horzinek MC, Lutz H. An update on feline infectious peritonitis. *Vet Sci Tomorrow* 2001;Jan:1–11.

Olsen CW. A review of feline infectious peritonitis virus: molecular biology, immunopathogenesis, clinical aspects, and vaccination. *Vet Microbiol* 1993;36:1–37.

Report from the International FIP/FECV Workshop. *Feline Pract* 1995;23:2–111.

Sparkes AH, Gruffydd-Jones TJ, Harbour DA. An appraisal of the value of laboratory tests in the diagnosis of feline infectious peritonitis. *J Am Anim Hosp Assoc* 1994;30:345–350.

Author: Fred W. Scott
Consulting Editor: Stephen C. Barr

chapter 42

Feline Leukemia Virus Infection

DEFINITION/OVERVIEW

- A viral infection that causes immunodeficiency and neoplastic disease in domestic cats.

ETIOLOGY/PATHOPHYSIOLOGY

- Retrovirus—gammaretrovirus.
- Early infection consists of five stages—(1) viral replication in tonsils and pharyngeal lymph nodes; (2) infection of a few circulating B lymphocytes and macrophages that disseminate the virus; (3) replication in lymphoid tissues, intestinal crypt epithelial cells, and bone marrow precursor cells; (4) release of infected neutrophils and platelets from the bone marrow into the circulatory system; and (5) infection of epithelial and glandular tissues, with subsequent shedding of virus into the saliva and urine.
- Adequate immune response—stops progression at stage 2 or 3 (4 to 8 weeks after exposure) and forces the virus into latency.
- Persistent viremia (stages 4 and 5)—usually develops 4 to 6 weeks after infection, but may take 12 weeks.
- Tumor induction—occurs when the DNA provirus integrates into cat chromosomal DNA in critical regions (oncogenes).
- Feline sarcoma viruses (mutants of FeLV)—arise by recombination between the genes of FeLV and host.
- Virus-host fusion proteins—responsible for the efficient induction of fibrosarcomas.
- Multiple systems affected—hemic/lymphatic/immune (anemia; blood cell dyscrasias; neoplasias originating in the bone marrow; immunosuppression, possibly resulting from neuroendocrine dysfunction; absolute decrease in CD4+ and CD8+ subsets of T cells; decreased CD4+:CD8+ ratio), nervous (degenerative myelopathy, neuropathy, neoplasias), other body systems (immunosuppression, with secondary infections or development of neoplastic disease).
- Cat-to-cat transmission—bites, close casual contact (grooming), shared dishes or litter pans.
- Perinatal transmission—fetal and neonatal death of kittens from 80% of affected queens.
- Transplacental and transmammary transmission—occurs in at least 20% of surviving kittens from infected queens.
- Neonatal kittens—most susceptible to persistent infection (70% to 100%).
- Older kittens—<30% susceptible by 16 weeks of age.

SIGNALMENT/HISTORY

- Distribution—worldwide.
- North America—2% to 3% incidence in healthy cats; 3 to 4 times greater in cats exhibiting clinical illness.
- Prevalence—highest between 1 and 6 (mean of 3) years of age.
- Male:female ratio—1.7:1.
- Most patients—live outdoor or in multicat households.
- Onset of FeLV-associated disease—usually occurs over a period of months to years after infection.
- Associated diseases—nonneoplastic or neoplastic.
- Most of the nonneoplastic or degenerative diseases result from immunosuppression or bone marrow disease.
- Clinical signs of FeLV-induced immunodeficiency—cannot be distinguished from those of FIV-induced immunodeficiency.
- FIV and FeLV—may occur concurrently.

CLINICAL FEATURES

- Depend—on the type of disease (neoplastic or nonneoplastic) and occurrence of secondary infections.
- Lymphadenomegaly—mild to severe.
- Upper respiratory tract—rhinitis, conjunctivitis, and keratitis.
- Persistent diarrhea—bacterial or fungal overgrowth, parasite-induced inflammation, direct effect of infection on crypt cells.
- Oral—gingivitis; stomatitis; periodontitis.
- Skin—chronic nonresponsive or recurrent infections of the external ear and skin.
- Fever.
- Wasting.
- Lymphoma (lymphosarcoma)—most common associated neoplastic disease; thymic and multicentric lymphomas highly associated; miscellaneous lymphomas (extranodal origin) most frequently involve the eye and nervous system.
- Erythroid and myelomonocytic leukemias—predominant nonlymphoid leukemias.
- Fibrosarcomas—in patients coinfected with mutated sarcoma virus, most frequently in young cats.
- Peripheral neuropathies—progressive ataxia.
- FeLV-positive queens—abortions, stillbirths, and fetal resorptions common.

DIFFERENTIAL DIAGNOSIS

- FIV.
- Other infections—bacterial, parasitic, viral, or fungal.
- Nonviral neoplastic diseases.

DIAGNOSTICS

- CBC—anemia (often severe, lymphopenia, neutropenia—may be in response to secondary infections, thrombocytopenia and immune-mediated hemolytic anemia)—may occur secondary to immune complexes.
- RBC macrocytosis.
- *Haemobartonella* spp. (RBC mycoplasmal) infections—often secondary.
- IFA—identifies FeLV p27 antigen in leukocytes and platelets in fixed smears of whole blood or buffy coat preparations.
- Positive IFA result indicates—productive infection in bone marrow cells.
- 97% of IFA-positive cats—remain persistently infected and viremic for life.
- IFA—p27 antigen can usually be detected by 4 weeks after infection, but may take up to 12 weeks to develop a positive test.
- IFA for leukopenic cats—use buffy coat smears rather than whole blood smears.
- IFA on bone marrow samples—may be positive when negative on peripheral blood.
- ELISA—detect soluble FeLV p27 antigen in whole blood, serum, plasma, saliva, or tears.
- ELISA—more sensitive than IFA at detecting early or transient infections.
- A single positive ELISA test—cannot predict which cats will be persistently viremic; retest in 12 weeks (many veterinarians test with IFA at this point).
- False-positive ELISA results—more common when whole blood rather than serum or plasma is used; positive tests with saliva or tears should be checked with whole blood (IFA) or serum (ELISA).
- A few cats have persistently ELISA-positive test results and IFA-negative results—recently, FeLV proviral genetic material has been detected in circulating blood cells from some of these cats; demonstrates infection despite no detectable viremia.
- Neither test detects FeLV-vaccinated cats—because the vaccine induces antibodies against gp70 antigen, not p27 antigen.
- Bone marrow aspiration or biopsy—with erythroblastopenia (nonregenerative anemia), bone marrow often hypercellular owing to an arrest in differentiation of erythroid cells; true aplastic anemia with hypocellular bone marrow may be seen; some cases of anemia result from myeloproliferative disease; myelofibrosis in some.

THERAPEUTICS

- Outpatient for most cats.
- Inpatient—may be required with severe secondary infections, anemia, or cachexia until condition stable.
- Blood transfusions—emergency support; multiple transfusions may be necessary; passive antibody transfer reduces level of FeLV antigenemia in some cats; thus immunization of blood donor cats with FeLV vaccines is useful.
- Management of secondary and opportunistic infections—primary consideration.
- Supportive therapy (e.g., parenteral fluids and nutritional supplements)—may be useful.

Drugs of Choice

- AZT or Zidovudine (Retrovir or Retrovis [Glaxo SmithKline, Philadelphia, PA])—direct antiviral agent; clinical improvement but does not clear virus; monitor for bone marrow toxicity.
- Immunomodulatory drugs—alleviate some clinical signs:
  - Human recombinant α-interferon (Roferon [Roche, Nutley, NJ])—may increase survival rates and improve clinical status.
  - *Propionibacterium acnes* (ImmunoRegulin [Neogen, Lansing, MI]).
  - Acemannan (Carrisyn, [Carrington Labs, Irving, TX])—freeze-dried extract from aloe vera plant.
  - *Staphylococcus* protein A (Prozyme [Sigma, St. Louis, MO])
  - *HaemobartonellaI* spp. (RBC mycoplasmal) infections—suspect in all cats with regenerative hemolytic anemias; oxytetracycline (Terramycin [Pfizer, Exton, PA]) or doxycycline (Vibramycin [Pfizer, Exton, PA]); short-term use of oral glucocorticoids in severe cases (*Table 42-1*).
- Lymphosarcoma—managed successfully with standard combination chemotherapy protocols; periods of remission average 3 to 4 months; some cats may remain in remission for much longer.
- Myeloproliferative disease and leukemias—more refractory to treatment.
- Yearly vaccination—for respiratory and enteric viruses with inactivated vaccines recommended.
- Vaccines against FeLV—most commercial vaccines induce virus-neutralizing antibodies specific for gp70; reported efficacy ranges from <20% to almost 100%, depending on the trial and challenge system; test cats for FeLV before initial vaccination; if prevaccination testing is not done, clients should be aware that the cat may already be infected.

TABLE 42-1. Drugs Used to Manage Cats with Feline Leukemia Virus Infections

Drug	Dose (mg/kg)	Route	Interval (Hours)	Duration (Days)
AZT (Retrovir)	5–15	PO	12	a
Human rα-interferon (Roferon)	30[b]	PO	24	7[c]
Propionibacterium acnes) (Immunoregulin)	0.5[d]	IV	Once or twice	Weekly
Acemannan (Carrisyn)	100[e]	PO	24	28
Staphylococcus protein-A	0.01	IP	Twice, 1st week	f
Oxytetracycline	15	PO	8	10
Doxycycline	5–10	PO	24	10

a Until a response is seen.
b International unit total dose per cat.
c Repeat every other week.
d Milliliter total dose per cat.
e Milligram total dose per cat.
f After first week, treat once monthly.

- FeLV vaccines—administer SC distally on the hind limb due to possibility of producing a vaccine-induced fibrosarcoma.
- One FeLV vaccine (Purevax [Merial], Iselin, NJ) is adjuvant-free in a canarypox vector (reducing risk of fibrosarcoma formation); administered in a small volume (0.25 ml) using a transdermal vaccination system (removing needle use and disposal).

Precautions/Interactions

- MLV—may cause disease in immunosuppressed cats.
- Systemic corticosteroids—use with caution because of the potential for further immunosuppression.
- AZT—can cause anemia, which is reversible with discontinuation of the drug.

 COMMENTS

- Discuss importance of keeping cats indoors and separated from FeLV-negative cats to protect them from exposure to secondary pathogens and to prevent spread of FeLV.
- Should be aggressive in dental tooth extraction if needed.
- Prevent contact with FeLV-positive cats; quarantine and test incoming cats before introduction into multicat households.
- More than 50% of persistently viremic cats succumb to related diseases within 2 to 3 years after infection.
- Zoonotic potential is probably low, but controversial; studies report conflicting results of antibodies to FeLV in humans and of correlation between certain human leukemias and exposure to cats.

Abbreviations

AZT, azidothymidine; CBC, complete blood count; DNA, deoxyribonucleic acid; ELISA, enzyme-linked immunosorbent assay; FLeV, feline leukemia virus; FIV, feline immunodeficiency virus; IFA, immunofluorescent antibody; MLV, modified live virus; RBC, red blood cell.

Suggested Reading

Levy JK. FeLV and non-neoplastic FeLV–related disease. In: Ettinger SJ, Feldman EC, eds. *Textbook of Veterinary Internal Medicine*, 5th ed. Philadelphia: WB Saunders; 2000:424–432.

Wolf AM. CVT update: feline leukemia virus. In: Bonagura JD, ed. *Kirk's Current Veterinary Therapy XIII: Small Animal Practice*. Philadelphia: WB Saunders; 2000:280–284.

Sparkes AH. Feline leukemia virus: a review of immunity and vaccination. *J Small Anim Pract* 1997; 38:187–194.

Author: Margaret C. Barr
Consulting Editor: Stephen C. Barr

chapter 43

Feline Lungworm (*Aelurostrongylus*)

DEFINITION/OVERVIEW

- A helminth infection in cats causing a spectrum of disease from asymptomatic to severe respiratory distress with weight loss.

ETIOLOGY/PATHOPHYSIOLOGY

- *Aelurostrongylus abstrusus*—a metastrongyloidae parasite.
- Adult worms—curl within the lung parenchyma, producing small grayish-white subpleural nodules.
- Adults worms—lay eggs within the alveoli of the lungs, where they develop to L1 larvae that hatch and ascend the trachea to be swallowed and eventually appear in the feces.
- L1 larvae—enter snails and slugs, where they develop to L3, which are infective to cats.
- Cats—also probably become infected by eating paratenic hosts (birds and rodents).
- PPP = 5 to 6 weeks.

SIGNALMENT/HISTORY

- Outdoor cats that hunt birds and rodents have a higher incidence.

CLINICAL FEATURES

- Most cats—asymptomatic.
- Coughing—most consistent sign.
- Respiratory distress—occasional sign.
- Severe infections—can produce lethargy and weight loss, especially in young cats.
- Pleural effusion—rare consequence of infection.

■ **Fig. 43-1** L1 larvae of *Aelurostrongylus abstrusus* in feces of a cat (Baermann's technique). Note the kinked tail and long esophagus typical of this larva.

DIFFERENTIAL DIAGNOSIS

- Allergic (asthma), other parasitic (heartworm disease), and cardiac disease.
- Although less likely, trauma (diaphragmatic hernia), pleural disease (pyothorax, chylothorax), neoplasia, and inflammatory diseases should be considered.
- Differentiated from other possible causes by finding L1 larvae in feces.

DIAGNOSTICS

Diagnostic Feature
- **L1 larvae in the feces—Baermann's technique is very reliable** *(Fig. 43-1).*
- L1 larvae—may also be found in a transtracheal wash, along with many eosinophils.
- CBC—eosinophilia is consistently present.
- Thoracic radiographs—show bronchial pattern with alveolar infiltrates and some increased interstitial densities *(Fig. 43-2).*

THERAPEUTICS

- Many cases will spontaneously regress after 2 to 3 months without treatment.
- Treatment is very effective in resolving clinical signs and larval shedding in the feces.
- Thoracic radiographic changes may worsen after treatment as the lesions consolidate and become more obvious *(Fig. 43-3).*
- Glucocorticoids may help alleviate clinical signs but may also interfere with parasitologic cure.
- Bronchodilators may alleviate clinical signs.

Drugs of Choice

- Ivermectin—very effective.
- Fenbendazole—effective but difficult to administer in cats *(Table 43-1).*

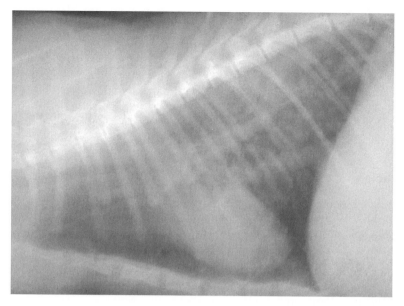

■ **Fig. 43-2** Lateral thoracic radiograph showing diffuse interstitial alveolar pattern in a cat with lungworm infestation.

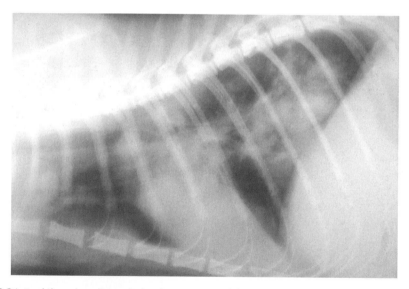

■ **Fig. 43-3** Lateral thoracic radiograph showing more consolidated interstitial alveolar pattern in a cat 1 week after treatment for lungworm. Even though clinical signs and larvae in the feces disappear, radiographic lesions look worse immediately post-treatment.

TABLE 43-1. Drug Therapy for Feline Lungworm (*Aelurostrongylus abstrusus*)				
Drug	**Dose (mg/kg)**	**Route**	**Interval (Hours)**	**Duration (Days)**
Ivermectin	0.4	PO, SC	Once	—
Fenbendazole	20	PO	24	5[a]

[a] Repeat this course of fenbendazole after 7 days.

COMMENTS

Precautions/Interactions

- The use of glucocorticoids may interfere with parasitologic cure.
- Thoracic radiographic changes look much worse up to a week post-treatment, even though clinical signs abate.
- Prognosis for complete cure in treated animals is excellent.

Abbreviations

CBC, complete blood count; PPP, prepatent period.

Suggested Reading

Reinemeyer CR. Parasites of the respiratory system. In: Bonagura JD, ed. *Kirk's Current Veterinary Therapy*. 12th ed. Philadelphia: WB Saunders; 1995;895–898.

Author: Stephen C. Barr
Consulting Editor: Stephen C. Barr

chapter 44

Feline Panleukopenia

DEFINITION/OVERVIEW

- An acute, enteric, viral infection of cats characterized by sudden onset, depression, vomiting and diarrhea, severe dehydration, and a high mortality rate.

ETIOLOGY/PATHOPHYSIOLOGY

- FPV—infects only mitotic cells, causing acute cell cytolysis of rapidly dividing cells.
- Affects organs containing rapid dividing cells—mainly the hemic/lymphatic/immune (severe panleukopenia; atrophy of the thymus), and GI systems (intestinal crypt cells of the jejunum and ileum).
- Death of crypt cells—results in shortened blunt villi with poor absorption of nutrients, acute enteritis with vomiting and diarrhea, dehydration, and secondary bacteremia.
- In utero infection—leads to fetal death, fetal resorption, abortion, stillbirth, or fetal mummification.
- Infections of neonatal kittens—affect the rapidly dividing granular cells of the cerebellum and retinal cells of the eye, causing cerebellar hypoplasia with ataxia and retinal dysplasia.
- Distribution—worldwide.
- The most severe and important feline infectious disease in unvaccinated populations—routine vaccination provides almost total control of this disease.
- Extremely contagious and stable virus—survives for years on contaminated premises.
- CPV-2a and CPV-2b—recently isolated from cats with feline panleukemia.
- Properties of CPV—like those for FPV.

SIGNALMENT/HISTORY

- History of recent exposure (e.g., adoption from shelter).
- Newly acquired kitten.
- Kittens 2 to 6 months of age are most susceptible (once passively transferred maternal immunity is lost).

- No vaccination history or last vaccinated when <12 weeks of age.
- Sudden onset of vomiting, diarrhea, depression, and complete anorexia.
- Owner may suspect poisoning.
- Cat may have disappeared or hidden for 1 day or more before being found.
- Owner may report cat hangs head over water bowl or food dish but does not eat or drink.

 CLINICAL FEATURES

- Depression—may be mild to severe.
- Typical "panleukopenia posture"—sternum and chin resting on floor, feet tucked under body, and top of scapulae elevated above the back.
- Dehydration—appears rapidly, may be severe.
- Vomiting and diarrhea—may occur; less likely to occur in older cats.
- Body temperature—usually mild to moderately elevated or depressed in the early stages of disease.
- Body temperature—becomes severely subnormal as affected cat becomes moribund.
- Abdominal pain—may be elicited on palpation.
- Small intestine—either turgid and hoselike or flaccid.
- Retina—retinal degeneration (discrete focal gray areas with dark margins) in kittens with neurologic signs or seen as an incidental finding in clinically normal cats (*Fig. 44-1*).
- Subclinical or mild infections—few or no clinical signs common, especially in adults.
- Ataxia from cerebellar hypoplasia (kittens infected in utero or neonatally)—signs evident at 10 to 14 days of age and persist for life: hypermetria; dysmetria; incoordination

■ **Fig. 44-1** Focal areas of retinal degeneration seen in a cat after recovery from panleukopenia virus infection (courtesy Dr. R. Riis, Cornell University).

with a base-wide stance and an elevated "rudder" tail; alert, afebrile, and otherwise normal; retinal dysplasia sometimes seen.

 # DIFFERENTIAL DIAGNOSIS

- Panleukopenia-like syndrome of FeLV infection—chronic infection; chronic enteritis; chronic panleukopenia; often anemia; patient positive for FeLV antigen in the blood and/or saliva.
- Salmonellosis—usually subclinical infection; severe gastroenteritis; total WBC counts usually high.
- Acute poisoning—similar to acute or fulminating disease; severe depression; subnormal temperature; total WBC count not severely depressed.
- Many diseases of cats can cause mild clinical signs that are hard to differentiate from those of mild feline panleukemia—total WBC count is always low during the acute infection with feline panleukemia, even in subclinical infections.

 # DIAGNOSTICS

- CBC—panleukopenia (most consistent finding); leukocyte counts usually between 500 and 3,000 cells/dl during the acute disease.
- Serum biochemical profile—reflects dehydration and electrolyte loss from vomiting and diarrhea.

Diagnostic Feature
- **CPV antigen fecal immunoassay (CITE Canine Parvovirus Test Kit [IDEXX Labs, Westbrook, ME])—not licensed for feline panleukemia; will detect FPV antigen in feces.**
- Chromatographic test strip—feces for FPV and CPV.
- Unknown if vaccination with MLV vaccine against FPV will cause a false positive test result 5 to 15 days postvaccination, as can happen for CPV in dogs.
- Serologic testing—paired serum samples (acute and convalescent); detects rising antibody titer.
- Viral isolation—from feces or affected tissues (e.g., thymus, small intestine, spleen).
- Electron microscopy of feces—detects parvovirus particles, presumably FPV.

 # THERAPEUTICS

- Main principles of treatment:
  - Rehydration.
  - Reestablishment of electrolyte balance.
  - Supportive care until the patient's immune system produces antiviral antibodies that neutralize the virus.
  - Protection against secondary bacterial infection.

- Inpatient—severe cases; hydration and replacement electrolyte therapy.
- Plasma transfusions—if plasma protein <4 g/dl.
- Whole blood transfusions—rarely required because cats do not get that anemic.
- Outpatient—mild cases.

Drugs of Choice

- Broad-spectrum antibiotics (ampicillin/gentamicin combination)—to counter secondary bacterial infection from GI tract flora.
- Vaccination—completely preventable by routine vaccination of kittens; vaccination after the development of clinical signs is contraindicated.
- Vaccinations—MLV or inactivated parenteral vaccines and MLV intranasal vaccine.
- Immunity—long duration, perhaps even for life.
- Kittens—vaccinate at 8 to 10 weeks of age; then after 12 weeks of age when maternally derived immunity has waned.
- Boosters—after 1 year; repeat every 3 years to provide excellent immunity.

Precautions/Interactions

- Chronic enteritis—due to vilus blunting and overgrowth with fungal infection or other pathogens not usually affected by antibiotics (protozoa, fungal, yeast).
- Teratogenic effects (cerebellar hypoplasia resulting in ataxia for life)—virus infection of fetus.
- Monitor renal function closely if administering gentamicin—do not administer to dehydrated animals.

 COMMENTS

- Inform client that all current and future cats in the household must be vaccinated against FPV before exposure—the virus will remain infectious on the premise for years unless environment can be adequately disinfected.
- Disinfection—can be achieved with 1:32 dilution of household bleach.
- Recovered cats are immune against FPV infection for life—do not require further vaccination.
- Prognosis—most cases acute, lasting only 5 to 7 days; if death does not occur during the acute disease, recovery is usually rapid and uncomplicated.
- Recovery—may take several weeks for the patient to regain weight and body condition.
- Prognosis—guarded during the acute disease, especially if the total WBC count is <2000 cells/dl.

Abbreviations

CBC, complete blood count; CPV, canine parvovirus; FeLV, feline leukemia virus; FPV, feline parvovirus; GI, gastrointestinal; MLV, modified live virus; WBC, white blood cell.

Suggested Reading

Barr MC, Olsen CW, Scott FW. Feline viral diseases. In: Ettinger SJ, Feldman EC, eds. *Veterinary Internal Medicine*. Philadelphia: WB Saunders; 1995:409–439.

Elston T, Rodan I, Flemming D, et al. Report of the American Association of Feline Practitioners and Academy of Feline Medicine Advisory Panel on Feline Vaccines. *J Am Vet Med Assoc* 1998; 212: 227–241.

Greene CE, Scott FW. Feline panleukopenia. In: Greene CE, ed. *Infectious Diseases of the Dog and Cat*. 2nd ed. Philadelphia: WB Saunders; 1998:52–57.

Pollock RVH, Postorino NC. Feline panleukopenia and other enteric viral diseases. In: Sherding RG, ed. *The Cat: Diseases and Clinical Management*. New York: Churchill Livingstone; 1994:479–487.

Author: Fred W. Scott

Consulting Editor: Stephen C. Barr

Feline Rhinotracheitis Virus Infection

chapter 45

DEFINITION/OVERVIEW

- A viral infection of domestic and exotic cats characterized by sneezing, fever, rhinitis, conjunctivitis, and ulcerative keratitis.

ETIOLOGY/PATHOPHYSIOLOGY

- FHV-1—causes an acute cytolytic infection of respiratory or ocular epithelium after oral, intranasal, or conjunctival exposure.
- Affects:
  - Respiratory tract—rhinitis with sneezing and serous to purulent nasal discharge; tracheitis may occur; chronic sinusitis may be a sequela.
  - Eyes—conjunctivitis with serous or purulent ocular discharge, ulcerative keratitis, or panophthalmitis.
  - Reproductive tract—in utero infection due to infection of pregnant queens may result in severe herpetic infections in neonates.
  - Dermis—herpes dermatitis may occur near the nasal openings.
- Common worldwide—especially in multicat households or facilities.
- Perpetuated by latent carriers—harbor the virus in nerve ganglia, especially in the trigeminal ganglion.

SIGNALMENT/HISTORY

- Kittens most susceptible, but cats of all ages can be affected.
- Kittens born to carrier queens infected at about 5 weeks of age.
- Acute onset of paroxysmal sneezing.
- Blepharospasm and ocular discharge.
- Anorexia from high fever, general malaise, or inability to smell.
- Signs can be recurrent (carriers).
- Abortion.

CLINICAL FEATURES

- Fever—up to 106°F (41°C).
- Rhinitis—serous, mucopurulent, or purulent nasal discharge.

■ **Fig. 45-1** Serous to mucopurulent ocular and nasal discharge in a kitten infected with rhinotracheitis virus (courtesy of Dr. Ron Riis, Cornell University).

- Conjunctivitis—serous, mucopurulent, or purulent ocular discharge *(Fig. 45-1)*.
- Chronic rhinitis/sinusitis—chronic purulent nasal discharge.
- Keratitis—ulceration, descemetocele, or panophthalmitis *(Figs. 45-2 and 45-3)*.

DIFFERENTIAL DIAGNOSIS

- Feline calicivirus infection—less sneezing, conjunctivitis, or ulcerative keratitis; may cause ulcerative stomatitis, pneumonia.
- Feline chlamydiosis—more chronic conjunctivitis, which may be unilateral; pneumonitis; intracytoplasmic inclusions in conjunctival scrapings; responds to tetracyclines or chloramphenicol.

■ **Fig. 45-2** Chronic keratitis and corneal ulceration in a cat infected with rhinotracheitis virus (courtesy of Dr. Ron Riis, Cornell University).

■ **Fig. 45-3** Corneal ulceration as shown by uptake of fluorescene stain on a cornea of a cat infected with rhinotracheitis virus (courtesy of Dr. Ron Riis, Cornell University).

- Bacterial infection (*Bordetella*, *Haemophilus*, or *Pasteurella* spp.)—less nasal and ocular involvement.
- Bacterial infections—often respond to antibiotics.

DIAGNOSTICS

- CBC—transient leukopenia followed by leukocytosis may occur.
- Skull radiologic examination—shows no lesions during acute disease.
- Open mouth and skyline radiographic views of the skull—may reveal presence of chronic disease in the nasal cavity and frontal sinuses (increased fluid densities and erosion of nasal turbinates).
- Skull radiographs—cannot be reliably distinguished from neoplasia, inflammatory polyps, or chronic rhinotracheitis infection.
- IFA—nasal or conjunctival scrapings; viral detection.
- Viral isolation—pharynxgeal swab sample.
- Stained conjunctival smears—detect intranuclear inclusion bodies.

THERAPEUTICS

- Outpatient—keep patient indoors to prevent environmentally induced stress, which may lengthen the course of the disease.
- Inpatient—nutritional and fluid support to anorectic cats.
- Isolate within hospital—to prevent contagion (especially during acute phase).
- Fluids—intravenous or subcutaneous to correct and prevent dehydration and to keep nasal secretions thin.

- Diet—entice to eat by feeding foods of appealing tastes and smells.
- Enteral feeding for anorectic cats—esophageal or PEG tube.
- Nose—clean off nasal secretions from around external nares.
- Routine vaccination with an MLV or inactivated virus vaccine—prevents development of severe disease.
- MLV—does not prevent infection and local viral replication with virus shedding.
- Vaccinations—at 8 to 10 weeks of age, at 12 to 14 weeks of age, and with boosters every 3 years.
- Endemic multicat facilities or households—vaccinate kittens with a dose of an intranasal vaccine at 10 to 14 days of age; then parenterally at 6, 10, and 14 weeks of age; isolate the litter from *all* other cats at 3 to 5 weeks of age; then use kitten vaccination protocol to prevent early infections.
- Vaccinations—queens at least 2 weeks before breeding.

Drugs of Choice

- Broad-spectrum antibiotics—amoxicillin; for secondary bacterial infections.
- Antibiotics—can use amoxicillin in combination with enrofloxacin.
- Lysine (available at health food stores)—may have some virucidal effect.
- Ophthalmic antibiotics—for keratitis.
- Ophthalmic antivirals—vidarabine (Vira-A, Parke-Davis, Morris Plains, NJ); for herpetic ulcers; must be instilled every 2 hours for significant effect.
- Therapeutic vaccination—conjunctival vaccination with an intranasal FHV-1 vaccine may improve chronic keratitis.
- Human recombinant interferon (Roferon, Roche, Nutley, NJ):

  - Some efficacy in controlling the viral aspect of chronic infectious nasal discharge.
  - To help prevent the effects of early exposure to FHV-1 in kittens (*Table 45-1*).

Precautions/Interactions

- Do not use MLV in pregnant queens.
- Systemic corticosteroids may induce relapse in chronically infected cats.

TABLE 45-1. Drug Therapy for Cats Infected with Feline Rhinotracheitis Virus

Drug	Dose (mg/kg)	Route	Interval (Hours)	Duration (Weeks)
Amoxicillin	22	PO	12	2–4
Enrofloxacin	2.5–5	PO	12	1–2
Lysine	250 mg[a]	PO	24	4
Interferon (Roferon)—chronic	30 U[a]	PO	24	2[b]
Early exposure	2 U[a]	PO	24	5[c]

[a] Total dose.
[b] Follow by 1 week on, 1 week off.
[c] Begin dosing when 3 to 8 weeks of age.

- Ophthalmic corticosteroids may predispose to ulcerative keratitis.
- Nasal decongestant drops 0.25% oxymetazoline HCl; decrease nasal discharge; contraindicated because some cats object and some experience rebound rhinorrhea.
- Enrofloxacin has been associated with blindness in some cats at high doses; avoid use in kittens because it can produce arthropathies.
- Amoxicillin may cause anorexia, vomiting, and diarrhea in some cats.

 COMMENTS

- Essential to monitor appetite closely—hospitalize for tube feeding and fluid therapy if anorexia develops.
- Inform client—of the contagious nature of the disease.
- Discuss with client—proper vaccination protocols and early vaccination of cats in multicat facilities and households.
- Inform client—early weaning and isolation from all other cats, except littermates, may prevent infections.
- Warn owners—chronic rhinosinusitis with lifetime sneezing and nasal discharge, herpetic ulcerative keratitis, and permanent closure of the nasolacrimal duct with chronic ocular discharge are consequences of chronic infection.
- Warn owners—pregnant cats that develop disease may transmit FHV-1 to kittens in utero, resulting in abortion or neonatal disease.
- Prognosis—acute disease; usually 7 to 10 days before spontaneous remission, if secondary bacterial infections do not occur.
- Prognosis generally good—if fluid and nutritional therapy are adequate.

Abbreviations

CBC, complete blood count; FHV-1, feline herpesvirus type 1; IFA, immunofluorescense assay; MLV, modified live virus; PEG, percutaneous endoscopic gastrostomy.

Suggested Reading

Barr MC, Olsen CW, Scott FW. Feline viral diseases. In: Ettinger SJ, Feldman EC, eds. *Veterinary Internal Medicine*. Philadelphia: WB Saunders; 1995:409–439.

Ford RB. Role of infectious agents in respiratory disease. *Vet Clin North Am Small Anim Pract* 1993;23:17–35.

Ford RB, Levy JK. Infectious diseases of the respiratory tract. In: Sherding RG, ed. *The Cat: Diseases and Clinical Management*. New York: Churchill Livingstone; 1994:489–500.

Gaskell R, Dawson S. Feline respiratory disease. In: Greene CE, ed. *Infectious Diseases of the Dog and Cat*. Philadelphia: WB Saunders; 1998:97–106.

Author: Gary D. Norsworthy
Consulting Editor: Stephen C. Barr

chapter 46

Feline Syncytium-Forming Virus Infection

DEFINITION/OVERVIEW

- A viral infection of cats that causes little or no pathologic effect.

ETIOLOGY/PATHOPHYSIOLOGY

- Retrovirus (spumavirus).
- Worldwide distribution.
- Estimated prevalence is 10% to 70% or greater.
- Present in some nondomestic feline populations.
- Infection linked statistically with chronic progressive polyarthritis.
- Disease has not been reproduced by experimental infection.
- Transmission primarily by bites from other cats.
- Free-roaming cats are at greater risk of infection.
- Transmitted efficiently from infected queens to their offspring, probably in utero.

SIGNALMENT/HISTORY

- Prevalence of virus—low in kittens; increases with age.
- Males—more likely than females to be infected.
- Chronic progressive polyarthritis—occurs predominantly in males aged 1.5 to 5 years.

CLINICAL FEATURES

- Most affected cats remain healthy.
- Coinfections of FeSFV with FIV and FeLV—fairly common, probably because of shared transmission modes and risk factors.
- Statistical links with myeloproliferative disease and chronic progressive polyarthritis—may actually reflect coinfection with FIV.
- Chronic progressive polyarthritis—swollen joints; abnormal gait; lymphadenopathy.
- Has been implicated in the etiology of feline lower urinary tract disease.

DIFFERENTIAL DIAGNOSIS

- Signs of chronic progressive polyarthritis—test for FIV, FeLV, and septic joint disease.

DIAGNOSTICS

- CBC, UA, and serum biochemical profile—normal.
- Serologic testing for FeSFV antibodies and virus isolation—not readily available and not particularly useful because correlation between FeSFV infection and disease is so tenuous.
- Joint fluid cytologic examination (chronic progressive polyarthritis)—may reveal high numbers of neutrophils and large mononuclear cells.

THERAPEUTICS

- Treat chronic progressive polyarthritis.
- No vaccine available.

Drugs of Choice

- Prednisolone.
- Cyclophosphamide (*Table 46-1*).

Precautions/Interactions

- Immunosuppressive drugs—take care when using in patients coinfected with FIV or FeLV.
- Cyclophosphamide—may cause myelosuppression and/or sterile hemorrhagic cystitis.

TABLE 46-1. Drugs Used to Treat Chronic Progressive Polyarthritis Caused by Feline Syncytium-Forming Virus Infection				
Drug	Dose (mg/cat)	Route	Interval (Hours)	Duration (Weeks)[a]
Prednisolone	10–15	PO	24	4
Cyclophosphamide	7.5	PO	24[b]	4

[a] Treat for 4 weeks or until improvement of clinical signs then taper doses.

[b] Treat for 4 days each week.

COMMENTS

- Infection with FeSFV alone—adverse consequences unlikely.
- Chronic progressive polyarthritis—often difficult to control.
- Prognosis—poor for long-term recovery.

Abbreviations

CBC, complete blood count; FeLV, feline leukemia virus; FeSFV, feline syncytium-forming virus; FIV, feline immunodeficiency virus; UA, urine analysis.

Suggested Reading

Greene CE. Syncytium-forming virus infection. In: Greene CE, ed. *Infectious Diseases of the Dog and Cat*. Philadelphia: WB Saunders; 1998:106–107.

chapter 47

Fleas and Flea Control

DEFINITION/OVERVIEW

- Flea allergy dermatitis—hypersensitivity reaction to antigens in flea saliva, with or without evidence of fleas and flea dirt.
- Flea infestation—large number of fleas and a large amount of flea dirt, with or without a flea allergy dermatitis.

ETIOLOGY/PATHOPHYSIOLOGY

- FBH—caused by a low molecular weight hapten and two high molecular weight allergens that help initiate the allergic reaction.
- High molecular weight allergens—increase binding to dermal collagen; when bound, form a complete antigen necessary for eliciting FBH.
- Flea saliva—contains histamine-like compounds that irritate skin.
- Intermittent exposure favors FBH; continuous exposure is less likely to result in hypersensitivity.
- Both IgE and IgG antiflea antibodies have been noted.
- Hypersensitivity reactions—immediate and delayed have been noted.
- Late-phase IgE-mediated response—part of FBH reaction; occurs 3 to 6 hours after exposure.
- Cutaneous basophil hypersensitivity—part of FBH reaction; an infiltration of basophils into the dermis; mediated either by IgE or IgG; subsequent exposures cause the basophils to degranulate; manifests as immediate and delayed hypersensitivity.

SIGNALMENT/HISTORY

- Dogs and cats.
- FBH—any breed; most common in atopic breeds.
- FBH—rare <6 months of age; average age range, 3 to 6 years, but may be seen at any age.
- FBH—intermittent exposure to fleas increases the likelihood of development; commonly seen in conjunction with atopy.

Historical Findings

- Compulsive biting.
- Chewing (corncob nibbling).
- Licking—primarily in the back half of the body, but may include the antebrachial regions.
- Cats—scratching around the head and neck.
- Signs of fleas and flea dirt.

CLINICAL FEATURES

- Depends somewhat on the severity of the reaction and the degree of exposure to fleas—seasonal versus year-round).
- Finding fleas and flea dirt is beneficial, although not essential, for the diagnosis of FBH—sensitive animals require a low exposure and tend to overgroom, making identification of the parasites difficult.
- Dogs—lesions concentrated in a triangular area of the caudal-dorsal-lumbosacral region; caudal aspect of the thighs, lower abdomen, inguinal region, and cranial forearms usually involved; primary lesions are papules; secondary lesions (e.g., hyperpigmentation, lichenification, alopecia, and scaling) common in uncontrolled FBH; secondary folliculitis and furunculosis may be seen.
- Cats—several patterns are seen; most common is a miliary crusting dermatitis in a wedge-shaped pattern over the caudal dorsal lumbosacral region and often around the head and neck; other presentations are alopecia of the inguinal region with or without inflammation or eosinophilic plaques and other forms of eosinophilic granuloma complex.
- Exposure to other animals and previous flea treatment should be ascertained.

DIFFERENTIAL DIAGNOSIS

- Food allergy.
- Atopy.
- Sarcoptic mange.
- Cheyletiellosis.
- Primary keratinization defects.

DIAGNOSTICS

- Cats—hypereosinophilia may be detected.
- Skin scrapings—negative.
- Flea combings—fleas or flea dirt, but often nothing is found.
- RAST and ELISA—variable accuracy; both false positive and false negative results reported.
- Diagnosis—usually based on historical information and distribution of lesions.

- Fleas or flea dirt—is supportive but is often quite difficult to find, especially in cats.
- Identification of *Dipylidium caninum* segments—is supportive.
- Intradermal allergy testing with flea antigen—positive immediate reactions in 90% of flea-allergic animals; delayed reactions (24 to 48 hours) may sometimes be observed in allergic animals that show no immediate reaction.
- The most accurate test may be response to appropriate treatment.

Biopsy

- Superficial perivascular dermatitis.
- Eosinophilic intraepidermal microabscesses strongly suggest FBH.
- Eosinophils as a major cellular component of the dermis is supportive of FBH.
- Histopathologic evaluation cannot accurately differentiate FBH from atopy, food allergy, or other hypersensitivities.

 THERAPEUTICS

- Corticosteroids—anti-inflammatory dosages for symptomatic relief while the fleas are being controlled.
- Antihistamines—symptomatic relief.
- Fipronil (GABA antagonist)—monthly spot treatment for cats and dogs and spray treatment for dogs; activity against fleas and ticks; resistant to removal with water; excellent safety and efficacy profile.
- Imidacloprid—monthly spot treatment for cats and dogs; excellent safety and efficacy profile.
- Systemic treatments—limited benefit because they require a flea bite that has already initiated FBH; may help animals with flea infestation; primarily licensed for use in only dogs; lufenuron, a chitin inhibitor, available as an oral formulation for cats and dogs and as an injection for cats; permethrin available as a spot treatment and reputed to have some repellent activity; imidacloprid (flea adulticide) available as a spot treatment for cats and dogs.
- Sprays—usually contain pyrethrins and pyrethroids (synthetic pyrethrins) with an insect growth regulator or synergist; generally effective <48 to 72 hours; advantages are low toxicity and repellent activity; disadvantages are frequent applications and expense.
- Indoor treatment—fogs and premises sprays; usually contain organophosphates, pyrethrins, and/or insect growth regulators; apply according to manufacturer's directions; treat all areas of the house; can be applied by the owner; advantages are weak chemicals and generally inexpensive; disadvantage is labor intensity; premises sprays concentrate the chemicals in areas that most need treatment.
- Professional exterminators—advantages are less labor intensive, relatively few applications, sometimes guaranteed, disadvantages are strength of chemicals and cost; specific recommendations and guidelines must be followed.
- Inert substances—boric acid, diatomaceous earth, and silica aerogel; treat every 6 to 12 months; follow manufacturer's recommendations; very safe and effective if applied properly.

- Outdoor treatment—concentrated in shaded areas; sprays usually contain pyrethroids or organophosphates and an insect growth regulator; powders are usually organophosphates; product containing nematodes (*Steinerma carpocapsae*) is very safe and chemical-free.

Precautions

- Insecticidal sprays and dips—should not be used on dogs and cats ≤3 months of age, unless otherwise specified on the label.
- Pyrethrin/pyrethroid-type flea products—adverse reactions include depression, hypersalivation, muscle tremors, vomiting, ataxia, dyspnea, and anorexia.
- Organophosphates—adverse reactions include hypersalivation, lacrimation, urination, defecation, vomiting, diarrhea, miosis, fever, muscle tremors, seizures, coma, and death.
- All pesticides—must be applied according to label directions.
- Toxicity—if any signs are noted, the animal should be bathed thoroughly to remove any remaining chemicals and treated appropriately.
- Rodents and fish—are very sensitive to pyrethrins.

Possible Interactions

- Organophosphate treatments—do not use more than one form at a time.
- Topical organophosphates—avoid in cats, very young animals (<3 months of age), and sick or debilitated animals.
- Straight permethrin sprays or spot-ons—do not use in cats.
- Cythioate—contraindicated in heartworm-positive dogs and greyhounds.
- Piperonyl butoxide—do not use in concentrations >1% in cats.

Alternative Drugs

- Powders—usually contain organophosphates or carbamates; advantage is high residual effectiveness; disadvantages are dry skin and toxicity; organophosphates and carbamates should be avoided in cats.
- Dips, sprays, powders, and foams—dips usually contain organophosphates and synthetic pyrethrins and should not be used more than once per week; follow manufacturer's instructions for safest and best results; after repeated use, these agents can be drying or irritating; newer, safer spot treatments have essentially replaced these products.

 COMMENTS

- Inform owners—there is no cure for FBH.
- Advise owners—flea-allergic animals often become more sensitive to flea bites as they age.
- Inform owners—controlling exposure to fleas is currently the only means of therapy; hyposensitization has not worked satisfactorily.
- Pruritus—a decrease means the FBH is being controlled.

- Fleas and flea dirt—absence is not always a reliable indicator of successful treatment in very sensitive animals.
- Year-round warm climates—year-round flea control.
- Seasonally warm climates—begin flea control in May or June.
- Allergy—approximately 80% of atopic dogs are also allergic to flea bites.
- Organophosphates—use with utmost caution in old animals; not recommended for use in very young animals (<3 months of age).
- In areas of moderate to severe flea infestation—humans can be bitten by fleas; usually papular lesions are located on the wrists and ankles.
- Corticosteroids and organophosphates—do not use in pregnant bitches and queens.
- Carefully follow the label directions for each individual product—to determine its safety.

Abbreviations

ELISA, enzyme-linked immunosorbent assay; FBH, flea bite hypersensitivity; GABA, gamma-aminobutyric acid; Ig, immunoglobulin; RAST, radioallergosorbent test.

Suggested Reading

Bevier-Tournay DE. Fleas and flea control. In: Kirk RW, Bonagura JD, eds. *Current Veterinary Therapy X*. Philadelphia: WB Saunders; 1989:586–591.
Griffin CE, Kwochka KW, MacDonald JM. *Current Veterinary Dermatology*. St. Louis: Mosby, 1993.

Author: Karen A. Kuhl and Jean S. Greek
Consulting Editor: Karen Helton Rhodes

Giardiasis

DEFINITION/OVERVIEW

- Enteric protozoan infection that can cause small bowel diarrhea in dogs and cats, but usually asymptomatic.

ETIOLOGY/PATHOPHYSIOLOGY

- Several species—*Giardia lamblia* (humans), *G. canis* (dogs), and *G. felis* (cats), but cross-infection occurs.
- Zoonosis—*G. canis* is not considered zoonotic, but *G. lamblia* cysts that infect humans have been identified in dogs (although rarely) and are considered zoonotic.
- Transmission—ingestion of cysts, which are usually water-borne, but also auto-transmission (cysts survive well adhered to the perianal region and in a pet's contaminated environment) common.
- Flagellated tachyzoites released (from cysts)—in GI tract attach to small intestinal enterocytes.
- Causes malabsorption syndrome—sugars, vitamin B_{12}, folate, triglycerides.
- Specific histologic changes—not identified, but blunting of intestinal villi can ensue.
- Cysts—found in feces, but also trophozoites (especially in animals with diarrhea).
- Cysts—survive for months in moist cool environment outside host.
- Trophozoites—do not survive outside host and are not infective.
- PPP = 5 to 12 days (dogs) and 5 to 16 days (cats).

SIGNALMENT/HISTORY

- Clinical signs—mainly seen in young dogs and cats.
- Older animals—rarely show signs unless there is an underlying problem (overcrowding stress, diet, concurrent GI tract disease).
- Prevalence.
  - Dogs—varies greatly from 10% in client-owned single-single household pets, to 100% in kennels.
  - Cats—usually between 1% and 10%.

CLINICAL FEATURES

- Usually excrete cysts with no signs.
- Diarrhea often small bowel (young animals); rancid odor, soft, frothy, pale, and steatorrheic.
- May show intermittent or chronic diarrhea with occasional vomiting.

DIFFERENTIAL DIAGNOSIS

- Anything that causes acute small bowel diarrhea, including dietary indiscretion; IBD; neoplasia (especially GI tract lymphoma); drugs (antibiotics); toxins (lead); parasites (cryptosporidiosis, trichomoniasis, whipworms); infectious agents (parvovirus, FIP, salmonellosis, rickettsia, GI bacterial overgrowth, clostridia, histoplasmosis, leishmaniasis, other rare infections—pythiosis); systemic organ dysfunction (renal, hepatic, pancreatic, cardiac); metabolic (hypoadrenocorticism, hyperthyroidism of cats).

DIAGNOSTICS

- Finding cysts (*Fig. 48-1*) in an animal with diarrhea—does not always mean the diarrhea is caused by *Giardia*.
- Direct fecal smear—to identify trophozoites (reasonably sensitive in cats with diarrhea) or cysts; a drop of feces mixed with a drop of Lugol's iodine kills the trophozoites and stains them brown so morphology can be examined (under 40× magnification).
- Differentiate *Giardia* trophozoites (*Fig. 48-2*) from *Tritrichomonas fetus* (only other organism it can be confused with in cats)—*T. fetus* has a smoother rolling motion, no concave ventral disc, a single nucleus, an undulating membrane.
- ZSCT—three tests performed on sequential fecal samples is nearly 100% sensitive.
- Sucrose concentration techniques—distort cysts.
- Commercial ZSCT (if do not include centrifugation)—lower specificity in comparison to techniques that include concentration by centrifugation.
- Commercial ELISA kits (ProSpecT/Giardia ELISA kit [Alexon Inc., Mountain View, CA])—have a false negative rate of 31.6% and high specificity (95.7%) compared to ZSCT; can use frozen or formaldehyde-fixed feces.
- Commercial direct immunofluorescence test (Merifluor Cryptosporidium/Giardia Direct Immunofluorescence Assay [Meridian Diagnostics, Cincinnati, OH])—may be more sensitive and specific for detecting low cyst numbers, and for use in stored feces compared to the ZSCT.

Diagnostic Feature

- **ZSCT is still considered the gold standard of *Giardia* diagnosis, but ELISA and immunofluorescence assays are gaining in popularity and efficacy.**

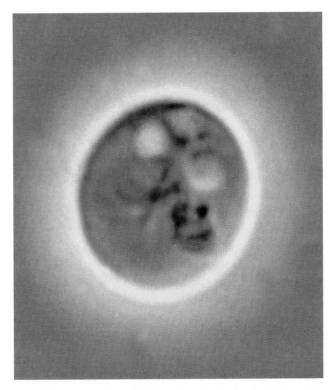

■ **Fig. 48-1** *Giardia* cyst characterized by two circular structures within.

■ **Fig. 48-2** *Giardia* trophozoites characterized by the comical "eyes," mouth, and long flagella.

- Duodenal aspiration—rarely identifies *Giardia* over and above ZSCT.
- Peroral nylon string test (Entero-test [HDC Corp., San Jose, CA])—not safe or effective in diagnosing *Giardia* infection in dogs.

 ## THERAPEUTICS

- If diarrhea is severe, treat supportively.
- Many recent studies suggest that when controlling diarrhea in animals with giardiasis, antigiardiacidal drug treatment must be coupled with measures to clean cysts from the animal's environment and coat.
- QUAT (Roccal [Winthrop Labs, New York, NY]; Totil [Calgon Corp., St. Louis, MO])—inactivate cysts within 1 minute of contact at room temperature; must clean up organic material first; can use on coat of animals as a rinse (allowing contact for 1 minute, then thoroughly rinse off) after washing the coat with a pet shampoo first to remove organic matter, then dry coat well (cysts very susceptible to drying).

Vaccination

- *Giardia* vaccine (GiardiaVax for cats and dogs [Fort Dodge Animal Health, Fort Dodge, IA])—made of chemically inactivated trophozoites.
- Pups and kittens (7-week-old and naïve to *Giardia* exposure)—receiving one vaccine and a booster 3 weeks later, were immune to a *Giardia* challenge 6 and 12 months later.
- Older dogs—vaccination reduced the duration of cyst shedding and the number of cysts shed.
- The vaccine has been used as an immunotherapeutic agent in dogs; 13 dogs that failed to be cured of giardiasis using chemotherapeutic measures showed clinical cures and cessation of fecal cyst shedding between 3 to 10 weeks postvaccination (some required up to 3 vaccines); suggests that vaccine might have a place in the treatment of some chronically infected dogs in which chemotherapy and hygiene control methods have failed.
- Vaccination—in some studies, vaccination failed to prevent reinfection.
- Vaccination—anecdotal reports of asymptomatic infected dogs developing clinical symptoms of diarrhea after receiving the vaccine.
- Vaccination for cats—vaccinated 4, 6, and 10 weeks after experimentally infected failed to clear the infection, suggesting that the vaccine may not be efficacious in those cats already infected.
- Vaccine—little utility as a general vaccine for the control of giardiasis in the general population of dogs because most are exposed to the organism before vaccination.

Drugs of Choice

- No drug is registered for use against *Giardia* in North America.
- Fenbendazole and combination of febantel-praziquantel-pyrantel (Drontal Plus [Bayer Co., Shawnee Mission, KS]) are preferred because of the lack of side-effects and high efficacy.

- Fenbendazole (Panacur [Hoechst-Roussel Agri-Vet Co., Somerville, NJ])—over 90% efficacy; can be used in pregnant animals, unlike other benzimadazoles.
- Febantel-praziquantel-pyrantel (Drontal Plus [Bayer Co., Shawnee Mission, KS])—contains similar efficacy to fenbendazole in dogs; active ingredient is febantel (which is converted to fenbendazole and oxfendazole), which might also have a synergistic action with praziquantel.
- Oxfendazole (Dolthene [Merial Laboratories, Lyon, France])—in Europe, has been shown very effective when combined with control methods.
- Oxfendazole suspension—available in United States (Synanthic Bovine Dewormer Suspension 9.06% [Fort Dodge, Fort Dodge, IA]); not registered for use in dogs.
- Albendazole (Valbazen Cattle Dewormer [Pfizer Animal Health, Morris Plains, NJ]). Potentially toxic; may cause myelosuppression in both dogs and cats.
- Metronidazole (Flagyl, Pfizer, Exton, PA)—67% efficacious in dogs, but also has efficacy against other GI tract flora and possible immunologic effects on cell populations in the bowel.
- Metronidazole benzoate (only available for formulation in the United States)—recently found to be 100% efficacious in cats *(Table 48-1)*.
- Tinidazole, ipronidazole, quinacrine, and furazolidone—some have good efficacy but high side effects.

Precautions/Interactions

- Albendazole, but not fenbendazole, is suspected of being teratogenic and, therefore, should not be given to pregnant animals.
- At higher doses, albendazole can cause myelosuppression in both dogs and cats.
- Metronidazole at higher doses (>30 mg/kg) can produce neurologic signs, including anorexia and vomiting, with deterioration to pronounced generalized ataxia and vertical positional nystagmus.

TABLE 48-1. Drug Therapy for Giardiasis in Small Animals					
Drug	Species	Dose (mg/kg)	Route	Interval (Hours)	Duration (Days)
Fenbendazole (Panacur)	D	50	PO	24	3
	C	50	PO	24	5[a]
Febantel-praziquantel-pyrantel (Drontal Plus)	D	[b]	PO	24	3
Metronidazole (Flagyl)	D	20	PO	12	5
Metronidazole benzoate	C	25	PO	12	7[c]
Oxfendazole (Dolthene)	D	11.3	PO	24	3
Albendazole[d] (Valbazen)	D	25	PO	12	2
	C	25	PO	12	5

[a] Efficacy, 50%.
[b] Dose of each drug—febantel (26.8 to 35.2 mg/kg), praziquantel (5.4 to 7 mg/kg) and pyrantel (26.8 to 35.2 mg/kg).
[c] Efficacy, 100%.
[d] May cause myelosuppression.
C, cats; D, dogs.

COMMENTS

- Apparent failure of drugs to clear infections is probably because autoinfection can occur immediately after drugs stopped, and, with a PPP of 5 days, cyst excretion can occur in dogs within 5 days of stopping drugs.
- Control of diarrhea and chronic giardiasis is more likely achieved when drugs are used in association with hygiene methods, particularly in kennel situations.

Abbreviations

CBC, complete blood count; ELISA, enzyme-linked immunosorbent assay; FIP, feline infectious peritonitis; GI, gastrointestinal; IBD, inflammatory bowel disease; PPP, prepatent period; QUAT, quaternary ammonium-containing disinfectants; ZSCT, zinc sulfate concentration technique.

Suggested Reading

Barr SC, Bowman DD, Frongillo MF, et al. Efficacy of a drug combination of praziquantel, pyrantel pamoate, and febantel against giardiasis in dogs. *Am J Vet Res* 1998;59:1134–1136.

Keith CL, Radecki SV, Lappin MR. Evaluation of fenbendazole for treatment of *Giardia* infection in cats concurrently infected with *Cryptosporidium parvum. Am J Vet Res* 2003;64:1027–1029.

Payne PA, Ridley RK, Dryden MW. Efficacy of a combination febantel-praziquantel pyrantel product, with or without vaccination with a commercial *Giardia* vaccine, for treatment of dogs with naturally occurring giardiasis. *J Am Vet Med Assoc* 2002;220:330–333.

Scorza AV, Lappin MR. Metronidazole for the treatment of feline giardiasis. *J Feline Med Surg* 2004; 6:157–160.

Stein JE, Radecki SV, Lappin MR. Efficacy of *Giardia* vaccination in the treatment of giardiasis in cats. *J Am Vet Med Assoc* 2003;222:1549–1551.

Author: Stephen C. Barr
Consulting Editor: Stephen C. Barr

chapter 49

Haemobartonellosis (Erythrocytic Mycoplasmal Infections)

DEFINITION/OVERVIEW

- RBC destruction and anemia caused by parasite attachment to the external surface of RBCs and immune response by the host.

ETIOLOGY/PATHOPHYSIOLOGY

- *Haemobartonella felis* (cats) and *Haemobartonella canis* (dogs)—classified as rickettsial bacteria.
- Recently recognized to be mycoplasmal bacteria based on genetic determinations.
- Proposed new names:
  - *Mycoplasma haemofelis* for a large form of *H. felis*.
  - *Mycoplasma haemominutum* for the small form of *H. felis*.
  - *Mycoplasma haemocanis* for *H. canis* (dogs).
- The large species of mycoplasmal organisms infecting cats—generally causes more severe disease than small species.
- Cats—anemia more severe if FeLV infected.
- Dogs—likelihood of severe anemia greatly increased if splenectomized or with pathologic changes in the spleen.

SIGNALMENT/HISTORY

- Worldwide distribtution.
- Most common in adult (dogs and cats).
- More common in males (cats).
- No sex prevalence in dogs.

CLINICAL FEATURES

Cats

- Variable disease severity—ranges from inapparent infection to marked depression and death.
- Intermittent fever (50% of the time) during the acute phase.

■ **Fig. 49-1** Severe icterus in a cat infected with *Mycoplasma haemofelis*.

- Depression.
- Weakness.
- Anorexia
- Pale mucous membranes.
- Splenomegaly.
- Icterus—rare *(Fig. 49-1)*.

Dogs

- Mild or inapparent signs—pale mucous membranes and listlessness.
- In splenectomized dogs—signs more like cats.

 DIFFERENTIAL DIAGNOSIS

- Other causes of hemolytic anemia include IMHA, babesiosis (not in cats in the United States), cytauxzoonosis (cats only), Heinz body hemolytic anemia, microangiopathic hemolytic anemia, pyruvate kinase deficiency, phosphofructokinase deficiency (dogs only).
- Differentiated from IMHA—only by recognition of parasites in blood (stained blood film or PCR-based assays); both disorders may have a positive Coombs' test result.
- *Babesia* and *Cytauxzoon* spp.—differ in morphology from these mycoplasmal organisms.
- New Methylene Blue stain—used to identify Heinz bodies.
- Enzyme assays or specialized DNA tests—used to diagnose pyruvate kinase and phosphofructokinase deficiencies.

DIAGNOSTICS

- CBC:
  - Anemia—usually with reticulocytosis if regenerative.
  - Anemia—may appear poorly regenerative if a precipitous decrease in PCV has occurred early in the disease or if there are other concurrent disorders (e.g., FeLV or FIV infections in cats).
  - Autoagglutination—may be seen in feline blood samples after they cool to below body temperature.
  - Variable total and differential leukocyte counts of little diagnostic assistance.
  - Hemoglobinemia—rarely observed, so no hemoglobinuria reported.
- Biochemical profile:
  - Hyperbilirubinemia—seen in some cases but seldom severe.
  - Substantial bilirubinuria—seen in some dogs.
  - Abnormalities related to anemic hypoxia—may be shown by clinical chemistry profiles, but profile can be normal.
  - Hypoglycemia—possible in moribund cats (not specific to this disease).
  - Plasma protein concentrations—usually normal but may be increased.
- Routine blood stains (e.g., Wright's–Giemsa)—to identify organisms in blood films; examine before treatment is begun because treatment increases false negative results.
- Reticulocyte—stains cannot be used because punctate reticulocytes in cats appear similar to the parasites.
- Organisms must be differentiated from precipitated stain—refractile drying or fixation artifacts, poorly staining Howell-Jolly bodies, and basophilic stippling can confuse diagnosis.
- Feline organisms—small blue-staining cocci, rings, or rods on RBCs (*Figs. 49-2 and 49-3*).
- Canine organisms—commonly form chains of organisms that appear as filamentous structures on the surface of RBCs (*Fig. 49-4*).
- Parasitemia—cyclic, and thus organisms not always identifiable in blood (especially in cats).
- PCR-based assays—can detect parasites in blood below the number required to make a diagnosis from a stained blood film.
- Direct Coombs' test—may be positive.

 THERAPEUTICS

- Without therapy—mortality with the larger form may reach 30% in cats.
- Outpatient treatment—unless severely anemic or moribund.
- Blood transfusions—required when the anemia is considered life-threatening.
- IV administration of glucose-containing fluid—recommended in moribund animals.

■ **Fig. 49-2** Small blue-staining cocci with some ring forms typical of *Mycoplasma haemominutum* in a cat (courtesy Dr. Joanne Messick, Cornell University).

Drugs of Choice

- Doxycycline, tetracycline, or oxytetracycline—drugs of choice.
- Enrofloxacin—efficacious alternative for cats that do not tolerate tetracycline antibiotics.
- Prednisolone—may be given to severely anemic animals (to treat immune-mediated destruction of RBCs); gradually decrease dosage as the PCV increases (*Table 49-1*).

■ **Fig. 49-3** Small blue-staining cocci, sometimes multiple within in one red blood cell, typical of *Mycoplasma haemofelis* in a blood sample from a cat (courtesy Dr. Joanne Messick, Cornell University).

■ **Fig. 49-4** Blue-staining cocci often in chains on the surface of dog red blood cells with *Mycoplasma haemocanis* (courtesy Dr. Joanne Messick, Cornell University).

Precautions/Interactions

- Tetracycline antibiotics—may produce fever or evidence of GI disease in cats; use a lower dosage or a different drug, or discontinue drug therapy altogether.
- Doxycycline—may cause esophagitis and stricture in cats; give with food.
- Enrofloxacin—has been associated with blindness in cats; may cause arthropathy in young cats.
- Chloramphenicol—may be used in dogs; can cause dose-dependent erythroid hypoplasia in cats.

TABLE 49-1. Drug Therapy for Haemobartonellosis (Erythrocytic Mycoplasmal Infections) in Dogs and Cats

Drug	Dose (mg/kg)	Route	Interval (Hours)	Duration (Weeks)
Doxycycline	5	PO, SC	12	3
Tetracycline	22	PO	8	3
Oxytetracycline	22	PO	8	3
Enrofloxacin	5–10	PO, IM	12	1–2
Prednisolone	1–2	PO	12	2[a]

[a] Gradually decrease dose as anemia improves; taper in 50% decrements every 2 weeks.

COMMENTS

- Examine animal after 1 week of treatment—to confirm that PCV has risen.
- Alert owner—cats may remain carriers even after completion of treatment but seldom relapse with disease once PCV returns to normal.
- Prognosis usually excellent in cats—if treated early in disease.

Abbreviations

CBC, complete blood count; DNA, deoxyribonucleic acid; IMHA, immune-mediated hemolytic anemia; FeLV, feline leukemia virus; FIV, feline immunodeficiency virus; GI, gastrointestinal; PCR, polymerase chain reaction; PCV, packed cell volume; RBC, red blood cell.

Suggested Reading

Harvey JW. Haemobartonellosis. In: Greene CE, ed. *Infectious Diseases of the Dog and Cat.* 2nd ed. Philadelphia: WB Saunders; 1998:166–171.

Harvey JW. *Haemobartonella* infection in cats. *Proc Am Assoc Feline Pract* 2001;18–22.

Jensen WA, Lappin MR, Kamkar S, et al. Use of a polymerase chain reaction assay to detect and differentiate two strains of *Haemobartonella felis* in naturally infected cats. *Am J Vet Res* 2001; 62:604–608.

Author: John W. Harvey
Consulting Editor: Stephen C. Barr

chapter 50

Heartworm Disease: Cats

DEFINITION/OVERVIEW

- Parasitic disease of cats affecting the heart and lungs.

ETIOLOGY/PATHOPHYSIOLOGY

- *Dirofilaria immitis*—adults infect pulmonary arteries.
- Unlike in dogs—worms are physically smaller, have a shorter life span (~2 years); lower worm burden (1 to 3 worms/cat).
- Microfilaria—uncommon (<20%).
- Prevalence—one-tenth that of unprotected dogs.

SIGNALMENT/HISTORY

- No age or breed predisposition.
- Males—more commonly infected.
- Historically—cats present with coughing, dyspnea, and vomiting.
- Sudden death—occurs due to acute respiratory failure from PTE.
- Vomiting and respiratory signs—predominate in chronic disease.

CLINICAL FEATURES

- Usually normal
- Increased bronchovesicular sounds with murmur or gallop rhythm—should increase suspicion of primary cardiac disease.

DIFFERENTIAL DIAGNOSIS

- Asthma—different radiographic signs; heartworm antibody/antigen negative.
- Cardiomyopathy—differentiate on radiography and cardiac ultrasound.
- Chylothorax—heartworm disease can be associated.
- *Aelurostrongylus abstrusus* infection—larvae in feces.

- *Paragonimus kellicotti* infection—eggs in feces.
- Other causes of chronic vomiting—IBD, GI tract lymphoma, fur balls, food allergy, diaphragmatic hernia.

 DIAGNOSTICS

- CBC:
  - Mild nonregenerative anemia.
  - Eosinophilia inconsistent.
  - Basophilia should increase suspicion.
- Hyperglobulinemia—occasionally.
- Microfilaria (Modified Knotts, filter test)—low sensitivity, high specificity.
- Heartworm antigen tests (ELISA or immunochromatographic tests)—detect circulating adult HWAg; more specific than antibody tests; a positive antigen test result is strong evidence of heartworm disease but low worm burdens (fewer than five worms) and single-sex infections commonly result in false-negative results; negative result does not rule out heartworm disease; more than 40% of cats with adult infection are antigen-negative; risk of false-positive results increases with low prevalence (most of United States), so positive results in low-prevalence areas should be confirmed by other diagnostic criteria or second test.
- Heartworm antibody tests (ELISA or immunochromatographic tests)—detect circulating antibodies to immature and adult heartworms; the most sensitive tests for feline heartworm disease; a positive result documents exposure but does not always indicate mature or current infection (positive predictive value, 25%); the more intense the antibody response (higher titer or ABU level), the more likely it is that it is an adult infection; can detect male-only and immature infections; strength of test is to rule out infection; antibody test is currently the most logical screening test for asymptomatic cats.
- Radiographic/angiographic examination—will show enlarged pulmonary artery (if >1.6 times the width of the 9th rib, highly suggestive of infection); blunted, tortuous pulmonary arteries; patchy perivascular pulmonary infiltrates *(Fig. 50-1)*; pulmonary arterial truncation, obstruction and linear filling defects often best viewed with nonselective angiography *(Fig. 50-2)*.
- Echocardiographic examination—more sensitive in cats than dogs; will show dilated main pulmonary artery, see worms in heart or main pulmonary artery often as "double-lined echodensity" (most commonly, the right pulmonary artery); expertise and high index of suspicion increases sensitivity of test.

 THERAPEUTICS

- Administration of adulticide is controversial in cats—none are approved.
- Severe and fatal PTE—frequently occurs after treatment.

■ **Fig. 50-1** Thoracic radiograph of a cat with heartworm disease showing enlarged blunted, tortuous pulmonary arteries, and patchy perivascular pulmonary infiltrates.

- Spontaneous "cure"—probably much more common in cats than dogs (shorter heartworm life span).
- Stabilize symptomatic cases—treat clinical signs.

Drugs of Choice

- Initial stabilization—oxygen, theophylline (25 mg/kg, PO, q24h in evening; sustained release formulation).
- Prednisolone (1 to 2 mg/kg, PO, q24h for 10 to 14 days; then reduce gradually but use periodically if respiratory signs reoccur)—reduces severity of PTE.

■ **Fig. 50-2** Thoracic radiograph during nonselective angiography of a cat with severe heartworm disease showing dilated and truncated pulmonary arteries and mild thromboembolism.

Precautions/Interactions

- Thiacetarsamide (Caparsolate) and melarsomine (Immiticide)—not indicated in cats.
- If an adulticide is used—PTE likely to occur 5 to 10 days after administration; mortality rate around 30%.
- Aspirin therapy—no documented benefit.

 COMMENTS

- Serial evaluation of clinical response, thoracic radiographs, and heartworm antigen and antibody tests are most informative.
- With judicious use of prednisone—possible to control the symptoms while waiting for the heartworms to die naturally.
- Prevention—formulations currently approved for cats include:
  - Ivermectin (Heartgard for Cats [Merial, Iselin, NJ])—24 µg/kg, PO, every 30 days.
  - Selamectin (Revolution for Cats [Pfizer, Exton, PA])—6 to 12 mg/kg topically, every 30 days.
  - Milbemycin oxime (Interceptor [Novartis, Greensboro, NC])—2 mg/kg, PO, every 30 days.

Abbreviations

ABU, antibody unit; CBC, complete blood count; ELISA, enzyme-linked immunosorbent assay; GI, gastrointestinal; HWAg, heartworm antigen; IBD, inflammatory bowel disease; PTE, pulmonary thromboembolism.

Suggested Reading

Atkins CE, Ryan WG. Diagnosis and prevention of heartworm disease in cats. In: Bonagura JD, ed. *Kirk's Current Veterinary Therapy XIII: Small Animal Practice*. Philadelphia: WB Saunders; 2000; 782–787.

Dillon R. Feline heartworm disease. In: Tilley LP, Goodwin J-K, eds. *Manual of Canine and Feline Cardiology*. 3rd ed. Philadelphia: WB Saunders; 2001:235.

Miller MW. Feline dirofilariasis. *Clin Tech Small Anim Pract* 1998;13:99–108.

Author: Matthew W. Miller
Consulting Editor: Stephen C. Barr

chapter 51

Heartworm Disease: Dogs

DEFINITION/OVERVIEW

- Parasitic infection of the pulmonary arteries of dogs causing respiratory (pulmonary hypertension, embolization, allergic pneumonitis, eosinophilic granulomas), cardiac (myocardial hypertrophy and, in some animals, congestive heart failure due to high right ventricle afterload), and renal (immune complex glomerulonephropathy) disease.

ETIOLOGY/PATHOPHYSIOLOGY

- *Dirofilaria immitis*—adults (female worms up to 30 cm long) live in the pulmonary arteries of dogs, leading to endothelial damage and myointimal proliferation.
- Pulmonary artery damage—results in lobar arterial enlargement, tortuosity, and obstruction, causing pulmonary hypertension and thrombosis.
- Severity of disease—directly related to the number of worms, duration of infection, and host response.
- Female adult worms—release L1 (microfilaria) into circulation (can live there for 2 years).
- L1 in circulation—may infect mosquitoes feeding; develop to L3 in mosquito and injected back into dog to migrate to heart.
- PPP = 6 to 7 months.
- Prevalence—varies with geographic location, but widespread throughout North America, even into Alaska.
- Prevalence—virtually 100% in unprotected dogs living in highly endemic regions.
- Prevalence—common along the Atlantic and Gulf coasts and Ohio and Mississippi River basins.
- Numerous pockets of infection in otherwise low-prevalence regions—usually where mosquito vector is ubiquitous.

SIGNALMENT/HISTORY

- Medium to large-breed dogs that spend a lot of time outdoors—most susceptible.
- Endemic regions—all unprotected dogs at risk.

- Most affected animals—between 3 and 8 years old.
- Historically—most infected dogs are asymptomatic or exhibit minimal signs such as occasional coughing (Class I).

 CLINICAL FEATURES

- Class I—no abnormalities in an infected dog.
- Class II—cough, exercise intolerance, weight loss, pulmonary changes on thoracic radiography, PCV between 20 and 25.
- Class III—cachexia, exercise intolerance, syncope, tachycardia, ascites (right-sided heart failure), hepatomegaly, pulmonary and cardiac changes on thoracic radiography, PCV <20.
- Hemoptysis—occasionally occurs; indicates severe pulmonary thromboembolic complications.
- Vena cava syndrome—occurs when vena cava is obstructed by adult worms; hemoglobinuria due to acute hemolytic crisis (shock).

DIFFERENTIAL DIAGNOSIS

- Other causes of pulmonary hypertension and thrombosis—for example, hyperadrenocorticism.
- Other causes of pulmonary disease—allergic lung disease, COPD, neoplasia, parasitic lung disease, foreign body, pneumonia; thoracic radiologic examination and heartworm antigen tests should differentiate from heartworm disease.
- Other causes of ascites—dilated cardiomyopathy and other causes of heart failure, hypoproteinemia, hepatic disease, caudal caval or portal vein thromboembolism, neoplasia, pericardial effusion.

 DIAGNOSTICS

- CBC:
  - Anemia—mild in Class II, severe in Class III.
  - Eosinophilia and basophilia (variable)—together, are a sensitive indicator of heartworm disease.
  - Leukocytosis and thrombocytopenia—associated with thromboembolism.
- Serum biochemical profile and urinalysis:
  - Hyperglobulinemia—inconsistent finding.
  - Proteinuria—common in animals with severe and chronic infection; may be caused by immune-complex glomerulonephritis or amyloidosis.
  - Hemoglobinuria—acute hemolytic crisis during vena cava syndrome.
- Heartworm antigen tests—highly specific, sensitive serologic tests that identify adult female *D. immitis* antigen; widely available; standard tests for screening.

- Antigen tests—take 7 months after infection to develop a positive status; do not use in pups under 7 months, and test 7 months after the end of the previous transmission season.
- Annual testing—unnecessary if dog receiving monthly macrolide chemoprophylaxis appropriately (2- to 3-year testing interval sufficient).
- Microfilaria identification tests—include the modified Knott's test, filter tests, and direct smear *(Fig. 51-1)*; 20% to 25% of infected dogs will be missed if rely on these tests alone.
- Thoracic radiologic examination—should always perform not only as a diagnostic aid but also to predict class of infection and extent of thromboembolism.
- Thoracic radiologic examination—allows comparison between radiographs taken during treatment and recovery *(Figs. 51-2 and 51-3)*.
- Thoracic radiographic signs:
  - Main pulmonary artery segment—enlargement.
  - Lobar arterial enlargement and tortuosity—vary from absent (Class I) to severe (Class III).
  - Parenchymal lung infiltrates of variable severity (surround lobar arteries)—may extend into most or all of one or multiple lung lobes when thromboembolism occurs.
  - Diffuse, symmetrical, alveolar, and interstitial infiltrates—occasionally occur because of an allergic reaction to microfilaria.
- Echocardiography—often unremarkable and therefore not a cost-effective test.
- Echocardiogram—may show right ventricular dilation and wall hypertrophy; parallel linear echodensities produced by heartworms may be detected in the RV, RA, and PA (inconsistent finding in dogs).

■ **Fig. 51-1** Although rarely found because of the advent of monthly heartworm preventive agents, a blood smear may reveal *D. immitis* microfilaria in a dog with heartworm disease (wet preparation, 400×).

■ **Fig. 51-2** Lateral thoracic radiograph of a dog with severe heartworm disease showing dilated pulmonary arteries, pulmonary thromboembolism, and right ventricular enlargement.

■ **Fig. 51-3** Dorsoventral thoracic radiograph of a dog with severe heartworm disease showing right ventricular enlargement (*top arrow*) and enlarged truncated right caudal pulmonary artery (*lower arrow*).

- Angiography—of little practical clinical importance.
- ECG—usually normal; may reflect RV hypertrophy in dogs with severe (Class III) infection; heart rhythm disturbances rarely seen but may include atrial fibrillation (most common) in severe infection.

 ## THERAPEUTICS

- Hospitalization—some patients may need hospitalization during adulticide administration.
- Hospitalization—recommended for dogs experiencing thromboembolic complications.
- Severe restriction of activity—required for 4 to 6 weeks after adulticide administration.
- Cage confinement—recommended for 3 to 4 weeks after adulticide administration for severe (Class III) disease.
- Cage confinement for 7 days—recommended for dogs experiencing pulmonary thromboembolic complications.
- Class III disease—treat CHF until stable before administering adulticide; use diuretics, cage rest, and sodium restriction.
- Stabilize pulmonary failure—with antithrombotic agents (e.g., aspirin or heparin) and anti-inflammatory doses of corticosteroid; monitor using clinical and radiographic parameters.
- Dogs with vena cava syndrome—surgical removal of adult worms from right heart and PA via jugular vein by use of fluoroscopy and a long, flexible alligator forceps; highly effective for treating high worm burden when employed by an experienced operator.
- Determine justification of adulticide treatment in older dogs—outcome may be worse than not treating because benefit of treatment may not be realized in dog's lifetime.

Drugs of Choice

Treatment of Infected Dogs

- Melarsomine dihydrochloride (Immiticide [Merial, Iselin, NJ])—low toxicity (hepatotoxicity); good efficacy (>90%) against both sexes of adult worms; adverse effects include pulmonary thromboembolism (usually 7 to 30 days after therapy), anorexia (13% incidence), injection site reaction (myositis—32% incidence but mild and lasts 1 to 2 days), lethargy or depression (15% incidence); causes elevations of hepatic enzymes.
- Class I infection—two injections 24 hours apart are given into the epaxial muscles (first injection on one side, second injection on opposite side, using 22-gauge needles); apply pressure over the injection site during and after needle withdrawal; check antigen test 6 months later and, if positive, repeat treatment.
- Class II and Class III infections (after CHF stabilization)—use alternative dose schedule: first injection administered initially (40% kill rate); 1 month later, two injections 24 hours apart are recommended.
- Alternative dose schedule—spreads the adulticide killing effect and thromboembolism over 2 treatments.
- Alternative dose schedule—used by many veterinarians for treating Class I infections.

- Microfilaricide administration—indicated for most dogs with circulating microfilariae, 4 to 6 weeks after adulticide:
  - Milbemycin (Interceptor, Novartis, Greensboro, NC, 0.5 mg/kg) or ivermectin (multiple preparation, 50 μg/kg)—administered in the morning, and the patient observed for signs of microfilarial anaphylaxis (shock, vomiting, diarrhea, circulatory collapse) for the day and discharged in the evening.
  - Likelihood of shock developing—highest in dogs with high microfilaremias.
  - If shock occurs—administer high-dose glucocorticoids and shock doses of IV fluids; excellent prognosis if treated quickly.
  - Ivermectin—given as a prophylaxis (6 μg/kg, monthly) will eventually remove microfilaria after 8 months in most dogs.
- Begin monthly microfilaricide prophylaxis 4 weeks later—reinfection can occur in treated dogs.
- Perform an antigen test 4 to 6 months after adulticide treatment—if positive, repeat adulticide treatment.
- Some dogs with persistent adult infection—may not require re-treatment; determined by age, severity of infection, degree of improvement since the first treatment, strength of the positive antigen test result, concomitant disease.
- Heparin (75 U/kg, SC, q8h) or aspirin (5 to 7 mg/kg, PO, q24h) for 1 to 3 weeks before and during, and for 3 weeks after, adulticide administration—controversial recommendation for the most severe cases of Class III disease; therapy is combined with strict, extended cage confinement.
- Heparin (75 U/kg, SC, q8h)—recommended for dogs with pulmonary thrombosis, thrombocytopenia, or hemoglobinuria.

Prophylaxis of Noninfected Dogs
- Heartworm prophylaxis—should be provided for all dogs at risk.
- New patients starting on prophylaxis for the first time—a test to detect microfilaria may be indicated because some macrolide endectocides (milbemycin) may induce a shock syndrome within 24 hours of the first dose; antigen test before starting preventive treatment in such cases is indicated to rule out possible adult infection (if positive, consider adulticide treatment options but start prophylaxis treatment immediately as long as patient is microfilaremic negative).
- Ivermectin (Heartgard [Merial, Iselin, NJ])—highly effective monthly preventive; retroactive efficacy as long as 4 months after infection when monthly administration is continued for 12 months; when combined with pyrantel pamoate (Heartgard Plus [Merial, Iselin, NJ]), also controls hookworm and roundworm infection; can be given safely to microfilaremic dogs, including so-called ivermectin-sensitive dogs.
- Milbemycin oxime (Interceptor [Novartis, Greensboro, NC])—highly effective monthly preventive; also controls hookworms, roundworms, and whipworms; the preventive dosage is microfilaricidal; acute reactions may occur when given to microfilaremic dogs.
- Moxidectin (ProHeart tablets [Fort Dodge, Fort Dodge, IA])—a monthly preventive; can be given to microfilaremic dogs.
- Moxidectin (ProHeart6 injectable [Fort Dodge, Fort Dodge, IA])—prophylactic effective for at least 6 months after injection; currently not available in the United States.
- Selamectin (Revolution [Pfizer, Exton, PA.])—monthly topical preventive; also controls fleas, ear mites, sarcoptic mange, and some tick infestations.

- Macrocide endectocide preventives (milbemycin oxime, ivermectin, selamactin, and moxidectin)—provide retroactive efficacy of 100% for 1 month and at least 75% for 2 months; ivermectin may provide up to 4 months of protection if continued for 12 months thereafter.
- Diethylcarbamazine citrate (Filaribits [Pfizer, Exton, PA]; Nemacide [Boehringer Ingelheim, St. Joseph, MO])—daily administration (6.6 mg/kg) is required to ensure prophylaxis; cheaper than macrolides; need to continue dosing 2 months beyond the end of transmission season; if miss a few doses (which voids protection), administer one dose of a macrolide endectocide (ivermectin, milbemycin, etc.) at prophylaxis doses.
- All of the prophylactic drugs—can be administered safely to collies or collielike breeds at the appropriate preventive dosages.

 # COMMENTS

Precautions/Interactions

- Adulticide treatment—not indicated in patients with renal failure, hepatic failure, or nephrotic syndrome.
- Standard adulticide therapy in dogs with severe infection—associated with high mortality due to subsequent pulmonary thromboembolism.
- Prognosis in Class I—usually excellent.
- Prognosis in Class III—guarded, with a higher risk of complications.
- Old dogs—may not require treatment, because heartworm infection may not be the life-limiting factor.
- Zoonosis—heartworms represent no zoonotic potential.
- Adulticide treatment—should be delayed in pregnant animals.
- Transplacental infection by microfilaria—can occur.

Abbreviations

CBC, complete blood count; CHF, congestive heart failure; COPD, chronic obstructive pulmonary disease; ECG, electrocardiogram; PA, pulmonary artery; PCV, packed cell volume; PPP, prepatent period; RA, right atrium; RV, right ventricle.

Suggested Reading

Dillon R. Dirofilariosis in dogs and cats. In: Ettinger SJ, Feldman EC, eds. *Textbook of Canine and Feline Veterinary Internal Medicine*, 5th ed. Philadelphia: WB Saunders; 2000:937–963.

Authors: Clay A. Calvert and Clarence A. Rawlings
Consulting Editor: Stephen C. Barr

Helicobacter Infection

DEFINITION/OVERVIEW

- A bacterial cause of inflammatory changes or glandular degeneration in the stomachs of cats and dogs.

ETIOLOGY/PATHOPHYSIOLOGY

- *Helicobacter* spp. (specifically *H. felis*, *H. canis*, *H. bizzozeronii*, *H. salomonis*, and *Flexispira rappini* in cats and dogs)—microaerophilic, gram-negative, urease-positive bacteria ranging from coccoid to curved to spiral.
- *H. pylori*—most important species affecting humans, causing gastritis, peptic ulcers, and gastric neoplasia.
- Experimentally—*H. pylori* causes gastritis, lymphoid follicle proliferation, and humoral immune responses in dogs and cats, but role in disease is currently unknown.

SIGNALMENT/HISTORY

- Infection with gastric *Helicobacter* spp.—appears to be acquired at a young age.
- Asymptomatic *Helicobacter* infection—common.
- Vomiting, anorexia, abdominal pain, weight loss, and/or borborygmis—seen in dogs and cats with gastric *Helicobacter* spp.
- Diarrhea in dogs—may be associated with *H. canis* infection.
- Vomiting, weakness, and sudden death seen in one dog with hepatic *H. canis*.

CLINICAL FEATURES

- As well as the above historical signs—may have signs of dehydration from fluid and electrolyte loss (from vomiting or diarrhea).

DIFFERENTIAL DIAGNOSIS

- High *Helicobacter* spp. prevalence rates exist in dogs and cats—exclusion of other causes of gastric disease and a positive test for *Helicobacter* infection are necessary before a diagnosis of GI disease due to *Helicobacter* spp. infection can be made.
- Identify other causes of vomiting, diarrhea, or liver disease—because *Helicobacter* is ubiquitous, it requires a diagnosis by exclusion.

DIAGNOSTICS

- CBC and biochemical panel—nonspecific changes; reflect fluid and electrolyte abnormalities, secondary to vomiting and/or diarrhea, or hepatic disease.
- Impression smears from the gastric mucosa obtained during endoscopy (stained with May-Gruüwald-Giemsa, Gram's, or Diff-Quik stains)—sensitive and easy test to perform *(Fig. 52-1)*.
- Rapid-urease test—requires gastric biopsy specimen; easy to perform in animals that undergo gastroduodenoscopy.
- 13C-urea breath or blood test—shown to be reliable in identifying infected dogs.
- Culture—requires special techniques and media; low success rate.
- PCR of DNA extracted from biopsy specimens or from gastric juice—sensitive; not commercially available.
- Serology (ELISA) measure of circulating IgG in serum—cannot distinguish among different HLOs.

■ **Fig. 52-1** *Helicobacter* organisms bordering the lining of the stomach mucosa in a dog (Warthin Starry silver stain, 1,400×).

Diagnostic Feature

■ Endoscopy to obtain histopathology—enables definitive diagnosis of gastric *Helicobacter* infection; grossly, may see superficial nodules (suggest lymphoid follicle hyperplasia), diffuse gastric rugal thickening, mucosal flattening, punctate hemorrhages, and erosions.

 THERAPEUTICS

■ No unanimously accepted guidelines for treatment because pathogenicity remains unclear.
■ Currently no indication for treating asymptomatic animals.
■ Attempt eradication of gastric *Helicobacter* spp. in infected dogs and cats that have compatible clinical signs not attributable to other causes.
■ A triple therapy (combination of two antibiotics and one antisecretory drug for 2 to 3 weeks); effective in humans with *H. pylori* infection.
■ Triple therapy cure rates approach/exceed 90% in humans.
■ Combination therapy in dogs and cats is less effective in eliminating *Helicobacter* infection than in humans.

Drugs of Choice

■ Combination 1: metronidazole, amoxicillin, and famotidine—effectively eradicated *Helicobacter* infection in 6 of 8 dogs evaluated 3 days post-treatment; all dogs were recolonized by day 28 after completion of treatment.
■ Combination 2: metronidazole, clarithromycin, ranitidine, and bismuth—effective in eradicating *H. heilmannii* in 11 of 11 cats by 10 days; 2 cats were reinfected 42 days post-treatment.
■ Combination 3: amoxicillin, metronidazole, and omeprazole—transiently eradicated *H. pylori* in 6 cats; all were reinfected 6 weeks post-treatment *(Table 52-1)*.
■ Recurrent infection after therapy—unclear if due to reinfection or recrudescence of infection.

TABLE 52-1. Drug Therapy Combinations for the Treatment of Helicobacteriosis in Dogs and Cats

Regimen (SPECIES)	Drug	Dose (mg/kg)	Route	Interval (Hours)	Duration (Days)
1 (Dogs)	Metronidazole	15	PO	12	14
	Amoxicillin,	20	PO	12	14
	Famotidine	0.5	PO	12	14
2 (Cats)	Metronidazole	30[a]	PO	12	4
	Clarithromycin	30[a]	PO	12	4
	Ranitidine	20[a]	PO	12	4
	Bismuth	40[a]	PO	12	4
3 (Cats)	Metronidazole	10	PO	8	21
	Amoxicillin	20	PO	8	21
	Omeprazole	0.7	PO	24	21

[a] Total dose per cat.

Precautions/Interactions

- Avoid metronidazole and tetracycline in pregnant and young animals.
- High doses of metronidazole can cause neurologic toxicity.
- Avoid bismuth subsalicylate in cats.

 COMMENTS

- Explain to clients—the difficulty of establishing a diagnosis, the high prevalence rates of infections with HLOs in normal dogs and cats, the potential for recurrence, and the zoonotic potential of the disease.
- Serologic tests—not useful to confirm eradication of gastric HLOs; serum IgG titers may not decrease for up to 6 months after cleared infection.
- 13C-urea breath and blood test—has been evaluated to monitor the eradication of HLOs in dogs and cats; shows promise for routine application.
- If vomiting persists or recurs after cessation of combination therapy—may need to repeat endoscopic biopsy to determine whether the infection has been successfully eradicated.

Abbreviations

CBC, complete blood count; DNA, deoxyribonucleic acid; ELISA, enzyme-linked immunosorbent assay; GI, gastrointestinal; HLO, *Helicobacter*-like organism; PCR, polymerase chain reaction; TNF, tumor necrosis factor.

Suggested Reading

Crystal MA. *Helicobacter* infection. In: Norsworthy GD, Crystal MA, Fooshee Grace SK, et al, eds. *The Feline Patient: Essentials of Diagnosis and Treatment*, 2nd ed. Baltimore: Williams & Wilkins; 2003:254–258.

Fox JG. *Helicobacter*-associated gastric disease in ferrets, dogs and cats. In: Bonagura JD, ed. *Kirk's Current Veterinary Therapy XII: Small Animal Practice*. Philadelphia: WB Saunders; 1995:720–723.

Fox JG, Lee A. The role of *Helicobacter* species in newly recognized gastrointestinal tract disease of animals. *Lab Anim Sci* 1997;47:222–255.

Neiger R, Simpson KW. *Helicobacter* infection in dogs and cats: facts and fiction. *J Vet Intern Med* 2000;14:125–133.

Simpson KW, Neiger R, DeNovo RC, et al. The relationship of *Helicobacter* spp. infection to gastric disease in dogs and cats: ACVIM consensus statement. *J Vet Intern Med* 2000;14:223–227.

Authors: Jan S. Suchdolski and Jorg M. Steiner
Consulting Editor: Stephen C. Barr

chapter 53

Hepatozoonosis

DEFINITION/OVERVIEW

- A systemic tick-borne protozoal infection of mammalian carnivores (foxes, coyotes, hyenas, and large cats, including lions, leopards, and cheetahs), including dogs, and very rarely cats.
- Infection in dogs is mainly characterized by severe periosteal proliferation, but may affect multiple organ systems.

ETIOLOGY/PATHOPHYSIOLOGY

- *Hepatozoon americanum*—infects dogs in southern and southwestern United States (Texas to Georgia).
- Domestic cats—extremely rare (one case reported in Hawaii).
- Infection—ingestion of tick vector (*Amblyomma maculatum*) or by bite from tick.
- Vertical transmission to puppies—can occur.
- Complex pathogenesis—complicated by other factors affecting immune status.
- Factors include—concurrent infections, such as with distemper, parvovirus, *Babesia*, *Ehrlichia*, and *Leishmania*.
- Age at infection—an important determinant of clinical disease development.
- If infected young—more chance of developing periosteal bone proliferation.
- Experimental infections—develop bloody diarrhea 3 days postinfection (lasts 2 to 14 days), pyrexia (day 7 and lasting weeks), lymphadenopathy (by 3 weeks postinfection); leukocytosis with cachexia and ocular discharge present by 4 weeks postinfection.
- Amyloid deposits—occur in multiple organs, with vasculitis and glomerulonephritis developing in fatal cases.
- Humoral immunity—not protective and may even facilitate fatal immune complex disease.

SIGNALMENT/HISTORY

- Young dogs—most severely affected mainly during warmer months (coinciding with rising and falling parasitemias).

CLINICAL FEATURES

Dogs

- Usually subclinical.
- Clinically affected—chronic antibiotic-unresponsive fever and cachexia.
- Anorexia.
- Diarrhea.
- Paraparesis.
- Signs may vary between localities—bloody diarrhea seems to be a feature of dogs infected in Texas.
- Generalized muscle atrophy and hyperesthesia—causes stiffness and reluctance to move.
- Cervical and trunk rigidity—caused by periosteal pain.
- Ocular abnormalities—low tear production, focal retinal scarring, hyperpigmentation, papilledema, and uveitis have all been reported.
- Prolonged course of disease—with periods of apparent remission interspersed with periods of fever and pain.
- Periods of remission—longer in surviving cases; shorter in fatal cases.
- Cats—asymptomatic, with schizonts being found in tissues at necropsy.

DIFFERENTIAL DIAGNOSIS

Dogs

- Few other causes of persistent antibiotic-resistant fever, cachexia, periosteal bone proliferation, with profound leukocytosis in dogs in southern and southwestern United States.
- Other possible causes include leishmaniasis, chronic erhlichiosis, babesiosis, systemic mycotic infections, pyelonephritis (lumbar hyperesthesia), neoplasia, endocarditis, immune-mediated polyarthritis or polymyositis, diskospondylitis.

DIAGNOSTICS

- CBC—profound leukocytosis (sometimes as high as 200,000 cells/μl blood) with left shift; sometimes eosinophilia (up to 20%); mild normocytic, normochromic regenerative anemia; often a thrombocytosis (as opposed to thrombocytopenia, characteristic of *Erhlichia* infection).
- Serum chemistry—hypoalbuminemia, hyperglobulinemia, increased SAP activity.
- Profound hypoglycemia—probably artifact due to high neutrophil counts metabolizing glucose after sample collection.
- Elevated urine protein/creatine ratio—dogs with glomerulopathy.

■ **Fig. 53-1** Ventrodorsal radiograph of the pelvis of a dog infected with *Hepatozoon americanum* showing periosteal bone proliferation over the ileum and vertebrae.

- Radiology—periosteal bone proliferation, particularly at the attachment sites of muscles in all bones, with the usual exception of the head *(Fig. 53-1)*.
- Not all dogs develop bone proliferative lesion—more common in younger dogs (<1 year).

Diagnostic Features
- **Diagnosis—made by finding gamonts in neutrophils or monocytes in buffy coat blood smears (Giemsa stain best) *(Fig. 53-2)*.**
- **Gamonts—difficult to find in white blood cells (WBCs) in North American strains.**
- **Muscle biopsy—muscle cysts are more consistently found than gamonts in WBCs in North American infections *(Fig. 53-3)*.**

■ **Fig. 53-2** Gamont of *Hepatozoon americanum* in a neutrophil on a peripheral blood smear (Wright's-Giemsa stain, 1,000×).

 THERAPEUTICS

- Mostly palliative—complete recovery rare, with relapses occurring 3 to 6 months after treatment.
- Symptomatic palliative treatment—nonsteroidal anti-inflammatory agents provide best relief.

■ **Fig. 53-3** *Hepatozoon americanum* cyst in a muscle biopsy section from an infected dog (hematoxylin and eosin, 800×).

Drug	Dose (mg/kg)	Route	Interval (Hours)	Duration (Weeks)
Trimethoprim-sulfadiazine (Tribrissen)	15	PO	12	2[a]
Clindamycin (Antirobe)	10	PO	8	2[a]
Pyrimethamine (Daraprim)	0.25	PO	24	2[a]
Decoquinate (Deccox)	10–20	PO	12	33 months[b]

TABLE 53-1. Drug Therapy for Hepatozoonosis in Dogs

[a] Initial therapy.

[b] Long-term therapy; 1/4 oz of feed additive will medicate 20 to 40 kg body weight of dog.

- Glucocorticoids—provide short-term temporary relief, but must be avoided over the long term.
- Combinations of therapies—provide the best outcome.

Drugs of Choice

Initial Therapy (Give All Drugs Together)
- TMS (Tribrissen [Schering-Plough, Union, NJ]).
- Clindamycin (Antirobe [Pharmacia and Upjohn, Kalamazoo, MI]).
- Pyrimethamine (Daraprim [Burroughs Welcome, Triangle Park, NC]).

Long-Term Therapy
- Decoquinate (Deccox [Alpharma, Fort Lee, NJ] *(Table 53-1)*.
- Medicated feed additive for cattle.
- Supplied as a 6% (each pound contains 27.2 g of decoquinate) feed medication mixed in corn meal, soybean oil, lecithin, and silicon dioxide.

Precautions/Interactions

- TMS—may induce keratoconjunctivitis sicca, hepatotoxicity, immune-mediated polyarthritis, retinitis, glomerulonephritis, vasculitis, thrombocytopenia, erythema multiforme, toxic epidermal necrolysis, and other cutaneous drug eruptions.
- Do not use pyrimethamine in pregnant animals—may cause teratogenesis.
- TMS and pyrimethamine—may induce folate deficiency and augment myelosuppression.
- Folate deficiency—supplement with 5 to 15 mg/day, PO of folinic acid.
- Clindamycin—GI signs with vomiting and diarrhea.

  COMMENTS

- Improvement—best monitored by clinical signs, not organisms in peripheral blood or on muscle biopsy.
- Most cases—asymptomatic.
- Cases with severe periosteal disease—even symptomatic therapy may not be enough to improve an animal's quality of life.

- Avoid glucocorticoids if possible—often exacerbate clinical disease.
- Humans—have been reported to be infected with *Hepatozoon* spp.
- Role of the infected dog as a source of infection to humans—probably insignificant.

Abbreviations

CBC, complete blood count; GI, gastrointestinal; SAP, serum alkaline phosphatase; TMS, trimethroprim-sulfadiazine; WBCs, white blood cells.

Suggested Reading

Graig TM. Hepatozoonosis. In: Greene CE, ed. *Infectious Disease of the Dog and Cat*. Philadelphia: WB Saunders; 1998:458–465.

Macintire DK, Vincent-Johnson NA, Kane CW, et al. Treatment of dogs infected with *Hepatozoon americanum*: 53 cases (1989–1998). *J Am Vet Med Assoc* 2001;218:77–82.

Author: Johnny D. Hoskins
Consulting Editor: Stephen C. Barr

chapter 54

Histoplasmosis

DEFINITION/OVERVIEW

- Systemic fungal infection resulting in mainly intestinal tract disease in the dog, and respiratory disease in the cat, but affecting multiple organs (including liver, spleen, bone marrow, bone, lung and lymph nodes) in both species.

ETIOLOGY/PATHOPHYSIOLOGY

- *Histoplasma capsulatum*—mycelial form, which grows in bird manure or organically enriched soil produces infectious spores (microconidia).
- Microconidia—inhaled into terminal airways; spores germinate in lungs and develop into yeast form.
- Yeast form—phagocytized by macrophages and distributed throughout the body.
- Ingested organisms—may directly infect the intestinal tract, especially in dogs.
- Immune response—determines if disease will develop.
- Affected animals—often develop transient asymptomatic infection.

Dogs

- Main organs affected—intestinal tract, but also liver, lung, spleen, and lymph nodes.
- Systems less frequently affected—bones, bone marrow, kidneys, adrenals, oral cavity, tongue, eyes, and testes.

Cats

- Respiratory tract—mainly affected.
- Also often affected—bone, bone marrow, liver, spleen, skin, and lymph nodes.
- Systems less frequently affected—intestinal tract, eyes, kidneys, adrenals, and brain.

SIGNALMENT/HISTORY

- Low prevalence of clinically relevant cases.
- Endemic areas—Ohio, Missouri, Mississippi, Tennessee, St. Lawrence rive basins; also present in Texas, Oklahoma, southeastern United States, and occasionally the Great Lakes region.

Dogs

- Most often—young dogs affected, but all ages.
- Historically—weight loss, depression and large bowel diarrhea is most common.
- Cough and dyspnea—often noted by owner.
- Lameness, ocular and skin changes—noted less commonly by owner.

Cats

- Usually <1 yr of age, but also all ages.
- Historically—more insidious onset of anorexia, weight loss, dyspnea, and cough.
- Lameness, ocular discharge, diarrhea—noted less commonly by owner.

 CLINICAL FEATURES

Dogs

- Emaciation.
- Fever.
- Generalized lymphadenopathy.
- Hepatosplenomegaly.
- Pale mucous membranes.
- Easily elicited cough and harsh lung sounds.
- Icterus, rarely.

Cats

- Fever.
- Increased respiratory effort.
- Harsh lung sounds.
- Pale mucous membranes.
- Generalized lymphadenopathy.
- Lameness.
- Ocular signs.

 DIFFERENTIAL DIAGNOSIS

Dogs

- Severe chronic diarrhea and weight loss—GI lymphoma; IBD (lymphocytic plasma-cytic, eosinophilic), exocrine pancreatic insufficiency, and chronic parasitism (whipworms).
- Respiratory signs—a general differential diagnosis for respiratory signs and cough includes such categories as:
  - Cardiovascular (pulmonary edema; enlarged heart, especially the left atrium; left-sided heart failure; pulmonary emboli) and congenital (hypoplastic trachea).

- Allergic (bronchial asthma, chronic bronchitis, eosinophilic pneumonia or granulomatosis, pulmonary infiltrate with eosinophilia).
- Trauma (foreign body, irritating gases, collapsing trachea).
- Neoplasia (not only of the respiratory tree but also associated structures such as ribs, lymph nodes, muscles).
- Inflammatory (pharyngitis; tonsillitis; kennel cough from such agents as *Bordetella bronchoseptica*, parainfluenza virus, infectious laryngotracheitis virus, and mycoplasma; bacterial bronchopneumonia; chronic pulmonary fibrosis; pulmonary abscess or granuloma; COPD); other fungal agents (blastomycosis, cryptococcosis); pleural space diseases.
- Parasites (*Oslerus [Filaroides] osleri, Crenosoma vulpis, Capillaria aerophila, F. milksi, Paragonimus kellicotti, Dirofilaria immitis*—heartworm disease).
- Lymph node enlargement—similar to lymphosarcoma differentiated by lymph node aspirate cytology.

- Chronic large bowel disease with severe weight loss unresponsive to antibiotics and motility modifiers in young dogs from endemic regions suggests the diagnosis.

Cats

- Respiratory signs—differentiate from heart disease, feline asthma, parenchymal lung disease (pneumonia, parasitic lungworms, neoplasia, toxoplasmosis), and pleural disease (pyothorax, neoplasia).
- Lameness—differentiate from trauma, cat bite abscess, spinal lymphoma, and polyarthritis.
- Ocular disease—lymphoma, toxoplasmosis, and FIP.

DIAGNOSTICS

- CBC—usually moderate to severe nonregenerative anemia; usually normal leukocyte counts but can have leukocytosis (rarely leukopenia from bone marrow involvement); frequently see thrombocytopenia.
- Peripheral blood smears—may find *Histoplasma* organisms in monocytes or neutrophils (*Fig. 54-1*) or bone marrow aspirate (*Fig. 54-2*).
- Biochemical panel—elevated hepatic enzymes (liver involvement), hypoalbuminemia (intestinal tract involvement), hyperglobulinemia.
- AGID test—detects antibodies against *H. capsulatum*; supports diagnosis; positive result usually indicates active infection, although false positive result can occur (suggests past infection); false negative results are common.
- Coombs' test—may be positive because antibodies to *H. capsulatum* may cross-react with RBCs.
- Imaging:
  - Thoracic radiographs—diffuse interstitial-to-nodular pneumonia; enlarged tracheobronchial lymph nodes compressing the tracheal bifurcation (*Fig. 54-3*) in dogs (rare in cats).
  - Abdominal imaging—organomegaly (liver, spleen, lymph nodes).

■ **Fig. 54-1** Peripheral blood smear of a dog with systemic histoplasmosis, showing the organisms within a monocyte (may also be found in neutrophils and very rarely, eosinophils). Note the two extracellular organisms; these have been torn out of cells during the fixation procedure (Wright's stain, 1,000×).

- Bones—predominantly osteolytic lesions, usually distal to elbows and stifles (especially cats).

Diagnostic Feature
- **Definitive diagnostic method of choice—identify organism on cytology, histopathology, or culture; obtain samples by rectal scraping** *(Fig. 54-4)*, **lymph node aspirates, bone marrow aspirates, or lung aspirates; lung aspirates are best (tracheal wash relatively low yield).**

■ **Fig. 54-2** *Histoplasma* organisms can be identified in mononuclear cells within bone marrow aspirates from dogs systemically affected by the fungus. Note also that the same cell containing the organisms has phagocytosed two red blood cells, a common occurrence (Wright's stain, 1,000×).

■ **Fig. 54-3** Lateral thoracic radiograph of a dog with pulmonary histoplasmosis, showing diffuse interstitial and nodular lung infiltrates and markedly enlarged hilar lymph nodes.

■ **Fig. 54-4** Cytologic preparation of a rectal scraping from a dog with intestinal histoplasmosis, showing organisms within a macrophage (Wright's stain, 750×). This is the method of choice to definitively diagnose intestinal histoplasmosis in the dog.

- Rectal scraping—with gloved fingernail of index finger, scrape the dorsal wall of the rectum; smear scraping on microscope slide, air dry and stain (Wright-Giemsa).

 THERAPEUTICS

- Usually outpatient—if stable (use oral itraconazole).
- Inpatient—if administering intravenous amphotericin B (dogs with severe intestinal disease and malabsorption).
- Dogs receiving amphotericin B—monitor carefully for renal toxicity (examine urinary sediment for appearance of casts).
- Administer total parenteral nutrition—to reverse wasting until intestinal disease is resolved enough for adequate food absorption.
- Oxygen therapy—may be required for dogs in respiratory distress.

Drugs of Choice

Itraconazole (Sporanox [Janssen, Titusville, NJ])
- Drug of choice in animals with good intestinal absorption.
- Less expensive than fluconazole.
- Give with a fat-rich meal (canned dog food) for the first 3 days to achieve a therapeutic blood concentration as soon as possible.
- For cats have drug compounded (by an appropriate pharmacy) or open the 100-mg capsules containing pellets and mix with palatable food.

Amphotericin B (Fungizone [E. R. Squibb, New York, NY])
- Check for nephrotoxicity by monitoring urine for appearance of casts; discontinue when they appear and maintain hydration.
- Use liposomal or lipid complex formulations to reduce nephrotoxicity; more expensive.
- Use until patient begins to gain weight, and then switch to itraconazole.

Fluconazole (Diflucan [Pfizer, Exton, PA])
- Use in dogs that cannot receive amphotericin B.
- Penetrates all body cavities and tissues, including eye and CNS; use in cases with ocular and/or CNS involvement (*Table 54-1*).

Precautions/Interactions

- Renal failure—precludes the use of amphotericin B; may use less nephrotoxic formulations.
- Steroids—use with caution; will allow proliferation of *H. capsulatum*; life-threatening respiratory distress due to infiltrative lung disease or hilar lymphadenopathy justifies the use of dexamethasone (dosage: 0.2 mg/kg, IV or IM, q24h, for 2 to 3 days) to decrease inflammation while the patient receives antifungal treatment.
- Itraconazole and fluconazole—hepatic toxicity; temporarily discontinue if patient becomes anorexic or if serum ALT activity >300 U/L (check monthly); restart at half dose after appetite returns.

TABLE 54-1. Drug Therapy for Histoplasmosis in Dogs and Cats

Drug	Dose (mg/kg)	Route	Interval (Hours)	Duration (Months)
Itraconazole (Sporanox)	5–10	PO	12–24	3–6[a]
Amphotericin B (Fungizone)	0.25–0.5[b]	IV	48[c]	[d]
Fluconazole (Diflucan)	5	PO	12–24	3–6[a]

[a] Give with a fatty meal for a minimum of 3 months depending on response.
[b] Reconstituted in 5% dextrose (do not reconstitute in electrolyte solutions that precipitate the drug) and dilute to administer; if normal renal function, dilute in 60 to 120 ml 5% dextrose given over 15 minutes; if renal compromise, dilute in 0.5 to 1 liter 5% dextrose given over 3 to 4 hours to reduce further renal toxicity.
[c] Or 3 times a week.
[d] Administer until a total cumulative dose of 5 to 10 mg/kg in dogs and 4 to 5 mg/kg in cats is reached.

- Itraconazole—not teratogenic at therapeutic doses but is at high doses in rats (no dog or cat studies, but one dog delivered normal litter when given drug half way through pregnancy).
- Follow-up—obtain chest radiographs after 60 days of treatment, and stop treatment when infiltrates are clear or remaining lung lesions fail to improve (continue treatment for 1 month after there is no change observed on radiographs); monitor bone lesions by radiology; monitor ocular lesions.

COMMENTS

- Identify high-risk environments to inform owners of risk to them—no risk of spread from animals to humans (although veterinarians need to take care with needle sticks such as for aspirate cytology or necropsies on infected animals, because cuts can become infected).
- Duration of treatment is usually 4 months—warn owners of expense of drugs.
- Prognosis is good for stable patients without dyspnea when starting treatment—prognosis worsens in debilitated, emaciated animals or those with severe lung involvement.
- Recovered dogs are probably immune—recurrence is possible, requiring a second course of treatment.

Abbreviations

AGID, agar gel immunodiffusion; ALT, alanine aminotransferase; CBC, complete blood count; CNS, central nervous system; COPD, chronic obstructive pulmonary disease; FIP, feline infectious peritonitis; GI, gastrointestinal; IBD, inflammatory bowel disease; RBC, red blood cell.

Suggested Reading

Kerl ME. Update on canine and feline fungal disease. *Vet Clin North Am Small Anim Pract* 2003;33: 721–747.

Schulman RL, McKiernan BC, Schaeffer DJ. Use of corticosteroids for treating dogs with airway obstruction secondary to hilar lymphadenopathy caused by chronic histoplasmosis: 16 cases (1979–1997). *J Am Vet Med Assoc* 1999;214:1345–1348.

Wolf AM. Histoplasmosis. In: Greene CE, ed. *Infectious Diseases of the Dog and Cat.* Philadelphia: WB Saunders; 1998:378–383.

Author: Alfred M. Legendre
Consulting Editor: Stephen C. Barr

chapter 55

Hookworms

DEFINITION/OVERVIEW

- Nematode parasites—adults (and 4th-stage larvae) are voracious blood feeders while attached to the small intestinal tract of dogs and cats, causing blood loss anemia.

ETIOLOGY/PATHOPHYSIOLOGY

- *Ancylostoma tubaeforme*—cats.
- *A. caninum*—dogs.
- *A. braziliense* and *Uncinaria stenocephala*—cats and dogs.
- *A. caninum*—most widely distributed; subtropical and temperate regions.
- *A. braziliense*—tropical/subtropical; southern states of United States.
- *A. tubaeforme* and *U. stenocephala*—temperate states.
- Infection—ingestion of infective larvae or by skin penetration (except *A. tubaeforme* in cats).
- *A. braziliense*—also transmitted via colostrum to pups.
- Adults and 4th-stage larvae—cause blood-loss anemia and enteritis by ingesting large quantities of blood.
- Once detached—parasite bite wounds and anticoagulants cause continual seepage of blood and serum in bowel lumen.
- Neonates—particularly susceptible to peracute and acute blood loss.

SIGNALMENT/HISTORY

- Neonates and young puppies—acute disease.
- Mature dogs and cats—chronic blood loss anemia.

CLINICAL FEATURES

Dogs

- Peracute disease—as a result of transmammary infection.
- Pups that are healthy in the first week of life—deteriorate rapidly in the second week, with severe anemia; soft, liquid, tarry, bloody feces; and sudden death before eggs appear in feces.

- Acute disease—older puppies (and some mature dogs) exposed to large numbers of infective larvae.
- Develop signs of anemia.
- Weakness.
- Tarry stools—even before eggs appear in feces.
- Chronic (compensated) disease—usually asymptomatic but with anemia and eggs in feces.
- Secondary disease—older dogs with other conditions (usually with severe weight loss) causing debilitation, resulting in profound anemia.
- Other signs—dry cough from larval migration through lungs of pups (rare).
- Mild acanthosis.
- Hyperkeratinization over site of larvae entry in skin.

Cats

- Usually asymptomatic—only rarely develop signs of anemia and loose, tarry stools.

 ## DIFFERENTIAL DIAGNOSIS

- Other causes of loss of RBC mass, including:
    - Hemolysis—caused by toxins (zinc, acetaminophen, onion), immune-mediated hemolytic anemia, parasites (*Babesia*, *Haemobartonella* spp.), microangiopathic hemolysis (splenic torsion, vena caval syndrome), RBC cell disorders (pyruvate kinase deficiency), and drugs (propylthiouracil, gold salts).
    - Acute or chronic blood loss—bowel lumen (neoplasia, parasites, ulcers), from skin (external parasitism—fleas); chronic blood loss often results in iron deficiency anemia.

 ## DIAGNOSTICS

CBC

- Acute—regenerative anemia (regeneration may not be present in the very young because blood loss and death can occur before regeneration has time to occur).
- Chronic—iron deficiency anemia (microcytic hypochromic nonregenerative anemia).
- Eosinophilia.

Fecal Flotation

- Eggs in stools (*Fig. 55-1*); *A. caninum*—elongated ellipsoid (60 × 40 μm), thin-shelled (usually in eight-cell-stage); indistinguishable from *A. braziliensis*.
- *A. caninum* egg is smaller than *U. stenocephala*—(70 μm long).

■ **Figure 55-1** The eggs of hookworms (**A**) *Ancylostoma caninum*, found in dogs; (**B**) *Ancylostoma tubaeforme* found in cats; and (**C**) *Uncinaria stenocephala*, found in both dogs and cats.

 ## THERAPEUTICS

- Pups in a heavily contaminated environment—treat at 2-week intervals to weaning.
- Peracute—often too late, but administer anthelmintic first (pyrantel), then blood transfusion (in neonates, give intraosseous) and fluid support.
- Alert owners—to the potential of sudden death.
- Acute and chronic primary hookworm cases—respond rapidly to anthelmintics alone.

■ Animals with secondary disease—need supplementation (iron, vitamin, blood transfusion, high-protein diet), as well as regular anthelmintic therapy.

■ Hookworms constantly repopulate the bowel from larvae sequestered in tissues—can continue for months or even years.

■ Treat bitches from 14th day of gestation (fenbendazole) to the 14th to 28th day of lactation—kills reactivated hookworm larvae before they reach the pups and should prevent pup loss.

Drugs of Choice

Adult Larvae Anthelmintic Activity
■ Fenbendazole (Panacur Granules 22.2% [Intervet, Millsboro, DE]).
■ Milbemycin oxime (Interceptor or Sentinel [Novartis, Greensboro, NC]).

Adulticide Activity
■ Pyrantel (Nemex [Pfizer, Exton, PA]).
■ Praziquantel/pyrantel/febantel (Drontal Plus [Bayer, Shawnee Mission, KS]).
■ Praziquantel/pyrantel (Drontal [Bayer, Shawnee Mission, KS]).
■ Ivermectin and pyrantel (Heartguard Plus [Merial, Iselin, NJ]).
■ Dichlorvos (Task Tabs [Boehringer Ingelheim, St. Joseph, MO]) (*Table 55-1*).

TABLE 55-1. Drug Therapy for Hookworms in Dogs and Cats						
Drug	Parasite Stage	Species	Dose (mg/kg)	Route	Interval (Hours)	Duration (Days)
Fenbendazole (Panacur)	AL	D	50	PO	24	3
Milbemycin oxime (Interceptor)	AL	D	0.5	PO	Once	30[a]
Pyrantel pamoate (Nemex)	A	D	15	PO	Once	14[b]
	A	C	20–30	PO	Once	14[b]
Praziquantel/pyrantel/ febantel (Drontal Plus)	A	D	[c]	PO	Once	14[b]
Praziquantel/pyrantel (Drontal)	A	C	[d]	PO	Once	14[b]
Ivermectin/pyrantel (Heartgard Plus)	A	D	[e]	PO	Once	30[a]
Dichlorvos (Task Tabs)	A	B	11	PO	Once	14[b]

[a] Repeat every month.
[b] Repeat in 14 days.
[c] Dose for praziquantel (5 to 12 mg/kg), pyrantel (5 to 12 mg/kg), and febantel (25 to 62 mg/kg).
[d] Dose for praziquantel (5 mg/kg) and pyrantel (20 mg/kg).
[e] Dose for ivermectin (0.006 mg/kg) and pyrantel (5 mg/kg).
AL, adults and larvae; A, adults; B, both cats and dogs; C, cats, D dogs.

Adulticide Activity

DOGS

- Adult larvae dewormer (fenbendazole)—during third trimester of pregnancy to kill migrating larvae in somatic tissue and adult worms.
- Adult larvae dewormer—on daily or monthly basis for pups and mature dogs.
- Treat pups biweekly until weaning—if at high risk.

Adulticide Activity

CATS

- Adult larvae dewormer for queen—before breeding and after littering.
- Start adulticide dewormer—by 4 weeks of age for kittens.

Precautions/Interactions

- Do not give dichlorvos to animals with heartworm disease.
- Do not give dichlorvos concurrently with other organophosphates (e.g., insecticides).
- Pay particular attention to the manufacturer's recommendations regarding use of the drugs in pregnant animals and in puppies and kittens <4 weeks of age.

COMMENTS

- CLM ("creeping eruption")—*A. braziliense* most often causes these linear, tortuous, erythematous, pruritic eruptions on humans as a result of larval migration into the skin.
- Contaminated environments—*Ancylostom* (but not *Uncinaria* eggs) are destroyed by freezing, so a hard winter often stops clinical hookworm infections.
- Sodium borate (10 pounds/100 square feet) raked into ground destroys larvae (and vegetation as well).
- Paved areas—physically cleaned, then spray with 1% sodium hypochlorite (3 cups of bleach/gallon of water).

Abbreviations

CLM, cutaneous larval migrans; RBC, red blood cell.

Suggested Reading

Bowman DD, ed. In: *Georgis' Parasitology for Veterinarians,* 8th ed. Philadelphia: WB Saunders; 2003:183–189.

Author: Julie Ann Jarvinen
Consulting Editor: Stephen C. Barr

Infectious Canine Hepatitis Virus Infection

chapter 56

DEFINITION/OVERVIEW

- Viral disease of dogs and other Canidae affecting mainly the liver but also eyes and endothelium.

ETIOLOGY/PATHOPHYSIOLOGY

- CAV-1—serologically homogeneous but antigenically distinct from respiratory CAV-2.
- Oronasal exposure—leads to viremia (4 to 8 days).
- Virus—shed in saliva and feces.
- After viremia—virus initially dispersed to hepatic macrophages (Kupffer cells) and endothelium.
- Replicates in Kupffer cells—damage to adjacent hepatocytes and massive viremia when released.
- Adequate antibody response clears organs in 10 to 14 days—persists in renal tubules and may be shed in urine for 6 to 9 months.
- Chronic hepatitis—follows infection in dogs with only partial neutralizing antibody response.
- Cytotoxic ocular injury—anterior uveitis leading to classic "hepatitis blue eye."

SIGNALMENT/HISTORY

- No breed or sex predilections.
- Most common in dogs <1 year of age.

CLINICAL FEATURES

Peracute

- Fever.
- CNS signs.
- Vascular collapse.
- DIC.
- Death within hours.

Acute

- Fever.
- Anorexia.
- Lethargy.
- Vomiting.
- Diarrhea.
- Hepatomegaly.
- Abdominal pain.
- Abdominal effusion.
- Vasculitis (petechia, bruising).
- DIC.
- Lymphadenopathy, rarely.
- Nonsuppurative encephalitis.

Uncomplicated

- Lethargy.
- Anorexia.
- Transient fever.
- Tonsillitis.
- Vomiting.
- Diarrhea.
- Lymphadenopathy.
- Hepatomegaly.
- Abdominal pain.
- Late—20% of cases develop anterior uveitis and corneal edema 4 to 6 days postinfection; recover within 21 days; may progress to glaucoma and corneal ulceration.

 DIFFERENTIAL DIAGNOSIS

- Other infectious hepatopathies—leptospirosis.
- Granulomatous hepatitis.
- Toxic hepatitis.
- Fulminant infectious disease—for example, parvovirus, canine distemper.

 DIAGNOSTICS

- CBC—schistocytes; leukopenia during acute viremia, followed by leukocytosis with reactive lymphocytosis and nucleated RBCs.
- Biochemistry profile—hepatic enzyme activity high initially, begins declining within 14 days; low glucose and albumin reflect fulminant hepatic failure, vasculitis, and endotoxemia; low sodium and potassium levels reflect GI losses; hyperbilirubinemia.

- Urinalysis—proteinuria reflects glomerular injury; granular casts reflect renal tubule damage; bilirubinuria.
- Coagulation tests—reflect severity of liver injury and DIC.
- Serologic test for antibodies to CAV-1—fourfold rise in IgM and IgG; vaccine-induced antibodies confuse interpretation.
- Viral isolation—anterior segment of eye, kidney, tonsil, and urine.
- Isolation difficult in parenchymal organs (especially liver)—unless first week of infection.
- Abdominal radiography—normal or large liver; poor detail due to effusion.
- Abdominal ultrasonography—may observe hepatomegaly, hypoechoic parenchyma (multifocal or diffuse pattern), and effusion.

 ## THERAPEUTICS

- Usually inpatient—fluid therapy (balanced polyionic fluids; carefully monitor fluids to avoid overhydration in context of increased vascular permeability and hypoalbuminemia).
- In fulminant hepatic failure (acute/peracute presentation)—lactate may be contraindicated (inability to metabolize).
- Judicious potassium and magnesium supplementation—electrolyte depletion may augment hepatic encephalopathy (monitor serum electrolytes closely).
- Avoid neuroglycopenia—supplement fluids with dextrose (2.5% to 5.0%) if patient becomes hypoglycemic.
- Blood component or synthetic colloids—for coagulopathy and low colloidal osmotic pressure.
- Synthetic colloids—for low colloid oncotic pressure.
- With overt DIC—fresh blood products and low molecular weight heparin (e.g., enoxaparin 100 U/kg [1 mg/kg] q24h).
- Nutritional support—frequent small meals as tolerated; optimize nitrogen intake to patient; inappropriate protein restriction may impair tissue repair and regeneration.
- If oral feeding is not tolerated—provide partial parenteral nutrition (maximum of 5 days) or, preferably, total parenteral nutrition.
- MLV using CAV-2 at 6 to 8 weeks of age—two boosters 3 to 4 weeks apart until 16 weeks of age; booster at 1 year; highly effective vaccine; boosters may not be needed.
- MLV using CAV-1—produces lifelong immunity with one dose, but the virus can localize in the kidneys to produce subclinical nephritis and persistent shedding, as well as a small percentage developing severe keratitis ("blue eye") and uveitis (*Fig. 56-1*) when given subcutaneously.
- Maternal antibody—may protect some pups for first 8 weeks; depends on antibody concentration in bitch and on effective passive transfer.
- Vaccination of pups with high levels of passively acquired antibodies—successful at 14 to 16 weeks of age.

■ **Fig. 56-1** Diffuse corneal edema and keratitis ("blue eye") after vaccination with canine adenovirus-1 modified live vaccine (courtesy Dr. R. Riis, Cornell University).

Drugs of Choice

- Prophylactic antimicrobials (for anticipated transmural migration of enteric flora and endotoxemia in the context of hepatic failure)—ticarcillin combined with metronidazole (at a reduced dose).
- Antiemetics—for vomiting; metoclopramide or ondansetron.
- H_2-Receptor antagonists—famotidine.
- Gastric protectants—sucralfate for gastrointestinal bleeding.
- Ursodeoxycholic acid—choleretic and hepatoprotectant; give indefinitely for chronic hepatitis.
- Antioxidants—vitamin E and *S*-adenosylmethionine until hepatic enzymes normalize and dog fully recovers; indefinitely with chronic hepatitis (*Table 56-1*).

TABLE 56-1. Drugs Used in the Treatment of Infectious Canine Hepatitis Virus Infections

Drug	Dose (mg/kg)	Route	Interval (Hours)	Duration (Days)
Ticarcillin	33–50	PO	6–8	14
Metronidazole[a]	7.5	IV, PO	8–12	14
Metoclopramide	0.2–0.5	SC, PO	6–8	5[b]
Ondansetron	0.5–1	PO	12	5[b]
Famotidine	0.5	SC, IV, PO	12–24	7[b]
Sucralfate	0.25–1 g[c]	PO	8–12	7[b]
Ursodeoxycholic acid	10–15	PO	24	28[d]
Vitamin E	10 U/kg	PO	24	28[d]
S-Adenosylmethionine	20	PO	24	28[d]

[a] Use in combination with ticarcillin.

[b] Or for as long as needed to control vomiting.

[c] Total dose.

[d] Or indefinitely for chronic hepatitis.

Precautions/Interactions

■ Consider severity of hepatic injury, protein depletion, and age when calculating dosages of drugs.

 COMMENTS

■ Routinely monitor—fluid, electrolyte, acid–base, and coagulation status to adjust supportive measures; monitor for acute renal failure.
■ Prognosis: peracute—poor; death within hours.
■ Prognosis: acute—guarded to good.
■ Poor antibody response (titer 1:16 to 1:50)—chronic hepatitis may develop.
■ Good antibody response (titer >1:500 IgG)—complete recovery in 5 to 7 days possible.
■ Recovered patients—may develop chronic hepatic or renal disease.

Abbreviations

CAV, canine adenovirus; CBC, complete blood count; CNS, central nervous system; COPD, chronic obstructive pulmonary disease; DIC, disseminated intravascular coagulation; GI, gastrointestinal; MLV, modified live virus.

Suggested Reading

Greene CE. Infectious canine hepatitis and canine acidophil cell hepatitis. In: Greene CE, ed. *Infectious Diseases of the Dog and Cat.* 2nd ed. Philadelphia: WB Saunders; 1998:22–28.

Author: Sharon A. Center
Consulting Editor: Stephen C. Barr

Infectious Canine Tracheobronchitis (Kennel Cough)

chapter 57

DEFINITION/OVERVIEW

- Any contagious respiratory disease of dogs that is manifested by acute onset of paroxysmal coughing.

ETIOLOGY/PATHOPHYSIOLOGY

- Etiology—usually complex involving viral (canine distemper, CAV-2, CPI, CAV-1, canine reovirus, and canine herpes virus), bacterial (*Bordetella bronchiseptica* as a primary pathogen and other secondary pathogens, including *Pseudomonas* spp., *Escherichia coli*, *Klebsiella* spp., *Pasteurella* spp., and *Streptococcus* spp.), and mycoplasma.
- CAV-2 and CPI—may damage respiratory epithelium to such an extent that invasion by bacteria and mycoplasma causes severe airway disease.
- *Bordetella bronchiseptica*—a gram-negative bacterium with an incubation period of about 6 days, replicates on cilia of respiratory epithelium; produces a number of toxins that impair phagocytosis and cause ciliastasis; produces strong local immunity but may persist in the respiratory tract for up to 3 months.
- *Mycoplasma* spp.—endogenous to the nasopharynx, but not usually found in the lower respiratory tract; takes advantage of damaged mucosa (such as viral, or physical damage); infection leads to a purulent bronchitis.

SIGNALMENT/HISTORY

- All ages susceptible—puppies 6 weeks to 6 months of age most severely affected.
- Dogs with preexisting respiratory conditions—at higher risk for developing severe disease.
- History of exposure—often in kennel/boarding situation with high-density housing, where rapid spread from seemingly healthy dogs to others can occur.
- Signs—usually develop 4 to 7 days after exposure.
- Historically—in uncomplicated cases, cough develops in otherwise healthy animal.
  - Dry and hacking, soft and dry, moist and hacking or paroxysmal coughing followed by gagging or expectoration of white foamy mucus often worse after exercise (clients often complain that dog is vomiting up white foam).

- Severe complicated cases:
  - Anorexia.
  - Moist, productive cough.
  - Lethargy.
  - Dyspnea and exercise intolerance.

CLINICAL FEATURES

- Uncomplicated—cough readily induced with tracheal pressure; other physical examination findings, including lung sounds, usually normal.
- Severe—low-grade fever, tachypnea, dyspnea, cough, increased lung sounds, crackles, and wheezes (less frequently).
- Paroxysmal cough—easily elicited on tracheal palpation.

DIFFERENTIAL DIAGNOSIS

- A general differential diagnosis for cough includes such categories as:
  - Cardiovascular (pulmonary edema; pleural effusions; enlarged heart, especially the left atrium; pulmonary emboli).
  - Allergic (bronchitis, eosinophilic pneumonia or granulomatosis, pulmonary infiltrate with eosinophilis).
  - Trauma (foreign body, irritating gases, collapsing trachea).
  - Neoplasia (not only of the respiratory tree but also associated structures such as ribs, lymph nodes, muscles).
  - Inflammatory (pharyngitis, tonsillitis, bacterial bronchopneumonia, chronic pulmonary fibrosis, pulmonary abscess or granuloma, chronic obstructive pulmonary disease).
  - Parasites (*Capillaria aerophila, Oslerus* [*Filaroides*] *osleri, Filaroides hirthi, F. milksi, Paragonimus kellicotti, Dirofilaria immitis*—heartworm disease).
- Kennel cough—often a clinical diagnosis based on a history of sudden onset, recent exposure to likely pathogens (boarding), lack of recent vaccinations for the respiratory pathogens, lack of other clinical signs other than cough, and cough easily induced upon even slight tracheal palpation.

DIAGNOSTICS

- CBC—usually normal; in severe cases, leukocytosis with neutrophilia and left shift.
- Serum biochemical profile and urinalysis—normal.
- Thoracic radiography—normal or mild bronchial pattern; in severe cases and those complicated by bronchopneumonia, interstitial and alveolar lung pattern found, often with a cranioventral distribution typical of bacterial pneumonia.
- Transtracheal wash—perform only if resistant to initial therapy; to isolate organism by culture for antibacterial sensitivity studies; examine cytology for type of inflammation and other causes (parasitic).

THERAPEUTICS

- Strongly recommend—to treat uncomplicated cases as outpatients to prevent hospital contamination.
- Hospitalize—only those with pneumonia that require IV fluid support.
- Enforced rest—for at least 14 to 21 days (uncomplicated cases); 2 months in cases of pneumonia.
- Owner should be aware of infectivity of dog to other dogs—should be encouraged to isolate the patient from other dogs (even up to months after recovery because *B. bronchiseptica* can be present in respiratory tract for months after infection).
- Dogs with uncomplicated disease—should respond to treatment in 10 to 14 days.

Drugs of Choice

- Broad-spectrum antibiotics in uncomplicated cases—amoxicillin/clavulanic acid, doxycycline, or TMS.
- Severe cases that are resistant to first-choice antibiotic therapies above—combination therapy of an aminoglycoside (gentamicin or amikacin) with a cephalosporin (cefazolin). May use enrofloxacin as alternative to gentamicin.
- In severe cases (bronchopneumonia)—continue at least 2 weeks past radiographic resolution of signs.
- Resistant bacteria (*B. bronchiseptica* and others)—important to culture and establish the bacterial sensitivity; may need to deliver antibiotics by nebulization (kanamycin 250 mg; gentamicin 50 mg; polymixin B 333,000 IU) for 3 to 5 days.
- Cough suppressants—butorphanol (Torbutrol [Fort Dodge, Fort Dodge, IA] or hydrocodone bitartrate (Hycodan) [DuPont Pharma, Wilmington, DE]) often effective in suppressing a dry, nonproductive cough.
- Bronchodilators (theophylline or aminophylline)—offer little help but may relieve clinically apparent wheezing (*Table 57-1*).
- Vaccination—available for *B. bronchiseptica* and CPI; intranasal vaccines generally considered to offer superior protection because they induce both local and systemic immunity, they are not affected by maternal antibody, and they protect against challenge more rapidly than parenteral vaccines; vaccinate puppies intranasally as early as 2 to 4 weeks of age, followed by revaccination annually; may vaccinate mature dogs with a one-dose intranasal vaccination; a single booster at least 5 days before exposure in dogs not vaccinated in the previous 6 months is recommended.
- Best protection is achieved when both intranasal and parenteral vaccines given together or sequentially.

Precautions/Interactions

- Do not use cough suppressants in patients with pneumonia or productive coughs.
- TMS—multiple adverse reactions, including:
  - KCS—monitor tear production weekly throughout treatment.
  - Hepatotoxicity—anorexia, depression, icterus; monitor ALT—if prolonged therapy.

TABLE 57-1. Drug Therapy for Canine Infectious Tracheobronchitis (Kennel Cough)

Drug	Dose (mg/kg)	Route	Interval (Hours)	Duration (Days)
Amocicillin-clavulanic acid	12.5–25	PO	12	10–14
Doxycycline	5	PO	12	10–14
Trimethoprim-sulfadiazine	15	PO, IV	12	10–14
Gentamicin[a]	6	IV, SC, IM	24	14
Amikacin[a]	6.5	IV, SC, IM	8	14
Cefazolin[b]	20–35	IV, IM	8	14–28
Enrofloxacin[c]	2.5–5	PO, IV, IM	12	14–28
Butorphanol	0.55	PO	8–12	[d]
Hydrocodone bitartrate	0.22	PO	6–8	[d]
Theophylline	10	PO	8	[d]
Aminophylline	10	PO, IM, IV	8	[d]

[a] Use in combination with a cephalosporin or penicillin; monitor for nephrotoxicity by examining urine for cast formation.
[b] Use in combination with an aminoglycoside.
[c] Use as an alternative to aminoglycosides.
[d] Use for extended periods to suppress cough.

- Megaloblastic-folate acid deficiency anemia—especially in cats after several weeks; supplement with folinic acid (2.5 mg/kg/day).
- Immune-mediated polyarthritis, retinitis, glomerulonephritis, vasculitis, anemia, thrombocytopenia, urticaria, toxic epidermal necrolysis, erythema multiforme, and conjunctivitis—remove from drug.
- Renal failure and interference with renal excretion of potassium—leading to hyperkalemia.
- Salivation, diarrhea, and vomiting (cats).
- May interfere with thyroid hormone synthesis (dogs)—check T_3 and T_4 after 6 weeks.

■ TMS—use with caution in neonates and pregnant patients.
■ Fluoroquinolones—avoid use in pregnant, neonatal or growing animals (medium-sized dogs <8 months of age; large or giant breeds <12 to 18 months of age) because of cartilage lesions.
■ Fluoroquinolones and theophylline derivatives—used together may increase the plasma theophylline concentrations to toxic levels.
■ Intranasal vaccine—can induce a cough or nasal discharge 2 to 5 days postinoculation, whereas parenteral vaccination does not.

 COMMENTS

■ If infection is established in a kennel situation, evacuate the kennel for 1 to 2 weeks and disinfect with sodium hypochlorite (1:30 dilution), chlorhexidine, or benzalkonium.

- Uncomplicated cases should resolve within 10 to 14 days; if patient continues to cough beyond 14 days, question the diagnosis of uncomplicated disease.
- Dogs recovering from *B. bronchiseptica* infection are immune for at least 6 months.

Abbreviations

ALT, alanine aminotransferase; CAV, canine adenovirus; CBC, complete blood count; CPI, canine parainfluenza; KCS, keratoconjunctivitis sicca; TMS, trimethoprim-sulfadiazine.

Suggested Reading

Ellis JA, Krakowka GS, Dayton, et al. Effect of vaccination on experimental infection with *Bordetella bronchiseptica* in dogs. *J Am Vet Med Assoc* 2001;218:367–375.
Ford BB, Vaden SL. Canine infectious tracheobronchitis. In: Greene CE, ed. *Infectious Diseases of the Dog and Cat.* Philadelphia: WB Saunders; 1998:33–38.

Author: Johnny D. Hoskins
Consulting Editor: Stephen C. Barr

chapter 58

Kidney Worm (Dioctophyma)

DEFINITION/OVERVIEW

- A nematode parasite (the largest in existence), the adults of which are found in the abdominal cavity and renal pelvis of dogs (rarely infect cats).

ETIOLOGY/PATHOPHYSIOLOGY

- *Dioctyophyma renale*—mink are the definitive host (in which the adult worm is much smaller); occasionally found in dogs.
- Female worm (can reach 1 meter in length)—lays brownish, thick-shelled eggs with bipolar plugs.
- Eggs—passed in the urine; mature to larvated eggs (if enter water) over about a month.
- Larvated eggs—infect earthworms to hatch L1 that develop to L3.
- Dogs—become infected after ingesting paratenic hosts (intestines of fish or frogs) or earthworms containing the L3.
- L3 larvae—migrate through the stomach wall, cross the peritoneal cavity to enter the liver, where they molt to L4.
- L4 larvae—enter the peritoneal cavity, molt to adults before entering the renal capsule.
- Adult worms—migrate to the renal pelvis (usually of the right kidney).
- Exact mechanism of how adult worms destroy the renal parenchyma—unknown.
- Hydronephrosis and pyelonephritis may play a role in the pathogenesis.
- Histopathology—shows destruction of the renal tubules surrounded by chronic inflammation, with preservation of many glomeruli.
- Worms in the peritoneal cavity—produce a serofibrinous to chronic fibrinous peritonitis.
- Worms in close proximity to the liver—cause large erosions on the liver (and even severe hemorrhage from liver rupture)
- Eggs—often found within chronic granulomas within the peritoneal cavity.
- The severity of renal disease—depends on the number of parasites in the kidney, the number of kidneys infected, duration of infection, and the presence of concomitant renal disease.

SIGNALMENT/HISTORY

Dogs

- Exceptionally rare in the dog, given its relatively high prevalence in the wild.
- Usually dogs have a history of ingesting earthworms or the raw viscera of fish.

Cats

- Last natural infection—reported in the 1930s.

CLINICAL FEATURES

- Most cases—asymptomatic.
- Most infections—restricted to the abdominal cavity, producing a mild peritonitis.
- Infections involving the kidneys—hematuria, right renomegaly, and UTI.
- Renal failure—if both kidneys are infected (very rare).
- Renomegaly (especially right kidney)—on abdominal palpation.

DIFFERENTIAL DIAGNOSIS

- Other causes of hematuria with unilateral renomegaly:
  - Neoplasia (renal carcinoma, hemangiosarcoma).
  - Unilateral hydronephrosis.
  - Trauma.

DIAGNOSTICS

- Urinalysis—large (68×44 μm) brown, thick-shelled eggs with bipolar plugs.
- Urinalysis—occult blood, elevated protein, and RBCs and WBCs per high-power field too numerous to count, consistent with pyelonephritis or UTI.
- Serum biochemistry profile—usually normal unless in renal failure (BUN and creatine, low urine specific gravity).
- Abdominal ultrasound—coiled parasite within the pelvis of the right kidney; mild fibrinous peritonitis.
- Renal function tests—often show reduced function of the right kidney (if only one infected) and compensation of the left kidney.

■ **Fig. 58-1** A kidney removed surgically from a dog containing an adult *Dioctyphyma renale* worm (courtesy Dr. Carl A. Osborne, University of Minnesota).

 ## THERAPEUTICS

- If no biochemical signs of renal insufficiency exist, and infection is confined to one kidney—surgically remove that kidney *(Fig. 58-1)*.
- If both kidneys are infected, but renal function tests show good renal function—attempt to remove the worms from one renal pelvis by surgery.
- Examine abdominal cavity thoroughly for the presence of adult worms at the time of surgery.

Drugs of Choice

- None identified

 ## COMMENTS

- Although *D. renale* has been reported in humans (exceptionally rare), they cannot become infected by ingesting eggs passed in the urine of dogs.
- Dogs should be prevented from ingesting raw fish (especially their viscera) or earthworms.

Abbreviations

BUN, blood urea nitrogen; RBCs, red blood cells; UTI, urinary tract infection; WBCs, white blood cells.

Suggested Reading

Osborne CA, Stevens JB, Hanlon GF, et al. *Dioctyphyma renale* in the dog. *J Am Vet Med Assoc* 1969;155:605–620.

Author: Stephen C. Barr
Consulting Editor: Stephen C. Barr

Leishmaniasis

DEFINITION/OVERVIEW

- An uncommon protozoal infection of dogs affecting skin, liver, spleen, kidneys, eyes, and joints.
- Cats—rarely (skin).

ETIOLOGY/PATHOPHYSIOLOGY

- Protozoan—genus *Leishmania*.
- Acquisition—in the United States, dogs acquire infection in two different ways:
  - Overseas, usually from an infected vector—*L. donovani infantum* (Mediterranean basin, Portugal, and Spain; sporadic cases in Switzerland, northern France, and the Netherlands); *L. donovani* complex or *L. braziliensis* (endemic areas of South and Central America and southern Mexico).
  - Endemic—in the Foxhound population in North America (*L. donovani infantum*).
- Sandfly vector—transmit flagellated parasites into the skin of a host.
- Vector unknown in North America—transfusion of blood products, direct contact with other dogs, or transplacentally are other methods of transmission that can occur in dogs.
- Dogs—organism invariably spreads throughout the body to most organs.
- Renal failure—most common cause of death in dogs.
- Cats—organism often localizes in skin.
- Incubation period—1 month to several years.

SIGNALMENT/HISTORY

Dogs

- Virtually all develop visceral or systemic disease.
- 90% also have cutaneous involvement.
- No sex or breed predilection.

Cats

- Cutaneous disease is rare.
- No sex or breed predilection.

■ **Fig. 59-1** Hyperkeratosis, excessive epidermal scale, nodule, and some alopecia over the head of a dog with leishmaniasis.

 CLINICAL FEATURES

Dogs

- Exercise intolerance.
- Severe weight loss and anorexia.
- Fever (33% of patients).
- Splenomegaly (33% of patients).
- Diarrhea.
- Vomiting.
- Epistaxis and melena (less common).
- Generalized lymphadenopathy.
- Cutaneous lesions—hyperkeratosis most prominent finding, often bilaterally symmetrical over the head *(Fig. 59-1)*; excessive epidermal scale with thickening, depigmentation, and chapping of the muzzle and foodpads; dry brittle hair coat with hair loss; intradermal nodules and ulcers may be seen *(Fig. 59-2)*; abnormally long or brittle nails in some patients.
- Signs of renal failure terminally—polyuria, polydipsia, vomiting.
- Rare signs—neuralgia, polyarthritis, polymyositis, osteolytic lesions, and proliferative periostitis.

Cats

- Cutaneous nodules—especially on the ears.

 DIFFERENTIAL DIAGNOSIS

- Visceral—mycoses (blastomycosis, histoplasmosis); SLE; metastatic neoplasia; distemper; and vasculitis.
- Cutaneous—other causes of hyperkeratosis: primary idiopathic seborrhea and nutritional dermatoses (vitamin A responsive, zinc responsive); idiopathic nasodigital

■ **Fig. 59-2** Dermal ulcers over the hock of a dog with advanced leishmaniasis. Impression smear of such a lesion would easily demonstrate typical intracellular organisms.

hyperkeratosis, lichenoid-psoriasiform dermatosis, mucocutaneous syndrome, pemphigus foliaceus, epidermal dysplasia, and Schnauzer comedo syndrome are rare and breed specific.

- Skin biopsy—hyperkeratotic and nodular lesions; existence of organisms confirms diagnosis of leishmaniasis.
- Hyperglobulinemia—need to differentiate from chronic ehrlichiosis and multiple myeloma.

 ## DIAGNOSTICS

- Hyperproteinemia with hyperglobulinemia—100% of cases.
- Hypoalbuminemia—95% of cases.
- Proteinuria—85% of cases.
- High hepatic enzyme activity—55% of cases.
- Thrombocytopenia—50% of cases.
- Azotemia—45% of cases.
- Leukopenia with lymphopenia—20% of cases.
- Coombs', ANA, and lupus erythematosus cell tests—sometimes positive.
- Serologic diagnosis by IFA or ELISA available—most tests give cross-reaction to *Trypanosoma cruzi* (closely related organism); differentiate based on clinical signs, history, and likelihood of exposure.
- Culture of skin, spleen, bone marrow, or lymph node tissue—send to the CDC.

■ **Fig. 59-3** Bone marrow aspirate showing typical intracellular organisms containing both a nucleus and kine-doplast typical of *Leishmania* (Wright-Geimsa stain, 1,000×).

Diagnostic Feature

- **Cytology is diagnostic method of choice (same samples as cultured)—identify typical intracellular organisms *(Fig. 59-3).***

 THERAPEUTICS

- Outpatient.
- Use multiple drugs (if able to obtain them)—induce initially with amphotericin B or sodium stibogluconate (if available) and keep on allopurinol for entire life (maintenance).
- Emaciated, chronically infected animals—consider euthanasia; prognosis very poor.
- Diet—high-quality protein; special for renal insufficiency, if necessary.
- Cats—single dermal nodule lesions are best surgically removed.

Drugs of Choice

- Sodium stibogluconate (Pentostam [available from the CDC]); interferes with energy metabolism; expensive; excellent initial clinical response; relapses common months to years after stop treating.
- Allopurinol—organism hydrolyzes the drug to an aberrant isomer of inosine, which becomes incorporated into RNA and interferes with protein synthesis; cheap and nontoxic; produces clinical cure, but relapses occur; best when used in combination with other drugs for long-term maintenance; probably does not prevent transmission in endemic regions.
- Amphotericin B (Fungizone, BM Squibb, New York, NY)—poorly absorbed into bone, eyes and body cavities; nephrotoxic; when combined with allopurinol, has improved efficacy.

TABLE 59-1. Drug Therapy for Leishmaniasis in Dogs

Drug	Dose (mg/kg)	Route	Interval (Hours)	Duration (Months)
Sodium stibogluconate (Pentostam)	30–50	IV, SC	24	1
Allopurinol	7–10	PO	8	3–24[a]
Amphotericin B (Fungizone)	0.25–0.5[b]	IV	48[c]	[d]
Meglumine antimonite[e] (Glucantime)	100	IV, SC	24	1

[a] Or for rest of dog's life.
[b] Reconstituted in 5% dextrose (do not reconstitute in electrolyte solutions, which precipitate the drug) and dilute to administer; if normal renal function, dilute in 60 to 120 ml 5% dextrose given over 15 minutes; if renal compromise, dilute in 0.5 to 1 liter 5% dextrose given over 3 to 4 hours to reduce further renal toxicity.
[c] Or 3 times a week.
[d] Administer until a total cumulative dose of 5 to 10 mg/kg is reached.
[e] Not available in the United States.

- Meglumine antimonite (Glucantime, Merial, Iselin, NJ [not available in North America])—probably the most efficacious drug when combined with allopurinol (*Table 59-1*).

Precautions/Interactions

- Seriously ill dogs—start antimonial drugs at lower doses.
- Renal insufficiency—treat before giving antimonial drugs; prognosis depends on renal function at the onset of treatment.
- Sodium stibogluconate—pain at injection site; resistance has been identified in Europe due to underdosing of drug.
- Amphotericin B—nephrotoxicity needs to be monitored by examining renal sediment for casts; perivascular injection can cause severe phlebitis.
- Treatment efficacy—monitor by clinical improvement and identification of organisms in repeat biopsies.
- Relapses—a few months to a year after therapy; recheck at least every 2 months after completion of treatment.
- Relapses—identified by monitoring rise in blood globulins or reappearance of clinical signs in a dog previously in remission.
- Prognosis for a cure—very guarded, even when using best treatment (meglumine with allopurinol).

 COMMENTS

- Leishmaniasis is a notifiable disease—confirmed cases must be reported to the CDC.
- Advise client—potential zoonotic transmission of organisms in lesions to humans is possible.
- Inform client—organisms will never be eliminated, and relapses, requiring treatment, are inevitable.

Abbreviations

ANA, antinuclear antibody; CDC, Centers for Disease Control and Prevention; ELISA, enzyme-linked immunosorbent assay; IFA, immunofluorescence assay; RNA, ribonucleic acid; SLE, systemic lupus erythematosus.

Suggested Reading

Lindsay DS, Zajac AM, Barr SC. Canine leishmaniasis in American foxhounds: an emerging zoonosis? *Comp Cont Educ Pract Vet* 2002;24:304–312.

Schantz PM, Steurer FJ, Duprey ZH, et. al. Autochthonous visceral leishmaniasis in dogs in North America. *J Am Vet Med Assoc* 2005;226:1316–1322.

Author: Stephen C. Barr
Consulting Editor: Stephen C. Barr

Leptospirosis

DEFINITION/OVERVIEW

- A systemic bacterial infection of dogs (and very rarely, cats), causing mainly acute nephritis and hepatitis, vasculitis, and chronic carrier states.

ETIOLOGY/PATHOPHYSIOLOGY

- Pathogenic members of the genus *Leptospira*—main serovars causing disease in dogs include *L. pomona* and *L. grippotyphosa*, occasionally *L. autumnalis* and *L. bratislava*, and, rarely, *L. canicola* and *L. icterohaemorrhagiae*.
- Direct transmission—host-to-host contact via infected urine, postabortion discharge, infected fetus/discharge, and sexual contact (semen).
- Indirect transmission—exposure (via urine) to a contaminated environment (vegetation, soil, food, water, and bedding) under conditions in which *Leptospira* organisms can survive.
- *Leptospira* spp.—penetrate intact or cut skin or mucous membranes; rapidly invade bloodstream (4 to 7 days); spread to all parts of the body (2 to 4 days).
- Invasion—leads to transient fever, leukocytosis, transitory anemia (hemolysis), mild hemoglobinuria, and albuminuria; capillary and endothelial cell damage (occasionally results in petechial hemorrhages); liver necrosis and jaundice; acute nephritis with leptospiruria (organism replicates readily in tubular epithelial cell).
- Vasculitis—may cause interstitial pneumonia, anterior uveitis, myocardial damage and meningitis (rare), and abortions.
- Death—usually a result of interstitial nephritis, vascular damage, and renal failure; may result from acute septicemia or DIC.
- Usually one or more serovars account for endemic disease in a geographic area—overall reported incidence probably falsely low because most infections are inapparent (undiagnosed).
- Distribution—worldwide, especially in warm, wet climates or seasons.
- Standing water and neutral or slightly alkaline soil—promote presence in environment.
- Most cases—occur during late summer/fall in northeastern United States.

SIGNALMENT/HISTORY

- Dogs in rural habitat.
- Young dogs without passive maternal antibody are more likely to exhibit severe disease.
- Old dogs with adequate antibody titer levels seldom exhibit clinical disease unless exposed to a serovar not in the vaccine.
- Dense animal population (kennels and urban settings) increases chances of urine exposure, exposure to rodents, and other wildlife (hunting dogs).
- Historically:
  - Peracute/acute—fever, sore muscles, stiffness, weakness, anorexia, depression, acute onset of vomiting, rapid dehydration, diarrhea (occasional bloody), occasionally icterus, cough with mild respiratory distress if respiratory component severe, and polyuria/polydipsia progressing to anuria.
  - Chronic—usually no apparent illness; polyuria/polydipsia if chronic renal failure.

CLINICAL FEATURES

- Peracute/acute disease.
  - Tachypnea.
  - Tachycardia, sometimes with arrhythmias.
  - Poor capillary perfusion.
  - Hematemesis.
  - Hematochezia.
  - Melena.
  - Epistaxis.
  - Injected mucous membranes.
  - Petechial and ecchymotic hemorrhages.
  - Reluctance to move, stiff gait.
  - Paraspinal hyperesthesia.
  - Conjunctivitis, uveitis (*Fig. 60-1*), blepharospasm.
  - Hematuria.
  - Harsh respiratory sounds on auscultation.
  - Mild lymphadenopathy (occasionally).

DIFFERENTIAL DIAGNOSIS

Dogs

- Subacute/acute disease—any severe systemic disease involving mainly the liver or kidneys alone, or together: heartworm disease, immune-mediated hemolytic anemia, bacteremia/septicemia (bite wound, prostatitis, endocarditis, dental disease), infec-

■ **Fig. 60-1** Hyphema and uveitis in a dog with leptospirosis (courtesy Dr. R. Riis, Cornell University).

tious canine hepatitis virus, CHV, hepatic neoplasia, lupus, RMSF, ehrlichiosis, toxoplasmosis, acute nephritis, renal neoplasia, and renal calculi, trauma.
■ Reproductive failure—brucellosis, distemper, and herpes.

Cats

■ Much more rare; consider other causes of acute systemic hepatic and nephritic disease: haemobartonellosis, bacteremia/septicemia, FIV- and FeLV-associated diseases, cholangitis, toxoplasmosis, FIP, hepatic neoplasia, autoimmune disease (e.g., SLE), renal calculi, renal neoplasia, trauma, drugs (acetaminophen).

 DIAGNOSTICS

■ CBC—signs of dehydration (PCV and total plasma solids elevated), leukocytosis with left shift, thrombocytopenia.
■ Serum biochemistry profile—elevated BUN, creatine, and hepatic enzymes are main changes.
■ Other changes—due to dehydration or renal failure (electrolyte changes include hyponatremia, hypochloremia, hyperkalemia, hyperphosphatemia, hypoalbuminemia).
■ Urinalysis—proteinuria, isosthenuria usually, and casts.
■ Chronic carrier states—may only see isosthenuria, with few granular casts in urine.
■ Serologic examination—MAT; test in acute stage and 3 to 4 weeks later (convalescent serum); in unvaccinated patients, titers may be low initially (1:100 to 1:200), then

rise during convalescents (1:800 to 1:1600 or higher); several serovars usually show elevated titer but make serovar diagnosis based on highest titer.

- MAT titers in vaccinated dogs—vaccination causes elevation of MAT titer in most cases but usually only to serovars vaccinated against (no cross-reactivity); do get MAT titer elevations to *L. autumnalis* after vaccination with subunit vaccines against *L. grippotyphosa* and *L. pomona* (Fort Dodge).
- Dogs vaccinated with whole cell bacteria—usually develop higher MAT titers (up to 1:800) than subunit vaccines (negative to 1:400).
- MAT titers induced by vaccination—usually only last up to 4 months.
- MAT titers induced by infection—usually last over 12 months.
- Darkfield microscopy of urine—often inconclusive because it is difficult to read and requires fresh urine.
- FA test of urine—more conclusive because leptospires do not need to be viable; submit urine to laboratory on ice by overnight courier; pretreatment with furosemide (2 mg/kg, SC) 15 minutes before urine collection will increase success rate.
- PCR on urine—offered by some commercial laboratories; shown in 1 dog out of 8 to detect organisms in urine before development of serologic titer; needs more work in experimentally infected dogs before being well validated.
- Culture—usually unrewarding.

THERAPEUTICS

- Tissue diagnosis (kidney biopsy)—FA, immunohistochemistry, Warthin-Starry silver stain, and PCR are all effective.
- Inpatient for acute severe disease—extent of supportive therapy depends on severity; renal failure requires closely monitored diuresis, attention to DIC development; care must be taken not to overhydrate, because vasculitis of respiratory endothelium can lead to pulmonary edema during diuresis.
- Vaccines—bacterin and subunit vaccines available against *L. canicola* and *L. icterohaemorrhagiae*, and subunit vaccine available against *L. pomona*, *L. grippotyphosa*; most claim year efficacy except those subunit vaccines covering *L. pomona* and *L. grippotyphosa* (protect for 2 to 2½ weeks after booster); no cross protection outside of the serovars used in vaccine serogroup); revaccination at least yearly; vaccinate dogs at risk (hunter, show dogs, dogs with access to water/ponds) every 4 to 6 months, especially in endemic areas; does not protect against carrier state; associated with a high incidence of anaphylaxis (particularly bacterin vaccines) after booster doses occurring within 1 hour of booster.

Drugs of Choice

- Doxycycline (Vibramycin®, Pfizer, Exton, PA)—use alone to clear leptospiremia and leptospiruria, as well as carrier state.
- If doxycycline to be used, unnecessary to use penicillin.
- Penicillin compounds—may be used during acute leptospiremic phase if unable to administer doxycycline (*Table 60-1*).

TABLE 60-1. Drug Therapy for Leptospirosis in Dogs				
Drug	Dose (mg/kg)	Route	Interval (Hours)	Duration (Weeks)
Doxycycline	5	PO, IV	12	2
Penicillin G	25,000–40,000 U/kg	IM, SC, IV	12	2
Ampicillin	22	PO, SC, IV	6–8	2
Amoxicillin	22	PO	8–12	2

- Streptomycin—will clear organisms from kidneys but difficult to obtain and may potentiate renal insufficiency.

Precautions/Interactions

- If vomiting, use injectable doxycycline.

COMMENTS

- Inform client—of zoonotic potential from contaminated urine of affected dogs and their environment.
- Kennels—strict sanitation to avoid contact with infected urine; control rodents; monitor and remove carrier dogs until treated; isolate affected animals during treatment; disinfect premises, using iodine-based disinfectant or stabilized bleach solutions.
- Activity—limit access to marshy/muddy areas, ponds, low-lying areas with stagnant surface water, heavily irrigated pastures, and wildlife.
- Chronic active hepatitis and chronic interstitial nephritis—can occur as chronic disease.

Abbreviations

BUN, blood urea nitrogen; CBC, complete blood count; CHV, canine herpes virus; DIC, disseminated intravascular coagulation; FA, fluorescent antibody; FeLV, feline leukemia virus; FIP, feline infectious peritonitis; FIV, feline immunodeficiency virus; MAT, microagglutination titer; PCR, polymerase chain reaction; PCV, packed cell volume; RMSF, Rocky Mountain spotted fever; SLE, systemic lupus erythematosus.

Suggested Reading

Adin CA, Cowgill LD. Treatment and outcome of dogs with leptospirosis: 36 cases (1990–1998). *J Am Vet Med Assoc* 2000;216:371–375.

Birnbaum N, Barr SC, Center SA, et al. Naturally acquired leptospirosis in 36 dogs: serological and clinicopathological features. *J Small Anim Pract* 1998;39:231–236.

Harkin KR, Roshto YM, Sullivan JT. Clinical application of a polymerase chain reaction assay for diagnosis of leptospirosis in dogs. *J Am Vet Med Assoc* 2003;222:1224–1229.

Langston CE, Heuter KJ. Leptospirosis: a re-emerging zoonotic disease. *Vet Clin North Am Small Anim Pract* 2003;33:791–807.

Ward MP, Glickman LT, Guptill LE. Prevalence of and risk factors of leptospirosis among dogs in the United States and Canada: 677 cases (1970–1998). *J Am Vet Med Assoc* 2002;220:53–58.

Author: Patrick L. McDonough
Consulting Editor: Stephen C. Barr

L-form Bacterial Infections

DEFINITION/OVERVIEW

- Infections, usually at the site of entry (arthritis in dogs, bite wounds in cats), caused by bacteria that have lost their cell wall or that have a defective cell wall.

ETIOLOGY/PATHOPHYSIOLOGY

- Soft pleomorphic spherical and osmotically fragile organisms.
- Differ from mycoplasma by lack of sterols in their membranes.
- Grow and replicate by cell fission; yield daughter cells that vary in size, nucleic acid content, and amount of cytoplasm.
- Formed as spontaneous variants of bacteria or when cell wall synthesis is inhibited or impaired by antibiotics, specific immunoglobulins, or lysosomal enzymes that degrade cell walls.
- Virtually all gram-positive or gram-negative bacteria are capable of forming L-forms.
- Formation stimulated by antibiotic use, resistance of host, suitability of in vivo site in host for developing infective foci, and relatively low to moderate virulence of infecting bacterium.
- May revert to normal cell wall strain in a suitable host.
- Usually no pathogenicity.
- Can be isolated from humans, animals, and plants.

SIGNALMENT/HISTORY

- Sporadic in cats and dogs.
- Most common in free-roaming cats; all ages.

CLINICAL FEATURES

Dogs

- Arthritis.
- Fever.
- Local lymphadenopathy.

Cats

- Penetrating wounds (usually cat bites).
- Infected surgical sites.
- Cellulitis.
- Fever
- Arthritis.
- Synovitis.

DIFFERENTIAL DIAGNOSIS

Dogs

- Other causes of arthritis—immune-mediated disease; Lyme disease; mycoplasma; rickettsia; and fungal.

Cats

- Other causes of suppurative skin infections—wounds infected with bacteria; mycobacterium; yeast; and fungi.

DIAGNOSTICS

- CBC—neutrophilia with left shift; monocytosis; lymphocytosis; eosinophilia; occasionally, mild normocytic normochromic anemia (anemia of chronic disease).
- Cytologic examination of infected wound—nondiagnostic (suppurative inflammation).
- Joint fluid from infected joint—high neutrophil count.
- Radiologic examination of joint—shows periarticular joint swelling (nonspecific).

Diagnostic Feature
- **Culture—difficult; requires special medium (Hayflick) on which colonies appear as "fried-eggs" on solid agar.**
- Light microscopy—usually of no help.
- Electron microscopy—used to differentiate from mycoplasma.

THERAPEUTICS

- Gentle cleaning of the wound will degrade organisms.
- Allow open wounds to heal by secondary intention.

Drugs of Choice

- Variable antibiotic sensitivity.
- Tetracycline (dosage: 22 mg/kg, PO, q8h for 10 days after signs disappear).

Precautions/Interactions

- Antibiotics that interfere with cell wall synthesis (β-lactam antibiotics)—not effective.

 COMMENTS

- Usually, once tetracyclines are begun and wound is appropriately drained (if necessary)—fever will resolve in 24 to 48 hours.
- Public health significance of having an infected animal around humans—unknown.

Abbreviation

CBC, complete blood count.

Suggested Reading

Carro T. L-forms and mycoplasmal infections. In: August JR, ed. *Consultations in Feline Internal Medicine*. Philadelphia: WB Saunders;: 1994:13–20.

Author: J. Paul Woods
Consulting Editor: Stephen C. Barr

Liver Fluke Infection

chapter 62

DEFINITION/OVERVIEW

- A parasitic (trematode) infection of cats in Florida, Hawaii, and many other tropical parts of the world.

ETIOLOGY/PATHOPHYSIOLOGY

- *Platynosomum concinnum*—acquired from ingestion of an infected intermediate host (usually lizards or frogs).
- Endemic areas—15% to 85% of cats are infected.
- Adults parasites—reside in the bile ducts and gallbladder of infected cats.
- Embryonated eggs—passed in cat feces to be ingested by first intermediate host (land snails).
- Sporocysts emerge from eggs within the snail—ingested by second intermediate host (anole lizards, skinks, geckos, frogs, toads), which are then ingested by cats.
- Cats—cercariae are released in upper digestive tract before migrating to bile ducts.
- Cercariae mature to adults in bile ducts—shed eggs.
- PPP = 8 weeks.
- Adult parasites—if they cause disease, produce intrahepatic bile duct obstruction and hepatic necrosis.

SIGNALMENT/HISTORY

- Typical patient—6 to 24 months old feral cat with access to local fauna.

CLINICAL FEATURES

- Depend on severity of infection.
- Most affected cats show no clinical signs.
- Affected cats may show:
  - Jaundice.
  - Emaciation.
  - Anorexia.
  - Mucoid diarrhea.

- Hepatomegaly—abdominal distention.
- Vomiting.
- Malaise.

 DIFFERENTIAL DIAGNOSIS

- Cholangiohepatitis, hepatic lipidosis, bile duct carcinoma, hepatic lymphoma, pancreatitis, and any disorder causing major bile duct occlusion.
- Differentiated by examination of cytologic specimens from hepatic or bile aspirates.

 DIAGNOSTICS

- CBC—usually eosinophilia beginning 3 weeks after infection; persists for months.
- Serum biochemistry profile—elevated hepatic enzyme activities (especially ALT and AST; ALP may be normal or only slightly elevated) and bilirubinemia (markedly high in advanced severe disease).
- Urinalysis—bilirubinuria.
- Fasting/postprandial bile acid—increased (not necessary to perform if bilirubinemia present).

Diagnostic Feature
- **Definitive diagnostic test—identification of *P. concinnum* eggs** (Fig. 62-1) **using sedimentation (formalin-ether or sodium acetate most reliable; demonstrates eight times more eggs than direct fecal examination).**

■ **Fig. 62-1** *Platynosomum concinnum* eggs in the feces of a cat infected with the liver fluke (sodium acetate sedimentation, 400×).

- Fecal eggs—detected in only 25% of cats.
- Patients with few parasites (1 to 5 flukes)—may shed only 2 to 10 eggs/gram of feces that may not be found on fecal testing, making serial examinations necessary.
- Abdominal radiographic examination—nonspecific mild hepatomegaly.
- Abdominal ultrasonography—differentiates biliary obstruction from hepatocellular disease; shows one or more of the following:
  - Biliary obstruction—dilated gallbladder, common bile duct (>2 mm), and intrahepatic ducts.
  - Gallbladder—sediment with flukes (oval hypoechoic structures with an echoic center), mildly thick gallbladder wall with a double-layered appearance (cholecystitis).
  - Overall hypoechoic hepatic parenchyma—with prominent hyperechoic portal areas (ducts) associated with cholangiohepatitis.
- Cholecystocentesis—reveals fluke eggs.
- Histopathology of biopsied liver tissue—usually definitive.

THERAPEUTICS

- Outpatient versus inpatient—depends on severity of illness.
- Inpatient—balanced polyionic solution with potassium supplementation.
- Nutritional support—important to avoid development of hepatic lipidosis:
  - Feed—high-protein canned food.
  - Ensure—cat is taking in food.
  - If anorectic—use feeding tube (nasogastric initially, place esophageal or PEG once condition is stable).
  - Cats with severe clinical signs—partial parenteral nutrition (not >5 days) or total parenteral nutrition may be necessary.
  - Hepatic encephalopathy—rare, but may develop, necessitating protein restriction.
- B vitamin supplementation—important for anorectic and ill cats on fluid therapy (2 ml of B-soluble vitamins/liter fluids).

Drugs of Choice

- Praziquantel (Droncit injectable, 56.8 mg/ml solution [Bayer, Shawnee Mission, KS])—eggs may pass in feces for up to 2 months after treatment.
- Prednisolone—initial dose for cats showing eosinophilia to decrease eosinophilic infiltration around bile ducts in liver.
- Ursodeoxycholic acid—unless there is biliary obstruction.
- Broad-spectrum antibiotic (amoxicillin/clavulanic acid)—protect from retrograde biliary tree infection with enteric organisms introduced by parasite; growth permissively encouraged by parasite death in tissues.
- Antioxidant therapy (vitamin E and *S*-adenosylmethionine)—suggested by necrotic inflammatory tissue injury.
- Antiemetics (metoclopramice)—for vomiting (*Table 62-1*).

TABLE 62-1. Drug Therapy for Liver Flukes in Cats				
Drug	**Dose (mg/kg)**	**Route**	**Interval (Hours)**	**Duration (Days)**
Praziquantel (Doncit)	20	SC	24	3–5
Prednisolone	2	PO	24	2–4[a]
Ursodeoxycholic acid	10–15	PO	24	6[b]
Amoxicillin/clavulanic acid	10–20	PO	12	2
Vitamin E	10 U	PO	24	6[b]
S-Adenosylmethionine	20	PO	24	4[c]
Metoclopramide	0.2–0.5	PO, SC, IV	6–8[d]	1[b]

[a] Then taper in 50% decrements every 2 weeks.
[b] Or until clinical signs have resolved.
[c] Until hepatic enzymes normalize.
[d] Or by constant rate infusion.

Precautions/Interactions

- Watch for signs of biliary tree obstruction—from dying adult parasites after starting praziquantel.
- Avoid ursodeoxycholic acid—in cats with biliary obstruction.

COMMENTS

- Restrict outdoor access.
- Praziquantel prophylaxis—every 3 months, especially for outdoor cats in endemic, tropical climates.
- Uncomplicated recovery in most patients treated.
- Zoonosis—no records of it infecting humans.

Abbreviations

ALP, alkaline phosphatase; ALT, alanine aminotransferase; AST, aspartate aminotransferase; CBC, complete blood count; PEG, percutaneous endoscopic gastrostomy; PPP, prepatent period.

Suggested Reading

Bowman DD, Hendrix CM, Lindsay DS, et al. *Platynosomum concinnum.* In: Bowmann DD, ed. *Feline Clinical Parasitology.* Ames, Iowa: Iowa State University Press; 2002:148–150.

Tams TR. Hepatobiliary parasites. In: Sherding RG, ed. *The Cat: Disease and Management.* Philadelphia: WB Saunders; 1994:607–611.

Authors: Colin F. Burrows and Julie Corbet Pembleton
Consulting Editor: Stephen C. Barr

chapter 63

Lung Fluke Infection
(Paragonimus)

DEFINITION/OVERVIEW

- Trematode parasite found in pulmonary cysts in dogs and cats and other mammals, including humans and mink.

ETIOLOGY/PATHOPHYSIOLOGY

- *Paragonimus kellicotti*—female lays eggs in subpleural cysts that communicate directly with a bronchiole.
- Eggs—swept up the airways, swallowed, and passed in feces.
- Life cycle—requires two intermediate hosts; the first is an aquatic snail; the second is a crayfish.
- Dogs and cats—become infected when they eat an infected crayfish.
- PPP = 4 to 5 weeks.

SIGNALMENT/HISTORY

- No sex, breed, or age predisposition.
- Hosts must have eaten a crayfish at some stage.

CLINICAL FEATURES

- Usually clinically inapparent.
- Chronic cough unresponsive to antibiotics or other therapies.
- Hemoptysis, occasionally.
- Pneumothorax, rarely.

DIFFERENTIAL DIAGNOSIS

Dogs

- A general differential diagnosis for cough includes such categories as:
  - Cardiovascular (pulmonary edema; enlarged heart, especially the left atrium; left-sided heart failure; pulmonary emboli).
  - Allergic (bronchial asthma, eosinophilic pneumonia or granulomatosis, pulmonary infiltrate with eosinophilia).
  - Trauma (foreign body, irritating gases, collapsing trachea, hypoplastic trachea).
  - Neoplasia (not only of the respiratory tree but also associated structures such as ribs, lymph nodes, muscles).
  - Inflammatory (pharyngitis; tonsillitis; kennel cough from such agents as *Bordetella bronchiseptica*, parainfluenza virus, infectious laryngotracheitis virus, and mycoplasma; bacterial bronchopneumonia; aspiration pneumonia; fungal pneumonia; chronic pulmonary fibrosis; pulmonary abscess or granuloma; chronic obstructive pulmonary disease).
  - Parasites (*Oslerus* [*Filaroides*] *osleri, Crenosoma vulpis, Filaroides hirthi, F, milksi, Dirofilaria immitis*—heartworm disease).

Cats

- Principally—allergy (feline asthma), other parasites (*Aelurostrongylus abstrusus, Capillariasis* spp., feline heartworm disease), and cardiac disease.
- Consider—trauma (diaphragmatic hernia), pleural disease (pyothorax, chylothorax), neoplasia, and inflammatory diseases.

DIAGNOSTICS

Diagnostic Feature
- **Large, single, operculated eggs present in a fecal sample or occasionally in phlegm from the animal** (*Fig. 63-1*).
- Use centrifugal flotation (sucrose technique with specific gravity of 1.275 or ZSCT with specific gravity of 1.18).
- Thoracic radiographs may reveal multiloculated cysts in dogs and interstitial nodules in cats, usually within the caudodorsal lung fields (*Fig. 63-2*); pneumothorax may be present.

THERAPEUTICS

- Pneumothorax—usually mild, requiring little treatment; excellent prognosis.
- Tension pneumothorax—if present, institute continuous external drainage, which is usually successful; prognosis fair.

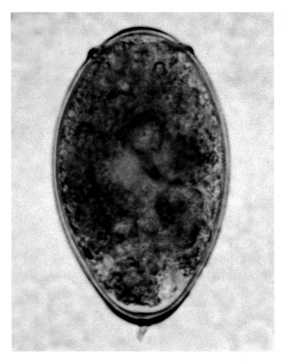

■ **Fig. 63-1** Single operculated egg of *Paragonimus kellicotti* from the feces of an infected dog.

■ **Fig. 63-2** Lateral thoracic radiograph of a dog with *Paragonimus kellicotti* infestation. Note the "coin" lesion in the dorsoventral lung fields typical of paragonimiasis.

TABLE 63-1. Drug Therapy for *Paragonimus kellicotti* in Dogs and Cats

Drug	Dose (mg/kg)	Route	Interval (Hours)	Duration (Days)
Praziquantel (Droncit)	25	PO	8	3
Fenbendazole (Panacur)	50	PO	24	10

- After 72 hours, if there is still constant flow of air into the pleural space—prognosis becomes very guarded and a thoracotomy may be the only hope of identifying and removing the lesion.

Drugs of Choice

- Praziquantel (Droncit [Bayer, Shawnee Mission, KS]); preferred treatment.
- Fenbendazole (Panacur [Intervet, Millsboro, DE]) (*Table 63-1*).

Precautions/Interactions

- Praziquantel—do not use in puppies under 4 weeks of age or kittens under 6 weeks of age.

COMMENTS

- Praziquantel—results in resolution of radiographic lesions within 8 weeks.
- Asymptomatic cases in which typical radiographic lesions have been found incidentally and eggs found on fecal examination—should be treated, because pneumothorax can occur at a later date.
- If lung biopsies are performed during thoracotomy—a large adult fluke may be extracted from the affected lung tissue (*Fig. 63-3*).

■ **Fig. 63-3** Adult *Paragonimus kellicotti* removed from a lung lesion during thoracotomy.

Abbreviations

PPP, prepatent period; ZSCT, zinc sulfate concentration technique.

Suggested Reading

Bowman DD, Frongillo MK, Johnson RC, et al. Evaluation of praziquantel for treatment of experimentally induced paragonimiasis in dogs and cats. *Am J Vet Res* 1991;52:68–71.

Harrus S, Nyska A, Colorni A, et al. Sudden death due to *Paragonimus kellicotti* infection in a dog. *Vet Parasitol* 1997;71:59–63.

Madden A, Pinckney RD, Forrest LJ. Canine paragonimosis. *Vet Med* 1999;94:783–792.

Author: Stephen C. Barr
Consulting Editor: Stephen C. Barr

chapter 64

Lyme Disease

DEFINITION/OVERVIEW

- A common bacterial tick-transmitted zoonotic diseases of dogs (rarely cats) causing recurrent arthritis with lameness and occasionally glomerulonephritis, cardiac, and neurologic disease.

ETIOLOGY/PATHOPHYSIOLOGY

- *Borrelia burgdorferi*—a spirochete.
- Acquisition—dogs acquire infection from an infected tick bite by hard ticks (*Ixodes*) (Fig. 64-1).
- Produces a generalized infection—predominantly of connective tissues, joint capsules, muscle, and lymph nodes.
- Incubation period in experimental dogs—2 to 5 months.
- Persistent *B. burgdorferi*—found in skin, muscle, connective tissues, joints, and lymph nodes.
- Rarely—found in body fluids (blood, CSF, and synovial fluid).
- Pathologic changes—with few exceptions, restricted to joints, local lymph nodes, skin at the tick bite site.
- In specific cases—pathology of the glomeruli of the kidney.
- Infection—only after tick (nymphal stage in spring or adult female in fall) is partially engorged; 24 to 48 hours after the initial infestation.
- *Ixodes* ticks—have a 2-year life cycle; larvae hatch in spring and become infected by feeding on white-footed mice (*Peromyscus leucopus*), which are persistently infected.
- Larvae molt into nymphs in the spring of the following year—stay infected or become infected by feeding on mice.
- Nymphs molt into adults in late fall of the second year—females engorge after mating on deer or other mammals, fall off, and hide under leaves until the following spring, when they each lay about 2,000 eggs.
- Male ticks—tend to stay on the deer.
- Seropositivity of dogs—varies greatly (5% to 80%) depending on tick exposure.
- Seropositivity of dogs—only about 5% of seropositive dogs in endemic areas ever develop clinical disease.
- Distribution—worldwide.
- United States—90% of cases occur in the northeast; also found in upper Mississippi region, California, and some southern states.

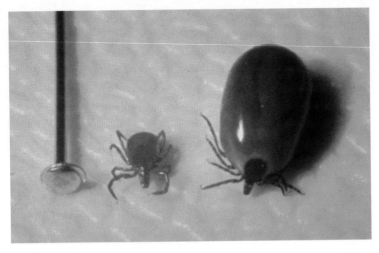

■ **Fig. 64-1** An unengorged and engorged adult *Ixodes* tick next to a pin shows the small size of these ticks.

SIGNALMENT/HISTORY

- Young dogs—appear more susceptible than older dogs.
- Historically—exposure to ticks; running in rural habitat.

CLINICAL FEATURES

- Recurrent acute arthritis with lameness—characteristic.
- Lameness—lasts for only 3 to 4 days; responds well to antibiotic treatment.
- Acute lameness—one or more joints may be swollen, warm, and painful on palpation.
- Affected dogs—may walk stiffly, with an arched back; sensitive to touch.
- Arthritis—may be accompanied by fever, anorexia, and depression.
- Superficial cervical and/or popliteal lymph nodes—may be swollen (*Fig. 64-2*).
- Cardiac—reported but rare; includes complete heart block.
- Neurologic complications—rare.
- Kidneys—reported glomerulonephritis with immune complex deposition in the glomeruli leading to fatal renal disease.
- Patients may present with renal failure due to advanced glomerulonephritis—vomiting, diarrhea, anorexia, weight loss, polyuria/polydipsia, peripheral edema, or ascites.

DIFFERENTIAL DIAGNOSIS

- Differentiate from other nonerosive inflammatory arthritides—infectious (RMSF, ehrlichiosis, histoplasma, *Cryptococcus* infection, blastomycosis, leishmaniasis, *Streptococcus* or *Staphylococcus* infection), immune-mediated diseases (idiopathic,

■ **Fig. 64-2** Swollen popliteal lymph node and a swollen stifle joint are typical of an acute arthritis seen in dogs infected with Lyme disease.

lupus erythematosus), non–immune-mediated diseases (hemarthrosis), specific breed diseases (Akita arthritis, sharpei fever).

■ Cytology and culture of the joint fluid, serologic assays, and immune testing (ANA, lupus erythematosus preparations, although low sensitivity)—to rule out other disorders.

 DIAGNOSTICS

■ CBC and serum biochemistry profile—unremarkable in dogs with arthritis only.
■ Dogs with protein-losing glomerulonephritis—uremia, proteinuria, hypercholesterolemia, hyperphosphatemia, and hypoalbuminemia usually occur.
■ Cytologic specimens from affected joints—acutely affected joints will have an increased volume of joint fluid, which will often be bloody *(Fig. 64-3)*; on smear, markedly increased WBC (mainly neutrophils) counts *(Fig. 64-4)*.
■ Serologic examination ELISA—positive titer indicates previous exposure or vaccination.
■ Western blot—used to differentiate between those with a positive vaccine titer and exposed dogs (cross-reactions with antibody responses to *Leptospira* spp. minimal).

■ **Fig. 64-3** An EDTA blood tube containing a joint aspirate from a stifle joint of a dog with Lyme disease arthritis. Note the increased volume and bloody color of the fluid.

- Canine Snap 3Dx Diagnostic Test (IDEXX Laboratories [Westbrook, ME])—an in-house snap test for antibodies against Lyme disease, *E. canis*, and heartworm antigen; measures antibody to the C6 *B. burgdorferi* protein; convenient test and eliminates antibody responses to Lyme vaccines; however, 10% false positive reactions were recently found with this test in field samples.
- PCR from skin biopsy specimens—*B. burgdorferi* frequently isolated or demonstrated; time-consuming and expensive (not practical).

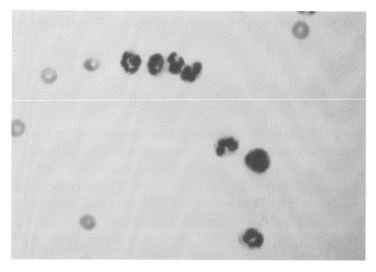

■ **Fig. 64-4** Cytology of joint fluid from a dog with Lyme arthritis showing an increased neutrophil count (Wright's stain, 400×).

TABLE 64-1. Drug Therapy for Lyme Disease in Dogs				
Drug	Dose (mg/kg)	Route	Interval (Hours)	Duration (Weeks)
Doxycycline	10	PO	12	4
Amoxicillin	20	PO	8–12	4

THERAPEUTICS

- Vaccine—two commercially available bacterins consisting of killed *B. burgdorferi* in adjuvant; one was shown to reduce the incidence of disease from 4.7% of seropositive dogs to about 1%; value still debated; single protein vaccine (OspA) protects dogs from infection and disease.
- Cage rest while lameness occurs—use pain medication or NSAIDs.

Drugs of Choice

- Doxycycline or amoxicillin are the drugs of choice (*Table 64-1*).
- Other drugs that are effective—include azithromycin, penicillin G, and chloramphenicol.
- Antibiotics do not eliminate persistent infection—significantly improve clinical signs and pathology.

Precautions/Interactions

- Doxycycline should not be used in very young pups—can cause teeth staining.

COMMENTS

- Inform client—may need to use antibiotic therapy to control arthritic reoccurrences because antibiotics are rarely totally curative.
- Acute arthritis—if no response within 3 days of starting antibiotics, reconsider diagnosis.
- Prevent tick engorgement—use repellents containing DEET or permethrin; tick collars; groom dogs daily.
- Controlling tick population in the environment—restricted to small areas; limited results from reducing deer and/or rodent population.
- Disease may be recurrent, with intervals of weeks to months—should respond again to antibiotic treatment.
- The nonresponsive chronic arthritis seen in humans—not known in dogs.
- Zoonosis—source of infection to man is ticks; experimentally.
- *B. burgdorferi* in the saliva or urine of affected dogs—not transmissible to humans.

- Dogs not a source of infected ticks to humans—once a tick starts feeding on a dog, it feeds to repletion and does not change hosts.
- No convincing evidence that *B. burgdorferi* infection is transmitted in utero in dogs—pregnant animals tolerate antibiotic treatment (do not use tetracyclines).

Abbreviations

ANA, antinuclear antibody; CBC, complete blood count; CSF, cerebrospinal fluid; ELISA, enzyme-linked immunosorbent assay; NSAIDs, nonsteroidal anti-inflammatory drugs; PCR, polymerase chain reaction; RMSF, Rocky Mountain spotted fever; WBC, white blood cell.

Suggested Reading

Appel MJG, Allan S, Jacobson RH, et al. Experimental Lyme disease in dogs produces arthritis and persistent infection. *J Infect Dis* 1993;167:651–664.

Dambach DM, Smith CA, Lewis RM, et al. Morphological, immunohistochemical, and ultrastructural characterization of a distinctive renal lesion in dogs putatively associated with *Borrelia burgdorferi* infection: 49 cases (1987–1992). *Vet Pathol* 1997;34:85–170.

Greene CE, Appel MJG, Straubinger RK. Lyme borreliosis. In: Greene CE, ed. *Infectious Diseases of the Dog and Cat*. Philadelphia: WB Saunders; 1998:282–293.

Liang ET, Jacobson RH, Straubinger RK, et al. Characterization of *Borrelia burgdorferi* VIsE invariable region useful in canine Lyme disease serodiagnosis by enzyme linked immunosorbent assay. *J Clin Microbiol* 2000;38:4160–4166.

Straubinger RK, Summers BA, Chang Y-F, et al. Persistence of *Borrelia burgdorferi* in experimentally infected dogs after antibiotic treatment. *J Clin Microbiol* 1997;35:111–116.

Author: Max J. G. Appel
Consulting Editor: Stephen C. Barr

chapter 65

Mycobacterial Infections

DEFINITION/OVERVIEW

- Rare systemic and/or cutaneous bacterial infections of dogs and cats causing a myriad of clinical entities and syndromes depending on the organism species, how the organism enters the body, and the immune function of the host.

ETIOLOGY/PATHOPHYSIOLOGY

- Mycobacteria—gram-positive, acid-fast bacteria (genus: *Mycobacterium*).
- Obligate or sporadic pathogens producing a wide range of syndromes in dogs and cats including those described in the following sections.

Tuberculosis

- *Mycobacterium tuberculosis* (humans), *M. bovis* (cattle and some wild mammals), and *M. microti* (voles).
- Dogs and cats—exposed to infected primary hosts sporadically infected.
- Dogs and cats—rare in developed countries.
- Disseminated or multiorgan disease—caused by obligate parasitic organism.

Leprosy

- *M. lepraemurium* (from rodents) and two unnamed leprosy organisms.

Cats
- Syndrome 1—affects young cats with localized nodular disease affecting limbs, with sparse to moderate numbers of acid-fast bacilli present in lesions (*M. lepraemurium*).
- Syndrome 2—affects old cats with generalized skin lesions with large numbers of acid-fast bacilli in lesions (unnamed species with affinity to *M. malmoense*).

Dogs
- Canine leproid granuloma syndrome caused by unnamed and uncultured *Mycobacterium* spp. identified by DNA sequencing.

Systemic or Noncutaneous Infection with Nontuberculosis Mycobacteria

- *M. chelonae-abscessus*, *M. avium* complex, *M. fortuitum*, *M. genavense*, *M. kansasii*, *M. smegmatis*, *M. thermoresistibile*, and *M. xenopi*.

- Sporadic infections in dogs and cats.
- Some patients with concurrent or immunosuppressing disease or the result of traumatic tissue introduction of saprophytic organism.
- Syndromes include pleuritis, localized or disseminated granulomas, disseminated disease, neuritis, bronchopneumonia.

Cutaneous/Subcutaneous Infections Due to Rapidly Growing Mycobacteria (Mycobacterial Panniculitis

- Saprophytic mycobacteria *M. fortuitum*, *M. chelonae-abcessus*, *M. smegmatis*, *M. phlei*, and *M. thermoresistibile*.

SIGNALMENT/HISTORY

Tuberculosis

- Cats and dogs of any age.
- Bassett hounds and Siamese cats reported as most susceptible—evidence unclear (possible statistical aberration).

Feline Leprosy

- Adult free-roaming cats and kittens.
- Kittens and young adult cats in syndrome 1.
- Older cats (average age 9 years) in syndrome 2.

Canine Leproid Granuloma

- Reported cases—mainly in mostly short-haired, outdoor-housed, large-breed dogs, especially boxers, and German shepherd dogs.

Systemic Nontuberculous Mycobacteriosis

- Sporadic diseas—can affect dogs and cats of any age.

Mycobacterial Panniculitis

- Adult cats and dogs.

CLINICAL FEATURES

Tuberculosis

- Correlated with the route of exposure.
- Major sites of involvement—oropharyngeal lymph nodes, cutaneous and subcutaneous tissues of the head and extremities, pulmonary system, GI system.

- Dogs—respiratory, especially coughing; dyspnea uncommon.
- Cats—from contaminated milk: weight loss, chronic diarrhea and thickened intestines; from predation: cutaneous nodules, ulcers, and draining tracts.
- Virtually all dogs and many cats—pharyngeal and cervical lymphadenopathy; retching, ptyalism, or tonsillar abscess; lymph nodes are visible or palpably firm, fixed, tender; may ulcerate and drain.
- Signs—Fever, depression, partial anorexia, and weight loss.
- Hypertrophic osteopathy—may occur.
- Disseminated disease—body cavity effusion, visceral masses, bone or joint lesions, dermal and subcutaneous masses and ulcers, lymphadenopathy and/or abscesses, CNS signs, sudden death.

Feline Leprosy

- Syndrome 1—initial localized nodules on limbs; progress rapidly, may ulcerate; aggressive clinical course; recurrence after surgical excision; widespread lesions develop in several weeks.
- Syndrome 2—initial localized or generalized skin nodules that do not ulcerate, slowly progressive over months to years.

Canine Leproid Granuloma

- One or more well-circumscribed painless nodules (2 mm to 5 cm) in dermis or subcutis; often on head or ear, but may be anywhere on the body; only very large lesions ulcerate (*Fig. 65-1*).

■ **Fig. 65-1** This well-circumscribed, painless dermal lump on the lateral thigh of this dog was caused by *M. phlei*.

■ **Fig. 65-2** A large, firm panniculitis-like lesion with pinpoint, deep draining ulcers covering the ventrum of a cat, caused by *M. smegmatis*.

■ No systemic signs of illness.

Systemic Nontuberculous Mycobacteriosis

■ Pulmonary and systemic infections with atypical mycobacteriosis are reported rarely in dogs—signs are as for TB.
■ With *M. avium* infection—disease is most often disseminated.

Mycobacterial Panniculitis

■ Cutaneous traumatic lesion that fails to heal with appropriate therapy.
■ Spreads locally in the subcutaneous tissue (panniculitis).
■ Original lesion enlarges, forming a deep ulcer that drains greasy hemorrhagic exudate.
■ Surrounding tissue becomes firm.
■ Satellite pinpoint ulcerations open and drain (*Fig. 65-2*).
■ Wound dehiscence at surgery sites
■ Systemic signs uncommon.

 DIFFERENTIAL DIAGNOSIS

Tuberculosis

■ Systemic mycoses, neoplasia (lymphoma), disseminated mast cell tumor, systemic histiocytosis, plague, nocardiosis, and other myobacterial infections.

Feline Leprosy

■ Plague, L-form bacterial infections, *Rhodococcus equi* infection, chronic bite wound abscess, neoplasia, mycetoma, dermatophyte pseudomycetoma, and other mycobacterial infections (especially cutaneous tuberculosis).

- If acid-fast organisms are identified on cytology/biopsy—consider tuberculosis or cutaneous nocardiosis, both of which can be fastidious and slow growing in culture, leading to the suspicion of an unculturable leprosy organism.

Atypical Mycobacteriosis

- Foreign body, bacterial abscess, L-form bacteria, feline leprosy, cutaneous tuberculosis, *Rhodococcus equi* infection, nocardiosis, sterile nodular panniculitis, deep pyoderma and cellulites, leishmaniasis, mast cell tumor, and sweat gland neoplasia.

 # DIAGNOSTICS

- CBC—nonregenerative normocytic normochromic anemia is common.
- Intradermal skin test with BCG—may produce false-positive results.
- Radiographs—thoracic, abdominal, or skeletal lesions suggest granulomatous infectious disease.
- No pathognomonic radiographic lesions for mycobacteriosis—pulmonary tuberculosis may become calcified or cavitated.

Diagnostic Feature
- **Definitive diagnosis—made on biopsy and culture results.**
- Ensure—biopsy uncontaminated by surface bacteria and incorporates the center of the granulomatous focus.
- Aspirate cytologic specimens—from lesions, transtracheal wash, rectal cytology, enlarged lymph nodes, or smears from affected tissue to detect acid-fast bacilli can be effective.
- Culture—submit heat-fixed smears and tissue; special media and techniques are required; isolate identification can take several weeks.

 # THERAPEUTICS

- Feline leprosy—cured by surgical excision of lesions.
- Subcutaneous atypical mycobacteriosis—may be aided by debulking surgery.
- Benefit of surgery in conjunction with aggressive medical treatment—undefined.

Tuberculosis

Primary
- Always—use double- or triple-drug oral therapy.
- Never—attempt single-drug therapy of any organism.
- Current recommendation—fluoroquinolone (e.g., enrofloxacin) combined with clarithromycin and rifampin for 6 to 9 months; enrofloxacin, orbifloxacin, ciprofloxacin.
- Rifampin (Rifadin [Marion Merrell Dow, Kansas City, MO])—reduce dosage in hepatic dysfunction or biliary obstruction; may cause hepatotoxicity, dermatologic signs in some cats (erythema, pruritus, dyspnea due to anaphylaxis.

- Clarithromycin (Biaxin [Abbott, Abbott Laboratories, Abbott Park, IL])—side effects include GI tract upsets, anorexia, diarrhea, but usually less likely to occur than with erythromycin.

Alternatives

- Isoniazid and rifampin combination—mainly used in past; little known about their use in cats; one recent report of treatment in a cat with isoniazid, rifampin, and dihydrostreptomycin for 3 months noted weight loss but eventual cure.
- Isoniazid (Laniazid, [Novartis, Greensboro, NC])—side effects include vomiting, hepatoxicity, and vitamin B_6 deficiency causing tonic/clonic seizures in dogs.
- Ethambutol (Myambutol [Lederle, Pearl River NY])—reduce dose by extending dosing interval in renal insufficiency.
- Pyrazinamide—instead of ethambutol.
- Dihydrostreptomycin—not available currently for small animal use.

Feline Leprosy

- Dapsone (Dapsone [Jacobus, Jacobus Pharmaceuticals, Princeton, NJ])—reduced dosage in renal failure; may cause skin eruptions, vomiting, diarrhea, CNS signs, and myelotoxicity.
- Clofazimine (Lamprene [Novartis, Greensboro, NC])—not to be used in pregnant animals; avoid in preexisting GI tract disease.
- Rifampin.

Atypical Mycobacteriosis

- Chemotherapy—may use in vitro sensitivity testing to choose drug.
- Antibiotics—macrolides, sulfonamides, tetracyclines, aminoglycosides and fluoroquinolones generally effective.
- Fluoroquinolone combined with clarithromycin—good empirical treatment; use same dosages as for tuberculosis; treat for 2 to 6 months; relapses during course of or after completion of treatment common.
- *M. avium*—clofazimine.
- Subcutaneous disease (*M. fortuitum*)—topical treatment with a 1:1 solution of 2.27% enrofloxacin in 90% DMSO has been used successfully in cats; applied 1 ml q12h for a total systemic dosage of 5 mg/kg; continue treatment for 2 to 6 months; relapses after stop treatment are common (*Table 65-1*).

Precautions/Interactions

- Traditional antituberculosis drugs—be alert for any adverse reactions; experience limited, especially in cats.
- Isoniazid—liver toxicity, seizures, neuritis, and drug eruption in humans.
- Ethambutol—optic neuritis in humans.
- Pyrazinamide—liver toxicity in humans.
- Rifampin—anorexia, vomiting, and liver toxicity.
- Dapsone—hemolytic anemia, other immune-mediated blood abnormalities, and liver toxicity.

TABLE 65-1. Drug Therapy for Mycobacterial Infections in Cats and Dogs

Syndrome	Drug	Dose (mg/kg)	Route	Interval (Hours)	Duration (Months)
Tuberculosis	Fluoroquinolone[a]	5–15	PO	24	6–9
	Clarithromycin	5–10	PO	24	6–9
	Rifampin	10–20	PO	24[b]	6–9
Feline leprosy	Dapsone[c]	1[d]	PO	12	1
	Clofazimine	2–8	PO	24	1[e]
	Rifampin	10–20	PO	24[b]	6
Atypical mycobacteriosis	Gentamicin	2	SC, IM	8–12	1[f]
	Kanamycin	5	SC, IM	12	1[f]
	Amikacin	5–10	SC, IM	8–12	1[f]
	Doxycycline	5–10	PO, IV	12	1–2
	TMS	15–30[g]	PO	12	1–2
	Enrofloxacin	5–15	PO	12–24	1–4
M. avium	Clofazimine	2–8	PO	24	1–2[e]
M. fortuitum subcutaneous disease	Enrofloxacin 2.27% topical[h]	1 ml[i]	Topical	12	2–6

[a] Enroflaxacin, orbifloxacin, or ciprofloxacin; use in combination with clarithromycin and rifampin.
[b] Or divided q12h to a maximal daily dose of 600 mg.
[c] Use in combination with clofazamine and rifampin.
[d] Up to a total dose of 50 mg/cat.
[e] After first month, every 3 to 4 days for 1 to 2 months.
[f] Four weeks is maximal treatment period (usually only 2 weeks needed); monitor for renal toxicity by examining urine for casts; combine with other nonaminoglycoside drugs.
[g] Use lower dose for cats (10 to 15 mg/kg).
[h] Topical solution in 90% DMSO at a 1:1 v/v ratio.
[i] Up to a total systemic dose of 5 mg/kg (each milliliter of solution contains approximately 12 mg).
TMS, trimethoprime-sulfadiazine.

- Clofazimine—orange discoloration of fat, diarrhea and/or weight loss, and hepatic enzyme elevation.
- Dihydrostreptomycin—hearing loss and renal toxicity.
- Antituberculosis and antileprosy drugs—examine at least monthly; monitor for anorexia and weight loss.

COMMENTS

- Monitor—hepatic enzymes monthly.
- Instruct clients—to report cutaneous lesions immediately.
- Clinicians aware of a human tuberculosis case in a household with dogs or cats—should counsel owners about the risk to the pets in the household.
- Tuberculosis—guarded prognosis, but currently undefined because experience of modern drug use is limited.
- Feline leprosy—fair prognosis, especially if lesions are amenable to surgical removal.

- Prognosis in subcutaneous atypical mycobacteriosis—good for survival but guarded for resolution; relapse after cessation of long-term antibiotic therapy occurs in >40% of cats treated with single-agent therapy.
- Prognosis in pulmonary and disseminated atypical mycobacteriosis—guarded, but may be improved with modern agents and double-drug treatment.
- Zoonosis—potentially.
  - Tuberculosis—affected pets pose a zoonotic threat to owners; public health authorities should be notified of any antemortum or postmortem diagnosis (required by law in some states); do not attempt treatment without concurrence of public health authorities.
  - *M. tuberculosis*—greatest potential for zoonosis, especially with draining cutaneous lesions.
  - Disease transmission between pets and humans—very rarely recorded; in recent outbreaks of tuberculosis in cats, no transmission to humans was reported.

Abbreviations

BCG, bacillus Calmette-Guérin; CBC, complete blood count; CNS, central nervous system; DMSO, dimethylsulfoxide; DNA, deoxyribonucleic acid; GI, gastrointestinal; TB, tuberculosis.

Suggested Reading

Greene CE. Mycobacterial infections. In: Greene CE, ed. *Infectious Diseases of the Dog and Cat.* Philadelphia: WB Saunders; 1998;313–325.

Author: Carol Foil
Consulting Editor: Stephen C. Barr

chapter 66

Mycoplasmosis

DEFINITION/OVERVIEW

- A variety of systemic illnesses (respiratory, urogenital, gastrointestinal, ophthalmic, and musculoskeletal) in dogs and cats caused by a small group of prokaryotic organisms.

ETIOLOGY/PATHOPHYSIOLOGY

- Fastidious, facultative anaerobic gram-negative rods—forming the smallest (0.2 to 0.3 μm) and simplest prokaryotic cells capable of self-replication (by binary fission).
- Lack a cell wall—makes them sensitive to lysis by osmotic shock, detergents, and alcohols.
- Ubiquitous in nature as parasites, commensals, or saprophytes in animals, plants, and insects—many are pathogens of humans, animals, plants, and insects.
- Often part of resident flora—commensals on mucous membranes of upper respiratory, digestive, and genital tracts.
- Pathogenicity and role in disease—often controversial and poorly understood.
- Frequent inhabitants of mucosal membranes—*Mycoplasma gateae* or *M. felis* found in oral cavity or urogenital tract of 70% to 80% of healthy cats.
- Rate of isolation in diseased dogs—much higher than in normal dogs (e.g., lung, uterus, prepuce).
- *Mycoplasma* spp.—show considerable host specificity.
- Require—direct contact with host cell to obtain nutrients.
- Induces primarily a humoral immune response—induces a fibrinous exudate, which protects organism from antibodies and antimicrobial drugs and contributes to chronicity of infection.
- Secondary bacterial invaders—common.

SIGNALMENT/HISTORY

- Commensals—occasionally cause systemic infection associated with immunodeficiency, immunosuppression, or cancer.
- Impaired resistance of the host—may allow organisms to cross the mucosal barrier and disseminate.

- Predisposing factors—stresses such as reproductive problems associated with overcrowded housing or local tissue injury (from urinary tract neoplasms or urinary calculi).
- Historical findings—reflect organ system involved.

 CLINICAL FEATURES

Dogs

- Respiratory (often associated with fever, malaise):
  - Pneumonia.
  - Upper respiratory tract infection.
- Urogenital—urinary and genital tract infections:
  - Balanoposthitis.
  - Urethritis.
  - Prostatitis.
  - Cystitis.
  - Nephritis.
  - Vaginitis.
  - Endometritis.
- Reproductive:
  - Infertility.
  - Early embryonic death.
  - Abortion.
  - Stillbirths or weak newborns.
  - Neonatal mortality.
- Musculoskeletal—arthritis.
- Gastrointestinal—colitis.

Cats

- Ophthalmic—conjunctivitis.
- Respiratory—pneumonia, uppper respiratory tract infection.
- Musculoskeletal—chronic fibrinopurulent polyarthritis and tenosynovitis.
- Urogenital—urinary tract infections.
- Reproductive—abortions and fetal deaths.
- Skin—chronic cutaneous abscesses.

 DIFFERENTIAL DIAGNOSIS

- Canine and feline upper respiratory tract infection—viruses (parainfluenza virus, canine distemper, herpes virus, feline calcivirus, reovirus); *Chlamydia psittaci*; bacteria (*Bordetella bronchiseptica*, staphylococci, streptococci, and coliforms).
- Canine and feline UTI—bacteria (staphylococci, streptococci, coliforms), fungi (*Candida* spp.), and parasites.
- Canine infertility, early embryonic death, abortion, stillbirths or weak newborns, and neonatal mortality—bacteria (*Brucella, Salmonella* spp., *Campylobacter* spp.,

Escherichia coli, streptococcus), viruses (CHV, canine distemper, CAV), *Toxoplasma gondii*, and endocrinopathies (progesterone deficiency, hypothyroidism).

- Canine prostatitis—bacteria (*E. coli*, *Brucella canis*) and fungi (*Blastomyces dermatitidis*, *Cryptococcus neoformans*).
- Canine and feline arthritis—immune-mediated; bacteria (staphylococci, streptococci, coliforms, anaerobes), bacterial L-forms, rickettsia (*Ehrlichia* spp.), *Borrelia burgdorferi*; fungi (*Coccidioides* spp., *Cryptococcus neoformans*, *Blastomyces dermatitidis*), protozoa (*Leishmania* spp.), viruses (FCV).
- Feline conjunctivitis—FHV, FCV, feline reovirus, *Chlamydia psittaci*, and bacteria.

 DIAGNOSTICS

- CBC—mild anemia, neutrophilic leukocytosis (polyarthritis, pneumonia).
- Serum biochemical profile—hypoalbuminemia, hyperglobulinemia (polyarthritis).
- Urinalysis—proteinuria resulting from immune-complex glomerulonephritis.
- Radiographic examination of arthritic joints—no radiographic changes.
- Serologic assays are available in some diagnostic laboratories—value of serology is controversial given that commensal organisms also produce a titer.
- PCR—only available on a research basis.

Diagnostic Feature
- **Diagnostic challenge is to distinguish between commensal organisms and those causing pathology.**
- Organisms are difficult to demonstrate in and from tissues—extremely pleomorphic, in smears (e.g., conjunctival scrapings) seen as coccobacilli, coccal forms, ring forms, spirals, and filaments; stain poorly (gram-negative), preferred staining method is by Giemsa or other Romanowsky stains.
- Scanning electron microscopy—demonstrates organism.
- Definitive diagnosis based on isolation and identification or detection of the *Mycoplasma* organisms in tissues by a fluorescent antibody procedure—submit cotton swabs placed in Hayflicks broth medium or use commercially available swabs (cool specimens and ship on ice if to arrive at lab in less than 24 hours; if longer, freeze samples and ship on dry ice).
- Culture—requires special medium (check that laboratory can perform culture before sending samples).

 THERAPEUTICS

Drugs of Choice

- Doxycycline—treat for extended periods (6 weeks).
- Tetracyclines.
- Chloramphenicol.

TABLE 66-1. Drug Therapy for *Mycoplasma* Infections in Cats and Dogs

Drug	Dose (mg/kg)	Route	Interval (Hours)	Duration (Weeks)
Doxycycline	5	PO, IV	12	4–6
Tetracycline	22	PO	8	4–6
Chloramphenicol	50	PO, IV, IM, SC	8–12	4–6
Erythromycin	10–20	PO	8–12	4–6
Enrofloxacin	5	PO	12–24	4–6

- Alternative drugs—gentamicin, kanamycin, spectinomycin, spiramycin, tylosin, erythromycin, nitrofurans, and fluoroquinolones (*Table 66-1*).
- Topical antibiotic—conjunctivitis.
- Resistant—to sulfonamides and β-lactams that inhibit peptidoglycan synthesis because organisms lack a cell wall.
- No standardized procedure for in vitro antimicrobial susceptibility tests.

Precautions/Interactions

- Improper use of topical steroid ointments with conjunctivitis—may prolong infection and predispose to corneal ulceration.
- Tetracycline and chloramphenicol should not be used in pregnant animals—use erythromycin instead.
- Chloramphenicol—may cause myelosuppression (reversible if stop drug); warn owners to only handle the drug while wearing gloves because it can cause fatal, irreversible idiosyncratic pancytopenia in some humans.
- Doxycycline—may cause esophagitis and esophageal stricture in some cats.
- Doxycycline—contraindicated in pregnant or lactating bitches.
- Tetracyclines—may cause dental discoloration in young animals; do not give to animals with renal failure.

 COMMENTS

- Organisms readily killed by drying, sunshine, or any chemical disinfectant.
- Not generally considered zoonotic.
- Suppurative mycoplasmal tenosynovitis has been reported in a veterinarian following a scratch from a cat being treated for colitis.

Abbreviations

CAV, canine adenovirus; CBC, complete blood count; CHV, canine herpes virus; FCV, feline calcivirus; FHV, feline herpes virus; PCR, polymerase chain reaction; UTI, urinary tract infection.

Suggested Reading

Greene CE. Mycoplasmal, ureaplasmal, and L-form infections. In: Greene CE, ed. *Infectious Diseases of the Dog and Cat*. Philadelphia: WB Saunders; 1998:174–178.

Author: J. Paul Woods
Consulting Editor: Stephen C. Barr

chapter 67

Nasal Capillariasis
(Eucoleus)

DEFINITION/OVERVIEW

- Nematode found in mucosa of nasal passages and sinuses of dogs.
- Usually asymptomatic but can cause chronic sneezing and nasal discharge.
- Often misidentified as *Eucoleus (=Capillaria) aerophilus* because eggs are nearly identical.

ETIOLOGY/PATHOPHYSIOLOGY

- *Eucoleus boehmi*—capillarid parasite.
- Life cycle—unknown but thought to be either direct or through earthworm paratenic hosts.
- Parasite produces—local inflammation and an allergic rhinitis.
- PPP = 1 month.

SIGNALMENT/HISTORY

- Few case reports but most described in young dogs.

CLINICAL FEATURES

- Most cases are asymptomatic.
- Chronic sneezing.
- Mucopurulent nasal discharge (occasionally bloody).
- Epistaxis.
- Face rubbing.

DIFFERENTIAL DIAGNOSIS

- Signs of sneezing with nasal discharge—other parasitic infections (*Pneumonyssoides caninum* and *Linguatula serrata*), other infections (bacterial, fungal such as aspergillosis), allergic rhinitis, nasal foreign body, dental disease, and neoplasia.

- Sneezing—more characteristic of parasitic infection or acute foreign body than neoplasia, which presents more often with nasal obstruction or discharge.
- Reverse sneezing—not usually accompanied by nasal discharge.

 ## DIAGNOSTICS

Diagnostic Feature
- **Bi-operculate eggs in feces need to be differentiated from those of *Eucoleus* (= *Capillaria*) *aerophilus*, *Pearsonema* (= *Capillaria*) *plica* (eggs usually in urine but can be passed in feces if ingested by dog or urine contaminates feces), or *Trichuris vulpis*** (Fig. 67-1).
- Eggs—if in nasal discharges, will only be E. *boehmi*, unless dog has E. *aerophilus* and has coughed up lower airway discharges through the nose.
- Nasal wash—diagnostic if contains bi-operculate eggs.

 ## THERAPEUTICS

- Ivermectin and fenbendazole are effective in alleviating clinical signs, but relapses may occur, so follow-up treatment may be necessary after a month of initial presentation.

Drugs of Choice
- Neither drug is registered for the treatment of E. *boehmi* in the dog.
- Ivermectin.
- Fenbendazole (*Table 67-1*).

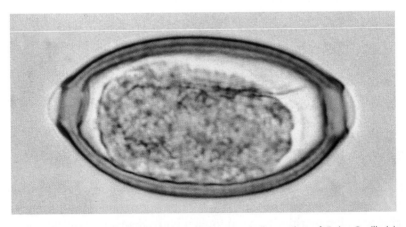

■ **Fig. 67-1** The bi-operculate egg of *Eucoleus boehmi* is very similar to that of *E.* (= *Capillaria*) *aerophilus*, which resides in the lungs. Both eggs can be found in the feces of infected dogs and differ only in that the surface of *E. boehmi* eggs are covered in small pits similar to a thimble, whereas the eggs of *E. aerophilus* are not.

TABLE 67-1. Drug Therapy for Nasal Capillariasis (*Eucoleus boehmi*) in Dogs				
Drug	Dose (mg/kg)	Route	Interval (Hours)	Repeat Interval (Months)
Ivermectin	0.2	PO, SC	Once	1
Fenbendazole	50	PO	10–14	1

Precautions/Interactions

- Ensure—dog does not have microfilaremia before administering ivermectin.
- Ivermectin-sensitive collie and collie-cross—dogs may show neurologic signs with this dose of ivermectin.

 COMMENTS

- The life cycle of E. *boehmi* is unknown; however, it is reasonable to expect it to be similar to *Capillaria* and therefore implement similar control methods used for urinary capillariasis.
- Dogs should be maintained away from soil, on wire-bottomed enclosures or impervious pavements or at least sand devoid of vegetation (where earthworms, the probably intermediate host, are unlikely to survive).
- Direct sunshine effectively kills eggs.

Abbreviation

PPP, prepatent period.

Suggested Reading

Campbell BG, Little MD. Identification of the eggs of a nematode (*Eucoleus boehmi*) from the nasal mucosa of North American dogs. *J Am Vet Med Assoc* 1991;198:1520–1523.
Schoning P, Dryden MW, Gabbert NH. Identification of a nasal nematode (*Eucoleus boehmi*) in greyhounds. *Vet Res Commun* 1993;17:277–281.

Author: Stephen C. Barr
Consulting Editor: Stephen C. Barr

chapter 68

Nasal Mites (Pneumonyssoides)

DEFINITION/OVERVIEW

- Arthropod found in the nasal cavity and sinuses of dogs, leading to sneezing, chronic nasal discharge, and epistaxis.

ETIOLOGY/PATHOPHYSIOLOGY

- *Pneumonyssoides caninum*—mite.
- Transmission—direct contact with an infested animal.
- The mite causes inflammation of the nasal mucosa (especially the olfactory area) possibly leading to a loss of sense of smell by the host.

SIGNALMENT/HISTORY

- Although not common in North America, the prevalence can be high in some northern European countries (20% in Sweden, 7% in Norway).
- No sex, breed, or age distribution, although dogs >3 years of age are more likely to be infested.
- Most clinically apparent infestations require large numbers (>50) of mites, whereas small numbers (<20) often cause no clinical signs.

CLINICAL FEATURES

- Sneezing—often reverse sneezing
- Epistaxis.
- Chronic nasal discharge.
- Signs of nasal irritation are pawing face, rubbing face against objects and the ground.
- May see mites on the outside of the nose (*Fig. 68-1*).
- One study suggests that nasal mite infestation predisposes large-breed dogs to gastric dilatation-volvulus because excessive aerophagia can occur during reverse sneezing.

■ **Fig. 68-1** Nose of an English bulldog covered in small white dots, which are the mites of *Pneumonyssoides caninum*.

 DIFFERENTIAL DIAGNOSIS

- Sneezing with nasal discharge need to be differentiated from:
  - Other parasitic infestations, including *Linguatula serrata* and *Eucoleus boehmi*.
  - Nasal foreign body.
  - Neoplasia.
  - Allergic rhinitis.
- Sneezing is more characteristic of parasitic infection or acute foreign body rather than neoplasia (which presents more often with nasal obstruction or discharge).
- Reverse sneezing is not usually accompanied by nasal discharge.

 DIAGNOSTICS

- Large (pin head sized) white mites visible to the naked eye—can be detected by rhinoscopy (or otoscope inserted into the nares), or in nasal flushings.
- Microscopy—mites have uncomplicated leg tips unadorned by suckers or hooks (Fig. 68-2).
- Rhinoscopy—mites scurry away from the bright light of the scope.

Diagnostic Feature
- **Mites dislike isoflurothane gas, so they will often appear at entrance of nares in anesthetized patient.**
- Mild eosinophilia may be present.

■ **Fig. 68-2** The *Pneumonyssoides caninum* mite is characterized by its large size and long legs without hooks or suckers.

Drugs of Choice

- Ivermectin (Ivermec [Merial, Iselin, NJ]).
- Milbemycin oxime (Interceptor [Novartis, Greensboro, NC]) *(Table 68-1)*.
- Both drugs should provide prompt improvement of clinical signs.
- Neither drug is registered for this use in dogs.

Precautions/Interactions

- Ensure that patients do not have microfilaremia before administering ivermectin.
- Ivermectin-sensitive collie or collie-cross dogs may show neurologic signs with this dose of ivermectin.

TABLE 68-1. Drug Therapy for *Pneumonyssoides caninum* in Dogs				
Drug	Dose (mg/kg)	Route	Interval (Weeks)	Duration (Weeks)
Ivermectin (Ivermec)	0.2	PO, SC	1	3
Milbemycin oxime (Interceptor)	0.5–1	PO	1	3

COMMENTS

- Treat all in contact animals.
- It is unlikely that mites survive in the environment for long.
- Keep dogs away from foxes, which can carry mites.

Suggested Reading

Bredal WP. *Pneumonyssoides caninum* infection: a risk factor for gastric dilatation-volvulus in dogs. *Vet Res Commun* 1998;22:225–231.

Bredal WP. An epidemiological survey of therapy and diagnostic procedures used by Norwegian small animal practitioners in cases of nasal mite (*Pneumonyssoides caninum*) infection in dogs. *Vet Res Commun* 1998;22:389–399.

Brendal WP, Vollset I. Use of milbemycin oxime in the treatment of dogs with nasal mite (*Pneumonyssoides caninum*) infection. *J Small Anim Pract* 1998;39:126–130.

Gunnarsson LK, Moller LC, Einarsson AM, et al. Clinical efficacy of milbemycin oxime in the treatment of nasal mite infection in dogs. *J Am Anim Hosp Assoc* 1999;35:81–84.

Author: Stephen C. Barr
Consulting Editor: Stephen C. Barr

chapter 69

Neosporosis

DEFINITION/OVERVIEW

- A protozoal (coccidian) disease causing tissue damage (by necrosis mainly of nerve tissue and muscle) from cyst rupture and tachyzoite invasion in dogs.

ETIOLOGY/PATHOPHYSIOLOGY

- *Neospora caninum*—tachyzoites and tissue cysts resemble *Toxoplasma gondii* under light microscopy.
- Dogs (and coyotes)—definitive host; excrete oocysts in feces.
- Oocysts sporulate to become infective after 24 hours—infective to other dogs and intermediate hosts, including cattle, goats, horses, sheep, and cats (experimentally).
- Of little clinical significance in intermediate hosts—except cattle, in which abortion and stillbirths can cause a loss of production in some herds.
- Transmission—transplacental, resulting in congenital infection.
- Transmission—ingestion of sporulated oocysts passed in feces of dogs or coyotes or tissue cysts in tissues of intermediate hosts (e.g., dogs ingesting infected bovine fetal membranes).

SIGNALMENT/HISTORY

- Natural infections occur in dogs, with hunting/farm dogs overrepresented.
- Serologic prevalence in farm dogs—usually >30%.
- Puppies (< 6 months of age)—overrepresented.
- Cats—no natural cases have been reported in cats.

CLINICAL FEATURES

- Similar to those of toxoplasmosis, except neurologic and muscular abnormalities predominate and are often more severe.
- Young dogs (<6 months of age):
  - Ascending paralysis is common.
  - Distinguished from other forms of paralysis by gradual muscle atrophy.
  - Stiffness of pelvic limbs; affected more than thoracic limbs.

■ **Fig. 69-1** Puppy affected with clinical neosporosis, showing pelvic limb muscle contracture forcing the limbs into rigid extension (courtesy Dr. A. Delahunta, Cornell University).

- Progresses to rigid contracture of limbs.
- Lower motor neuron paralysis (*Fig. 69-1*).
- Cervical weakness and dysphagia gradually develop, leading to death.
- Cerebellar atrophy with associated ataxia is reported, although rare (*Fig. 69-2*).
■ Older dogs:
  - Usually display CNS involvement (seizures, tremors).
  - Polymyositis and myocarditis reported.
  - Like toxoplasmosis, virtually any organ can be affected.
  - Head tremors.

■ **Fig. 69-2** Cerebellar atrophy can occur in young dogs from *Neospora caninum* infection (courtesy Dr. A. Delahunta, Cornell University).

- Postural deficits from cerebellar disease.
  - Horner's syndrome also reported.
- Generalized ulcerative and pyogranulomatous dermatitis reported in dogs on immunosuppressive therapy (mainly for SLE or lymphosarcoma)—large numbers of tachyzoites present in dermal lesions.

DIFFERENTIAL DIAGNOSIS

- Young dogs—other causes of peripheral multifocal neurologic signs, infectious diseases (toxoplasmosis, distemper), progressive polyradiculoneuritis, botulism, tick bite paralysis.
- Other causes of diffuse lower motor neuron muscular diseases—are rare in young dogs.
- Older dogs with CNS disease—other infectious diseases (fungal, rabies, pseudorabies), toxicity (lead, organophosphate, carbamate, chlorinated hydrocarbon, strychnine), nonsuppurative encephalitis, meningitis, GME, and metabolic disease (hypoglycemia, hepatic encephalopathy), and neoplasia.

DIAGNOSTICS

- CBC, biochemical panel, urinalysis findings—nonspecific, depending on organ systems involved.
- CK and AST activities—with muscle involvement.
- CSF—usually a slight increase in protein concentration and nucleated cell counts (usually mononuclear but neutrophils can be seen).
- Serologic testing (IFA)—CSF or serum; antibodies do not cross-react with *T. gondii* (ELISA available for testing cattle).
- PCR—described but not yet commercially available; differentiate *N. caninum* from *T. gondii* in CSF; another differentiates *N. caninum* from *Hammondia* cysts in fecal samples.

THERAPEUTICS

- Once muscle contracture or ascending paralysis has occurred—prognosis for clinical improvement is poor.
- Progression of clinical signs—may be arrested by treatment.

Drugs of Choice

- Clindamycin—continue for at least 2 weeks after clinical signs cleared or plateaued.
- TMS and pyrimethamine—may also be used (*Table 69-1*).

TABLE 69-1. Drug Therapy for Neosporosis

Drug	Dose (mg/kg)	Route	Interval (Hours)	Duration (Weeks)
Clindamycin	12.5–25	PO, IM	12	4[a]
Trimethoprim-sulfadiazine	15–20	PO	12	4[a]
Pyrimethamine[b]	1	PO	24	4

[a] Continue at least until 2 weeks after signs have plateaued.
[b] Use in combination with trimethoprim-sulfadiazine.

Precautions/Interactions

- Reduce dose of clindamycin in renal failure, hepatic dysfunction, or biliary obstruction from any cause.
- May cause GI signs (vomiting, diarrhea, anorexia), and transient diarrhea—temporarily discontinue dosing until signs stop, then reinstitute at half the dose, working up to full dose.

COMMENTS

- No zoonotic potential identified.
- Serologically test littermates and dam, along with any cattle if patient is from a farm.
- Prevent contamination of cattle feed with dog feces—prevent dog from eating bovine fetal membranes.
- Only way to prevent transmission cycle between dogs and cattle—remove dogs from the farm.

Abbreviations

AST, aspartate aminotransferase; CBC, complete blood count; CK, creatine kinase; CNS, central nervous system; CSF, cerebrospinal fluid; ELISA, enzyme-linked immunosorbent assay; GI, gastrointestinal; GME, granulomatous meningoencephalitis; IFA, immunofluorescent antibody; PCR, polymerase chain reaction; SLE, systemic lupus erythematosus; TMS, trimethoprim-sulfadiazine.

Suggested Reading

Condim LF, McAllister MM, Pitt WC, et al. Coyotes (*Canis latrans*) are definitive hosts of *Neospora caninum*. *Int J Parasitol* 2004;34:159–161.
Dubey JP. Review of *Neospora caninum* and neosporosis in animals. *Kor J Parasitol* 2003;41:1–16.
Schatzberg SJ, Haley NJ, Barr SC, et al. Use of a multiplex polymerase chain reaction assay in the antemortem diagnosis of toxoplasmosis and neosporosis in the central nervous system of cats and dogs. *Am J Vet Med Assoc* 2003;64:1507–1513.

Author: Stephen C. Barr
Consulting Editor: Stephen C. Bar

chapter 70

Nocardiosis

DEFINITION/OVERVIEW

- An uncommon bacterial infection of dogs and cats usually presenting as pyothorax, nonhealing cutaneous wounds, or systemic infection (although rarely).

ETIOLOGY/PATHOPHYSIOLOGY

- *Nocardia asteroides* (dogs and cats); *N. brasiliensis* (cats only); *Proactinomyces* spp. (rare).
- *Nocardia*—a soil saprophyte that enters the body through contamination of wounds or by respiratory inhalation.
- Compromised immune system—enhances likelihood of infection.

SIGNALMENT/HISTORY

- Dogs and cats—of any breed.
- Often animal is immunosuppressed—under treatment for neoplasia or immune-mediated disease.

CLINICAL FEATURES

- Depend on the site of infection.

Pleural

- Pyothorax.
- Dyspnea.
- Emaciation.
- Fever.

Cutaneous

- Chronic, nonhealing wounds.
- Fistulous tracts, which may result in local lymphadenopathy.

- Draining lymph nodes.
- Osteomyelitis.

Disseminated

- Most common in young dogs, usually originating in the respiratory tract.
- Lethargy.
- Fever, often cyclic.
- Weight loss.
- CNS may be affected, with diffuse neurologic signs.
- Pleural and abdominal effusion may also occur.

 DIFFERENTIAL DIAGNOSIS

Cutaneous

- Actinomycosis.
- Atypical mycobacteriosis.
- Leprosy.
- Fungal.
- Bite wound abscesses.
- Draining tracts resulting from foreign bodies.

Pleural

- Bacterial pyothorax.
- Thoracic neoplasia.
- Chronic diaphragmatic hernia.

Disseminated

- Systemic fungal infection.
- FIP.

 DIAGNOSTICS

- CBC—neutrophilic leukocytosis, nonregenerative anemia (of chronic disease).
- Biochemical panel—usually normal; hypergammaglobulinemia in long-standing infections.
- Radiographs—pleural or abdominal effusion, pleuropneumonia, or osteomyelitis.
- Cytology—pleural fluid, abscess discharge, or abdominal fluid.
- Stain with Romanowsky, Gram's, or modified acid-fast stains—reveals gram-positive, beaded, branching filamentous rods or cocci; sulfur granules (microaggregates) are infrequent in effusions; usually not able to differentiate from *Actinomyces* spp. (*Fig. 70-1*).

■ **Fig. 70-1** Impression smear of a chronic fistulous tract on the thorax of a cat containing aggregates of branching filamentous gram-positive rods of *Nocardia asteroides* (Gram's stain, 450×).

- Culture (definitive)—pleural fluid, abscess discharge, aspirated material from affected organ; grows under aerobic conditions on Sabouraud's medium.

 ## THERAPEUTICS

- Remove pleural effusion—usually by placing closed thorocostomy tube—through which to irrigate pleural cavity with warmed saline and remove any subsequent fluid accumulation.
- Supportive care—IV fluid therapy, with or without nutritional support.
- Antibiotic therapy.
- Remove thorocostomy tube when fluid becomes noninfected and minimal in volume.
- Fistulous tracts and abscesses—surgically drain and débride; long-term antibiotic therapy.

Drugs of Choice

- Antibiotics based on culture and sensitivity testing.
- While awaiting culture and sensitivity results, good first-choice drugs include sulfonamides (sulfadiazine or trimethoprim-sulfadiazine combination).
- Other effective drugs include gentamicin, amikacin, doxycycline, tetracycline hydrochloride, minocycline, and erythromycin alone or combined with ampicillin or amoxicillin (*Table 70-1*).
- Can use amoxicillin in combination with an aminoglycoside.
- Average treatment period is 6 weeks or for at least 2 weeks past the apparent remission of the disease.

TABLE 70-1. Drug Therapy for Nocardiosis

Drug	Dose (mg/kg)	Route	Interval (Hours)	Duration (Days)
Sulfadiazine	100[a]	IV, PO	12	42
Trimethoprim-sulfadiazine	15	PO	12	42
Gentamicin[b]	2–4	IM, SC	8	10[c]
Amikacin[b]	6.5	IV, IM, SC	8	10[c]
Doxycycline	5	PO, IV	12	42
Tetracycline hydrochloride	15–20	PO	8	42
Minocycline	5–12.5	PO	12	42
Erythromycin	10–20	PO	8	42
Ampicillin	20–40	PO	8	42
Amoxicillin	6–20	PO	8–12	42

[a] As initial loading dose, then reduce to 50 mg/kg.
[b] Use in combination with ampicillin or amoxicillin; monitor for renal toxicity.
[c] Or for short period if clinical response occurring.

Precautions/Interactions

- Tetracyclines may cause fever (especially cats); adjust dose (except doxycycline) in animals with renal insufficiency.
- Do not give aminoglycosides in poorly hydrated animals; monitor for renal tubular damage by monitoring urine sediment for the appearance of hyaline casts.
- Long-term use of sulfa drugs can cause polyarthritis, KCS, and blood dyscraisias.

COMMENTS

- Even after apparent clinical remission, the patient should be monitored carefully for the development of fever, weight loss, neurologic signs, dyspnea, and lameness during the first year postinfection because of the possibility of bone and CNS involvement.

Abbreviations

CBC, complete blood count; CNS, central nervous system; FIP, feline infectious peritonitis; KCS, keratoconjunctivitis sicca.

Suggested Reading

Edwards DF. Actinomycosis and nocardiosis. In: Greene CE, ed. *Infectious Diseases of the Dog and Cat.* Philadelphia: WB Saunders; 1998:303–313.

Author: Gary D. Norsworthy
Consulting Editor: Stephen C. Barr

chapter 71

Ollulanus Infection

DEFINITION/OVERVIEW

- A trichostrongyloid nematode—adult worms are found in the stomach wall of cats, causing chronic gastritis resulting in anorexia, vomiting, and weight loss.

ETIOLOGY/PATHOPHYSIOLOGY

- *Ollulanus tricuspis*—adults (only up to 1 mm in length) coil into the gastric mucosa, causing superficial erosions.
- Over time, gastric erosions can become severe, with marked inflammation, accumulation of lymphoid aggregates, and fibrous changes in the mucosa and submucosa.
- Eggs—hatch within female worms; larvae develop to infective L3 larvae.
- L3 larvae—passed into the stomach contents and vomited; infective to other cats.
- Adult male and female worms passed in the vomitus—can infect other cats.
- Distribution—throughout North America, Australia, New Zealand, Europe, Argentina, and Chile.
- Germany—up to 40% of free-roaming cats may be infected.

SIGNALMENT/HISTORY

- Colony cats—predisposed, probably because they have close access to other cats' vomitus.
- Stray cats living in urban areas heavily populated with cats—high incidence of infection.
- Captive cheetahs, lions, tigers, cougars—susceptible to infection.

CLINICAL FEATURES

- Chronic vomiting.
- Anorexia.
- Weight loss.
- Death from chronic gastritis.

DIFFERENTIAL DIAGNOSIS

- Other causes of vomiting including:
  - Dietary.
  - Toxins—lead, ethylene glycol.
  - Metabolic—diabetes mellitus, renal disease, hepatic disease, acidosis, heat stroke, hypoadrenocorticism, and hyperthyroidism.
  - Gastric abnormalities—IBD, neoplasia, obstruction, atrophic gastritis, ulcers, dilatation/volvulus, and parasitic, such as *Physaloptera*.
  - Gastroesophageal junction disorders—hiatal hernia.
  - Small intestine disorders—IBD disease, neoplasia, fungal, viral, obstruction, and paralytic ileus.
  - Large intestine disorders—colitis, obstipation, and IBD.
  - Abdominal disorders—pancreatitis, gastrinoma, peritonitis, steatitis, pyometra, diaphragmatic hernia, and neoplasia.
  - Neurologic disorders—psychogenic, motion sickness, vestibular lesions, head trauma, and brain neoplasia.
  - Miscellaneous—heartworm disease and heart disease.

DIAGNOSTICS

- Larvae (or eggs)—seldom found in feces, because they are digested within the GI tract.
- Vomitus—examine for L3 larvae.
- Vomiting can be induced in the cat using xylazine (0.5 mg/kg IV or 1 mg/kg IM)—successful in about 70% of cases.
- View worms through an endoscope *(Fig. 71-1)*—difficult due to size of worms.
- Gastric lavage—using saline collection followed by centrifugation to precipitate L3 larvae or use Baermann's technique.
- Histopathologic examination—gastric biopsy specimen occasionally shows parasites.

THERAPEUTICS

- Few treatments have been reported for this parasite.
- Fenbendazole, oxfendazole, and pyrantel pamoate have all been used but probably are ineffective.
- Although cats may improve clinically, parasites are not removed from stomach.

Drugs of Choice

- Tetramizole (give as a 2.5% formulation at 5 mg/kg, PO, once)—effective.
- Availability—tetramizole is available in virtually every country but the United States.

■ **Fig. 71-1** Adult *Ollulanus tricuspis* worms in the stomach of a cat at necropsy examination.

Precautions/Interactions

■ Tetramizole at this dose should not cause any side effects in cats.

                    COMMENTS

■ This author and others have successfully used tetramizole to treat *Ollulanus* infection in cats.

Abbreviations

GI, gastrointestinal; IBD, inflammatory bowel disease.

Suggested Reading

Bowman DD, Hendrix CM, Lindsay DS, et al. *Ollulanus tricuspis.* In: Bowman DD, ed. *Feline Clinical Parasitology,* Ames, Iowa: Iowa State University Press; 2002:262–265.
Hasslinger MA. *Ollulanus tricuspis,* the stomach worm of the cat. *Feline Pract* 1984;14:22–35.

Author: Stephen C. Barr
Consulting Editor: Stephen C. Barr

chapter 72

Physaloptera Infection

DEFINITION/OVERVIEW

- A spirurid nematode—adults and larvae are found attached to the gastric mucosa of cats (causing vomiting) and dogs (usually asymptomatic).

ETIOLOGY/PATHOPHYSIOLOGY

- *Physaloptera* (*P. praeputialis* is cat-specific).
- Adults (3 to 5 cm long)—attach by their anterior end to the gastric mucosa of their vertebrate host.
- Adults—pass ovoid eggs (50 × 35 μm) containing a fully formed larvae into the feces.
- L1 larvae—infect intermediate hosts (beetles, crickets, and cockroaches).
- Intermediate hosts—eaten by paratenic hosts (lizards, hedgehog).
- Cats and dogs—become infected by eating paratenic hosts.
- Distribution—worldwide.
- PPP = 4 to 5 months.

SIGNALMENT/HISTORY

- Cats usually have access to outdoors.
- No age, sex, or breed predilection.

CLINICAL FEATURES

Dogs

- Usually asymptomatic.
- Can cause intermittent vomiting, anorexia, and slight weight loss.

Cats

- Often asymptomatic.
- Chronic vomiting.

- Vomiting may continue for months.
- Vomiting occasionally coupled with melena.
- Vomitus can contain adult worms.

DIFFERENTIAL DIAGNOSIS

Cats

- Other causes of vomiting, including:
  - Dietary.
  - Toxins—lead, ethylene glycol.
  - Metabolic—diabetes mellitus, renal disease, hepatic disease, acidosis, heat stroke, hypoadrenocorticism, and hyperthyroidism.
  - Gastric abnormalities—IBD, neoplasia, obstruction, atrophic gastritis, ulcers, dilatation/volvulus, and parasitic, such as *Ollunanus*.
  - Gastroesophageal junction disorders—hiatal hernia.
  - Small intestine disorders—IBD, neoplasia, fungal, viral, obstruction, and paralytic ileus.
  - Large intestine disorders—colitis, obstipation, and IBD.
  - Abdominal disorders—pancreatitis, gastrinoma, peritonitis, steatitis, pyometra, diaphragmatic hernia, and neoplasia.
  - Neurologic disorders—psychogenic, motion sickness, vestibular lesions, head trauma, and brain neoplasia.
  - Miscellaneous—heartworm disease and heart disease.

DIAGNOSTICS

- CBC—blood-loss anemia (in cats with melena); eosinophilia reported.
- Vomitus—may contain adult parasites.
- Eggs—containing larvae present in fecal flotation (*Fig. 72-1*).
- Flotation—may require sodium dichromate or magnesium sulfate flotation to identify eggs.
- Endoscopy—reveals adult worms lying over the stomach wall (*Fig. 72-2*).

THERAPEUTICS

- Cats and dogs rarely require any additional therapeutics other than an anthelmintic to remove the parasites.

Drugs of Choice

- Pyrantel pomoate.
- Ivermectin (*Table 72-1*).

■ **Fig. 72-1** *Physaloptera praeputialis* eggs in a fecal flotation.

■ **Fig. 72-2** Adult *Physaloptera praeputialis* worms in the stomach of a cat at necropsy examination (courtesy Dr. J. King, Cornell University).

TABLE 72-1. Drug Treatment for *Physaloptera* Infection					
Drug	**Species**	**Dose (mg/kg)**	**Route**	**Interval (Hours)**	**Repeat (Weeks)**
Pyrantel pomoate (Strongid T)	B	5	PO	Once	3
Ivermectin (Ivomec 1% injectable)	B	0.2	SC, PO	Once	2

B, both dogs and cats.

Precautions/Interactions

- Ivermectin at this dose is not labeled for use in cats or dogs.

 COMMENTS

- Both pyrantel and ivermectin will stop clinical signs and egg shedding in 5 to 8 days post-treatment.

Abbreviations

CBC, complete blood count; IBD, inflammatory bowel disease; PPP, prepatent period.

Suggested Reading

Gustafson BW. Ivermectin in the treatment of *Physaloptera praeputialis* in two cats. *J Am Anim Hosp Assoc* 1995;31:416–418.

Theisen SK, LeGrange SN, Johnson SE, et al. *Pysaloptera* infection in 18 dogs with intermittent vomiting. *J Am Anim Hosp Assoc* 1998;34:74–78.

Santen DR, Chastain CB, Schmidt DA. Efficacy of pyrantel pomoate against *Physaloptera* in a cat. *J Am Anim Hosp Assoc* 1993;29:53–55.

Author: Stephen C. Barr
Consulting Editor: Stephen C. Barr

chapter 73

Plague

DEFINITION/OVERVIEW

- A systemic bacterial infection mainly of cats (dogs resistant).
- After skin inoculation, organisms rapidly migrate via lymphatics to regional lymph nodes to produce severe necrotic lymphadenopathy (buboes).
- Buboes—may rupture to the skin surface or cause septicemia.

ETIOLOGY/PATHOPHYSIOLOGY

- *Yersinia pestis*—a bipolar gram-negative staining rod found worldwide in wild rodents, squirrels, prairie dogs, rabbits, bobcats, and coyotes.
- Most U.S. cases—New Mexico, Arizona, California, Colorado, Idaho, Nevada, Oregon, Texas, Utah, Washington, Wyoming, and Hawaii.
- Common—May to October.
- Infection—vector (fleas) transmit organism in bite.
- After infection—organisms migrate from skin lymphatics to regional lymph nodes, multiply in phagocytic cells.
- After infection—disease characterized by fever, painful lymphadenopathy (buboes), and intermittent bacteremia; lymph nodes may rupture.
- Septicemia—can develop with or without lymph node involvement.

SIGNALMENT/HISTORY

- Cats—no sex, age, or breed predisposition.
- Dogs—naturally resistant.
- Outdoor (hunting) cats—increased risk.
- Cats heavily infected with fleas or living near heavy rodent infestations—increased risk.

CLINICAL FEATURES

Dogs

- Mild febrile signs with depression.

Cats

Bubonic Plague

- Most common form.
- Signs—develop 2 to 7 days after flea bite or after eating infected rodent.
- Buboes—mainly develop on the head and neck.
- Buboes—marked lymphadenopathy with hemorrhage, necrosis, and cellulitis.
- If survives long enough—lymph nodes abscess, rupture, and drain through skin.
- Signs of systemic illness—fever, depression, vomiting, diarrhea, dehydration, enlarged tonsils, anorexia, ocular discharge, weight loss, ataxia, coma, and oral ulcers.

Systemic Plague

- Rare—usually rapidly fatal.
- Septicemia—without lymphadenopathy or abscess formation.
- Cats—unique in that they can develop bubonic pneumonia.

DIFFERENTIAL DIAGNOSIS

Cats

- Lymphadenopathy:
  - Cat bite abscess formation.
  - Foreign body migration.
  - *Cuterebra* migration.
- Systemic illness:
  - Tularemia.
  - Cytauxzoonosis.
  - Other acute bacterial causes of septicemia.

DIAGNOSTICS

- CBC—leukocytosis with left shift and marked toxic changes in neutrophils.
- Thrombocytopenia—if DIC occurs late in disease.
- Biochemical profile—elevated hepatic enzyme activity and hyperbilirubinemia.
- Occasionally—organisms visible on a peripheral blood smear *(Fig. 73-1)*.
- Serology examination—performed by CDC and reference laboratories.
- Serologic examination—passive hemagglutination titers appear ~8 days post-infection; fourfold increase in titer between acute and convalescent serum samples.
- High titer—persists beyond a year in infected animals.

Diagnostic Feature

- **Culture—definitive technique on peripheral blood, affected lymph node or abscess aspirate, or tissue biopsy before treatment.**

■ **Fig. 73-1** *Yersinia pestis* organisms, the etiologic agent of the plague, in the blood of a patient with plague septicemia (Wright's-Giemsa stain, bar = 10 μm).

- Fluorescent antibody test—on same samples used in culture will often give a quicker result.

 THERAPEUTICS

- High mortality—if not treated early and aggressively.
- IV fluids and aggressive treatment of DIC—can save patient.
- Important to treat fleas quickly to prevent personal exposure—use imidacloprid (Advantage [Bayer, Shawnee Mission, KS]) for rapid flea kill.
- Cats with pneumonic form—should be euthanatized to reduce extreme zoonotic potential.

Drugs of Choice

- Tetracyclines (oxytetracycline, tetracycline, chlortetracycline)—25 mg/kg, PO, q8h for 10 days or parenterally 7.5 mg/kg, q12h.
- Doxycycline—effectiveness not established but probably effective.
- Chloramphenicol, gentamicin, TMS can be used if tetracyclines are contraindicated.

Precautions/Interactions

- Tetracyclines—may cause yellow staining of young animal's teeth.
- Tetracyclines—may produce GI upsets.
- Tetracyclines—use at reduced dose in animals with renal insufficiency.

 COMMENTS

- Control exposure of pet to wildlife in endemic areas and treat with monthly flea preventatives.
- Pay particular attention—to controlling rodents near housing in endemic areas.

- Pneumonic form is invariably fatal in cats—euthanasia is often advised to decrease zoonotic risk and because prognosis is so poor.

Abbreviations

CBC, complete blood count; CDC, Centers for Disease Control and Prevention; DIC, disseminated intravascular coagulation; GI, gastrointestinal; TMS, trimethoprim-sulfadiazine.

Suggested Reading

Gage KL, Dennis DT, Orloski KA, et al. Cases of cat-associated human plague in the Western US, 1997–1998. *Clin Infect Dis* 2000;30:893–900.

Monti DJ. Plague cases escalate again in New Mexico. *J Am Vet Med Assoc* 1999;213:192–193.

Author: Patrick L. McDonough
Consulting Editor: Stephen C. Barr

chapter 74

Pneumocystosis

DEFINITION/OVERVIEW

- An atypical fungal disease of dogs (asymptomatic in cats) characterized by respiratory difficulty from parenchymal lung disease progressing over 1 to 4 weeks.

ETIOLOGY/PATHOPHYSIOLOGY

- *Pneumocystis carinii*—saprophytic atypical fungus whose life cycle is completed in the alveolar spaces.
- Infection usually confined to the respiratory tract—but has been reported to disseminate throughout body.
- Transmission (by respiratory route)—occurs in susceptible hosts within a species (i.e., transmission does not appear to occur from dogs to humans or cats).

SIGNALMENT/HISTORY

- Most reported cases have occurred in dachshunds <12 months of age.
- Shetland sheepdogs, Cavalier King Charles spaniels, a beagle, and a Yorkshire terrier—also reported with the disease.
- Reduced immunity—may predispose to severe disease.
- Cats—can be infected but do not show clinical signs.

CLINICAL FEATURES

- Exercise intolerance (often primary complaint).
- Cough.
- Mild fevers.
- Gradual weight loss.
- May progress to cachexia, respiratory distress, and cyanosis with severe infections.
- Increased lung sounds on thoracic auscultation.
- Vomiting and diarrhea occasionally noted.

DIFFERENTIAL DIAGNOSIS

- Cardiovascular (pulmonary edema; enlarged heart, especially the left atrium; pulmonary emboli).
- Allergic (bronchial asthma, eosinophilic pneumonia or granulomatosis, pulmonary infiltrate with eosinophils).
- Trauma (foreign body, irritating gases, collapsing trachea, diaphragmatic hernia).
- Neoplasia (not only of the respiratory tree but also associated structures such as ribs, lymph nodes, muscles); unlikely in young animals.
- Inflammatory (pharyngitis; tonsillitis; kennel cough from such agents as *Bordetella bronchiseptica*, parainfluenza virus, infectious laryngotracheitis virus, and *Mycoplasma* spp.; bacterial bronchopneumonia; chronic pulmonary fibrosis; pulmonary abscess or granuloma; chronic obstructive pulmonary disease).
- Parasites (*Oslerus [Filaroides] osleri*, *Crenosoma vulpis*, *Filaroides hirthi*, *F. milksi*, *Paragonimus kellicotti*, *Dirofilaria immitis*—heartworm disease in the dog).
- Other infectious agents: systemic mycoses (blastomycosis, histoplasmosis, and cryptococcosis), toxoplasmosis, and bacterial pneumonias.

DIAGNOSTICS

- CBC, serum biochemical profile, urinalysis—changes nonspecific.
- Usually see leukocytosis—with neutrophilia and left shift, eosinophilia, and monocytosis.
- PCV—may be elevated due to chronic hypoxia.
- Arterial blood gas—reflects hypoxemia with ventilation-perfusion mismatch.
- Thoracic radiography—changes not specific for pneumocystosis; diffuse interstitial pattern with peribronchial infiltrates progressing to alveolar pattern; middle lung lobes more severely affected than cranioventral lobes; cor pulmonale may be present in severe long-standing infections.
- Serologic assays—unreliable.
- Diagnosis made by visualizing organism on a transtracheal wash, BAL, or lung aspirate cytologic examination (*Fig. 74-1*).
- Immunohistochemistry on lung biopsy or aspirate cytologic examination—definitive diagnosis.

THERAPEUTICS

- Inpatient—oxygen support for hypoxemic patients.
- Nutrition—may need to institute enteral nutrition in cachexic patients.
- Fluid therapy—may be needed while antimicrobial therapy is initiated.
- Cage rest or restricted exercise.

■ **Fig. 74-1** Cytology specimen from bronchoalveolar lavage in a dog with pulmonary *Pneumocystis carinii* infection. Note the small intracellular organisms within the mononuclear cell (Wright-Giemsa stain, 2,000×).

Drugs of Choice

- TMS—first-choice drug.
- Pentamidine isethionate (Pentam 300 injection [LyphoMed, Inc., Melrose Park, IL.])
- Carbutamide (*Table 74-1*).

Precautions/Interactions

- Pentamidine isethionate—potentiates renal insufficiency and hepatic dysfunction, hypoglycemia, hypotension, hypocalcemia, urticaria, hematologic disorders, and localized pain at injection site.

 COMMENTS

- Keep infected dogs away from other dogs, especially immunocompromised animals in an ICU.
- There is zoonotic potential reported.
- Human patients with HIV infection should be instructed to avoid contact with animals with pneumocystosis.

TABLE 74-1. Drug Therapy for Pneumocystosis

Drug	Dose (mg/kg)	Route	Interval (Hours)	Duration (Weeks)
Trimethoprim-sulfonamide	15	PO	6	3
Pentamidine isethionate	4	IM	24	2
Carbutamide	50	IM	12	3

Abbreviations

BAL, bronchoalveloar lavage; CBC, complete blood count; HIV, human immunodeficiency virus; ICU, intensive care unit; PCV, packed cell volume; TMS, trimethoprim-sulfadiazine.

Suggested Reading

Kirberger RM, Lobetti RG. Radiographic aspects of *Pneumocystis carinii* pneumonia in the miniature dachshund. *Vet Radiol Ultrasound* 1998:39;313–317.

Lobetti RG. Common variable immunodeficiency in miniature dachshunds affected with *Pneumocystis caninii*. 2000:12;39–45.

Author: Tania N. Davey
Consulting Editor: Stephen C. Barr

chapter 75

Pox Virus Infection

DEFINITION/OVERVIEW

- Rare orthopoxvirus that affects cats and causes a papular, crusted, and ulcerative dermatitis.

ETIOLOGY/PATHOPHYSIOLOGY

- Member of the genus *Orthopoxvirus*, family Poxviridae.
- Enveloped DNA virus, resistant to drying (viable for years) but readily inactivated by most disinfectants.
- Geographically limited to Eurasia.
- Relatively common.

SIGNALMENT/HISTORY

- Cats—domestic and exotic.
- No age, sex, or breed predisposition.
- Reservoir host—wild rodents.
- Infection thought to be acquired during hunting—most common in young adults and active hunters, often from rural environment.
- Lesions—often develop at the site of a bite wound (presumably inflicted by the prey animal carrying the virus).
- Most cases occur in autumn—when small wild mammals are at maximum population and most active.
- Severe cutaneous and systemic signs with poor prognosis—frequently associated with immunosuppression (iatrogenic or coinfection with FeLV or FIV).
- Cat-to-cat transmission—rare; causes only subclinical infection.
- Skin lesions—multiple, circular; dominant feature; usually develop on head, neck, or forelimbs.
- Primary lesions—crusted papules, plaques, nodules, crateriform ulcers, or areas of cellulitis or abscesses.
- Secondary lesions—erythematous nodules that ulcerate and crust; often widespread; develop after 1 to 3 weeks.
- Pruritus—variable.

- Systemic—20% of cases; anorexia, lethargy, pyrexia, vomiting, diarrhea, oculonasal discharge, conjunctivitis, and pneumonia.

DIFFERENTIAL DIAGNOSIS

- Bacterial and fungal infections.
- Eosinophilic granuloma complex.
- Neoplasia—particularly mast cell tumor; lymphosarcoma.
- Miliary dermatitis.

DIAGNOSTICS

- Serologic testing—demonstrate rising titers; hemagglutination inhibition, virus neutralizing, complement fixation, or ELISA; titers may remain high for months or years.
- Virus isolation from scab material—definitive diagnosis; 90% positive.
- Electron microscopy of extracts of scab, biopsy, or exudate—rapid presumptive diagnosis; 70% positive.
- Skin biopsy—characteristic histologic changes of epidermal hyperplasia and hypertrophy; multilocular vesicle and ulceration; large eosinophilic intracytoplasmic inclusion bodies.

THERAPEUTICS

- No specific treatment.
- Supportive (antibiotics, fluids) when necessary.
- Elizabethan collar—to prevent self-induced damage.
- Antibiotics—prevent secondary infections.
- Immunosuppressive agents (e.g., glucocorticoids and megestrol acetate)—absolutely contraindicated because they can induce fatal systemic disease.

COMMENTS

- Natural reservoir host is possibly small rodents; cats infected incidentally.
- Vaccines—none available; vaccinia virus may be considered for valuable zoo collections, but its effects in nondomestic cats have not been investigated.
- Most cats recover spontaneously in 1 to 2 months.
- Healing may be delayed by secondary bacterial skin infection.
- Prognosis is poor, with severe respiratory or pulmonary involvement.
- Rare human pox virus infections have been linked to contact with infected cats with skin lesions; use basic hygiene precautions (disposable gloves) when handling infected cats.

■ May cause painful skin lesions and severe systemic illness, particularly in the very young or elderly, people with a preexisting skin condition, and the immuno-deficient.

Abbreviations

DNA, deoxyribonucleic acid; ELISA, enzyme-linked immunosorbent assay; FeLV, feline leukemia virus; FIV, feline immunodeficiency virus.

Suggested Reading

Gaskell RM, Bennett M. Feline poxvirus infection. In: Chandler EA, Gaskell CJ, Gaskell RM, eds. *Feline medicine and therapeutics*. Oxford, UK: Blackwell Scientific; 1994:515–520.

Author: J. Paul Woods
Consulting Editor: Karen Helton Rhodes

Protothecosis

chapter **76**

DEFINITION/OVERVIEW

- Blue-green algae infection causing either localized infection (cats) of the skin and GI, or systemic disseminated infection (dogs).

ETIOLOGY/PATHOPHYSIOLOGY

- *Prototheca wickerhamii* (usually cats) and *P. zopfi* (usually dogs)—single-celled achlorophyllous blue-green algae.
- Algae live on raw and treated sewage—survive as contaminants of soil, water, and food.
- Occasionally isolated—from the feces of healthy individuals.

SIGNALMENT/HISTORY

- Dogs and cats—rare.
- Dogs—medium to large breeds, middle-aged females mostly affected.
- Depressed cell immunity may predispose dogs to infection—no known predisposing factors for cats.

CLINICAL FEATURES

Dogs

- Mainly affected by the GI form of the disease.
- Depends on the organ system involved, but signs can include:
  - Intermittent and chronic bloody diarrhea.
  - Chronic weight loss.
  - Blindness, with posterior segment disease with retinal granulomas and/or detached retinas.
  - Neurologic signs.
  - Cutaneous lesions, with ragged ulcers and crusts usually on extremities and mucosal surfaces.

405

Cats

- Chronic cutaneous or mucous membrane ulceration, with few if any systemic signs.
- Cutaneous lesions, usually localized, extend deep into the subcutaneous tissues (usually on limbs and/or face) and consist of granulomatous inflammation in which there are a large number of organisms.

DIFFERENTIAL DIAGNOSIS

- Systemic—systemic mycoses (histoplasmosis, blastomycosis).
- Cutaneous—systemic or cutaneous mycoses; mycobacteriosis.

DIAGNOSTICS

- CBC, biochemical profile, and urinalysis—usually normal but may reflect organ damage in systemic disease (normal in the cat).
- CSF tap—pleocytosis with mononuclear cells reported; elevated protein; may see organisms in CSF if CNS infected.

Diagnostic Feature

- **Cytology—most definitive diagnostic test to identify organism in skin lesions or organ aspirates (rectal or colonic mucosa, anterior chamber aspirations, or CSF); Wright-Giemsa best stain** *(Fig. 76-1).*
- Histopathologic examination—identify organism in biopsy of skin lesions (special stains: Gomori methenamine silver GMS), periodic acid–Schiff).
- Culture—grows on Sabouraud's dextrose agar at 25° to 37°C in 2 to 7 days.

■ **Fig. 76-1** Cytologic specimen of a rectal scraping from a dog with protothecosis. Organisms are identified by the halo and a thin cell wall and are of varying size (Wright's stain, 1,000×).

TABLE 76-1. Drug Therapy for Prototthecosis					
Drug	Species	Dose (mg/kg)	Route	Interval (Hours)	Duration (Weeks)
Amphotericin B	D	0.25–0.5	IV	3 times weekly	a
	C	0.25	IV	3 times weekly	b
Tetracycline	B	22	PO	8	c
Ketoconazole	B	10–15	PO	12–24	6
Itraconazole	B	5–10	PO	12	6
Fluconazole	B	2.5–5	PO	12	6

a Until total cumulative dose of 8 mg/kg or renal toxicity occurs.
b Until total cumulative dose of 4 mg/kg.
c Continue for as long as amphotericin B is administered.
D, dogs; C, cats; B, both dogs and cats.

THERAPEUTICS

- Dogs—require antimicrobials if systemically affected.
- Cutaneous lesions—excision is treatment of choice followed by systemic antifungal agents.

Drugs of Choice

- Amphotericin B—use for localized disease after surgical excision; lipid formulations are also effective and produce fewer side effects.
- Tetracyclines given concurrently with amphotericin B—may provide a synergistic effect; more effective for ocular disease.
- Oral antifungal agents such as ketoconazole, fluconazole, and itraconazole—may be used in conjunction with amphotericin B or as sole agent in non–life-threatening cases (*Table 76-1*).

Precautions/Interactions

- Amphotericin B—may cause toxic nephritis; monitor by examining urine for appearance of hyaline casts.
- Amphotericin B—may also cause severe phlebitis.
- Ketoconazole (and to a lesser extent itraconazole and fluconazole)—may induce hepatic enzymes and cause hepatotoxicity; monitor periodically.

COMMENTS

- The organism—difficult to eradicate with drug therapy.
- Prognosis in dogs—guarded to grave.
- Prognosis in cats—good if cutaneous lesions can be completely excised.
- No zoonotic potential has been recorded.

Abbreviations

CBC, complete blood count; CNS, central nervous system; CSF, cerebrospinal fluid; GI, gastrointestinal; GMS, Gomori methenamine silver.

Suggested Reading

Hollingsworth SR. Canine prototothecosis. *Vet Clin North Am Small Anim Pract* 2000:30;1091–1101.
Hosaka S, Hosaka M. A case report of canine prototothecosis. *J Vet Med Sci* 2004:66;593–597.

Author: Carol S. Foil
Consulting Editor: Stephen C. Barr

chapter 77

Pseudorabies Virus Infection

DEFINITION/OVERVIEW

- Rare but highly fatal viral disease of dogs and cats—usually have a history of contact with pigs.
- Characterized by sudden death, often without signs—if signs occur, they include hypersalivation, intense pruritus, and CNS signs.

ETIOLOGY/PATHOPHYSIOLOGY

- Pseudorabies virus (suid herpesvirus, Aujeszky's disease, mad itch of pigs)—an α-herpesvirus.
- Dogs and cats—become infected when they contact infected pigs, eat contaminated uncooked meat or offal from pigs, or eat infected rats.

SIGNALMENT/HISTORY

- Domestic and exotic dogs and cats of any age or breed—contact with a farm.
- May also be seen in other domestic species—cattle, sheep, goats, and pigs.

CLINICAL FEATURES

- Usually sudden death.
- Acute onset of:
  - Hypersalivation.
  - Dyspnea.
  - Fever.
  - Vomiting.
  - CNS signs, including depression, lethargy, ataxia, seizures, recumbency, coma, and death.
- Intense pruritus and self-mutilation are features of the disease.

DIFFERENTIAL DIAGNOSIS

- Rabies—in various forms; affected dogs and cats will attack anything that moves; there is usually no intense pruritus with rabies; sudden death is usually not a feature of rabies.
- Canine distemper—no hypersalivation, sudden death, or personality change; other multisystemic signs present.
- Toxicity exposure (organophosphate, lead, strychnine, inorganic arsenic)—no pruritus or personality changes; history of exposure; other signs consistent with exposure.

 DIAGNOSTICS

- CBC, serum biochemical profile, urinalysis—no characteristic changes.
- CSF—increased protein and mononuclear pleocytosis.
- Serologic assay—available, but antibodies develop after acute disease is over so may not be present at the time of death.
- Definitive diagnostic test—direct FA on brain tissue.
- Histologic examination—intranuclear inclusion bodies in glial and ganglion cells of brain.
- PCR—used in Japan to identify one case in a cat.
- Viral isolation at necropsy—from brain tissue.

 THERAPEUTICS

- No known effective treatment, except supportive care and prevention of self-mutilation.

Drugs of Choice

- No specific drugs available.

Precautions/Interactions

- Transmission from infected cats and dogs to other cats and dogs does not seem to occur, so should there should be no risk to other in-contact pets.

 COMMENTS

- Clinical course in cats typically lasts 24 to 36 hours, followed by death (60% of cases). Others (40%) last longer than 36 hours but also are invariably fatal.
- Mild potential for human infection; take precautions when treating infected animals and handling infected tissues and fluids.

Abbreviations

CBC, complete blood count; CNS, central nervous system; CSF, cerebrospinal fluid; FA, fluorescent antibody; PCR, polymerase chain reaction.

Suggested Reading

Vandevelde M. Pseudorabies. In: Greene CE, ed. *Infectious Diseases of the Dog and Cat.* Philadelphia: WB Saunders; 1998:126–128.

Author: Fred W. Scott
Consulting Editor: Stephen C. Barr

chapter 78

Pythiosis

DEFINITION/OVERVIEW

- An infectious disease causing primarily either a chronic pyogranulomatous lesion of the stomach or intestines, or nonhealing wounds and invasive masses that contain ulcerated nodules and draining tracts in the skin of dogs and cats.

ETIOLOGY/PATHOPHYSIOLOGY

- *Pythium insidiosum*—an aquatic pathogen.
- Infective form—thought to be a motile biflagellate zoospore.
- Zoospore is released into warm water and attracted chemotactically to damaged tissue and animal hair—animals likely infected when they enter or ingest contaminated water.
- Distribution—occurs mainly in tropical or semitropical regions of the world.
- Distribution—in the United States, occurs mainly in states bordering the Gulf of Mexico, but also reported in Oklahoma, Arkansas, Missouri, Kentucky, Tennessee, North and South Carolina, Virginia, Indiana, and New Jersey.
- Usually—only one body system (skin or GI tract) in any one patient affected at a time.
- Cats—skin usually affected; retrobulbar, periorbital, or nasopharyngeal regions and tail head or footpads.
- Dogs—skin and GI tract equally affected.
- GI tract—usually gastric outflow tract affected, including the proximal small intestine, but also the ileocolic junction and colon.
- Local thromboembolic events or vascular invasion—may lead to bowel wall ischemia and GI tract perforation or hemoabdomen (especially in dogs).
- Skin lesions—single or multiple cutaneous or subcutaneous lesions involving the extremities, tail head, ventral neck, perineum, or medial thigh (dogs).

SIGNALMENT/HISTORY

- Dogs more than cats; large-breed dogs (hunting, field trial breeds) working near water.
- Labrador retrievers—overrepresented.
- German shepherd dogs—may be predisposed to cutaneous form.

- Mainly—dogs <3 years of age.
- Sex distribution—more males affected than females.

 CLINICAL FEATURES

Gastrointestinal Tract Pythiosis

- Emaciation—common.
- Abdominal mass—often palpable.
- Affected dogs—often bright and alert, in spite of severe weight loss.
- Fever—occasionally.
- Systemic signs—may develop if intestinal obstruction, infarction, or perforation occurs (*Fig. 78-1*).

Cutaneous Pythiosis

- Nonhealing wounds—characterized by poorly defined nodules that ulcerate and drain a serosanguinous or purulent exudate from multiple tracts.

 DIFFERENTIAL DIAGNOSIS

Gastrointestinal Tract Pythiosis

- Intestinal mass and/or obstruction caused by foreign body, chronic intussusception, neoplasia (lymphosarcoma, carcinoma, other GI tract neoplasias), histoplasmosis; IBD; and other infections (protothecosis, basidiobolomycosis).

Cutaneous Pythiosis

- Other fungal infectious diseases (oomycotic pathogens such as *Lagenidium*, zygomycosis caused by *Basidiobolus* or *Conidiobolus* spp., cryptococcosis, coccidioidomycosis, sporotrichosis, eumycotic mycetoma, and phaeohyphomycosis).

■ **Fig. 78-1** Gross specimen of the gastric outflow tract of the stomach of a dog with pythiosis. Note the profound stomach wall thickening from the pylogranulomatous process.

- Bacterial diseases (actinomycosis, nocardiosis, leprosy, mycobacteriosis, botryomycosis, and brucellosis) and other infectious causes (protothecosis, nodular leishmaniasis).
- Noninfectious pyogranulomatous diseases (foreign body reactions, idiopathic nodular panniculitis, sebaceous nodular adenitis, and canine cutaneous sterile pyogranuloma/granuloma syndrome, cutaneous neoplasia).
- Systemic vasculitis and cutaneous embolic disease.

 DIAGNOSTICS

- CBC—eosinophilia, leukocytosis, and anemia of chronic disease may occur.
- Serum biochemical profile—hypoalbuminemia and hyperglobulinemia may occur in chronically affected animals.
- Electrolyte abnormalities (hypokalemia, hyponatremia, hypochloridemia, metabolic alkalosis)—in dogs with gastric outflow obstruction.
- Imaging—abdominal radiographs and ultrasound examination may reveal GI tract obstruction, bowel wall thickening, and mesenteric lymph node enlargement.
- Serology—ELISA (offered by Pythium Laboratory, LSU, Baton Rouge, Louisiana) is sensitive and specific.
- Histopathologic examination of biopsy specimen of GI tract and skin lesion—suggestive only but not definitive for pythiosis; need immunohistochemistry to confirm identity of hyphae in lesion.
- Culture—tissue samples; ship overnight at room temperature to experienced laboratory (LSU).
- PCR—is available to identify cultured organisms or organisms in tissue biopsy samples (LSU).

 THERAPEUTICS

- Treatment of choice—aggressive surgical excision of all infected tissues.
- Often not possible to remove all infected tissue—disease too advanced by the time a diagnosis is made.
- Dogs often improve after obstructive GI tract lesion is resected, even if significant disease is still grossly evident.
- After surgery—medical therapy with antifungal agents for 2 to 3 months will decrease likelihood of recurrence.

Drugs of Choice

- Itraconazole combined with terbinafine (Lamisil [Novartis Pharmaceuticals, Greensboro, NC])—drug protocol of choice; efficacy is 20% to 25% in nonresectable or partially resectable lesions; continue for 4 to 6 months.
- Amphotericin B lipid complex—shown to be effective in a limited number of dogs; recommended if patient cannot tolerate oral drugs (*Table 78-1*).

TABLE 78-1. Drug Therapy for Pythiosis

Drug	Species	Dose (mg/kg)	Route	Interval (Hours)	Duration (Months)
Itraconazole[a]	D	10	PO	24	4–6
Terbinafine (Lamisil)	D	5–10	PO	24	4–6
Amphotericin B lipid complex	D	2–3	IV	3 times weekly	1–4[b]
	C	0.5–1	IV	3 times weekly	1–4[b]

[a] Used in combination with terbinafine.
[b] To a total dose of 25 to 30 mg.
D, dogs; C, cats.

Precautions/Interactions

- Azole drugs—should not be given to animals with hepatic disease; monitor for hepatic toxicity by monitoring ALT monthly throughout treatment course.
- Amphotericin B lipid complex—can cause nephrotoxicity (monitor urine repeatedly for the appearance of hyaline casts); other side effects include fever, anorexia, vomiting during infusion.

 COMMENTS

- Reevaluation of ELISA serology 2 to 3 months after surgery or 3 months after medical management; excellent prognostic indicator.
- Examination for reoccurrence of GI tract lesion with abdominal ultrasound is useful.
- Prognosis—guarded to poor unless a complete resection is possible.
- Fewer than 25% of affected animals are cured with medical therapy alone.
- No zoonotic potential, although humans can become infected (very rare) from a common environmental source; no evidence of direct transmission from animals to humans.

Abbreviations

ALT, alanine aminotransferase; CBC, complete blood count; ELISA, enzyme-linked immunosorbent assay; GI, gastrointestinal; IBD, inflammatory bowel disease; LSU, Louisiana State University; PCR, polymerase chain reaction.

Suggested Reading

Grooters AM. Pythiosis, lagenidiosis, and zygomycosis in small animals. *Vet Clin North Am Small Anim Pract* 2003:33;695–720.

Author: Amy Grooters and Joseph Taboada
Consulting Editor: Stephen C. Barr

chapter 79

Q Fever

DEFINITION/OVERVIEW

- A systemic infection causing abortion in cats and CNS disease in dogs.

ETIOLOGY/PATHOPHYSIOLOGY

- *Coxiella burnetii*—zoonotic rickettsia.
- Infection—most commonly by inhalation or ingestion of organisms while feeding on infected body fluids (urine, feces, milk, or parturient discharges), tissues (especially placenta), or carcasses of infected animal reservoir hosts (cattle, sheep, goats).
- Can occur after tick exposure (many species of ticks implicated).
- Lungs—main portal of entry to systemic circulation.
- Organism replicates in vascular endothelium, causing widespread vasculitis.
- Vasculitis results in necrosis and hemorrhage in lungs, liver, and CNS.
- Severity—depends on the pathogenicity of the strain of organism.
- An extended latent period exists after recovery until chronic immune complex phenomena develop.
- Organism reactivated out of the latent state during parturition, resulting in large numbers entering the placenta, parturient fluids, urine, feces, and milk.
- Endemic worldwide.

SIGNALMENT/HISTORY

- Cats and dogs.
- History of contact with farm animals or ticks.

CLINICAL FEATURES

- Fever.
- Lethargy.
- Depression.
- Anorexia followed by ataxia, seizures, and other neurologic signs (dogs).
- Abortion, especially in cats.

DIFFERENTIAL DIAGNOSIS

Dogs

- Differentiate from granulomatous meningoencephalomyelitis, protozoal encephalitis (toxoplasmosis, neosporosis), distemper, cryptococcosis or other infectious agents (meningitis, ehrlichiosis, RMSF), pug dog encephalitis, toxicities (lead poisoning, organophosphate, carbamate, strychnine), and neoplasia.

Cats

- Other causes of abortion—infections (viral rhinotracheitis; panleukopenia; FeLV; toxoplasmosis; bacteria, including coliforms; streptococci; staphylococci; salmonellae), fetal defects, maternal problems (nutrition, genital tract abnormalities), environmental stress, and endocrine disorders (hypoluteidism).

DIAGNOSTICS

- CBC, biochemical profile, urinalysis—nonspecific findings.

Diagnostic Feature

- **Definitive diagnosis—made by isolation of organism or serology.**
- Organism identification—collect 2 to 3 ml of serum, refrigerate, and send on ice to test laboratory (New Mexico Department of Agriculture, Veterinary Diagnostic Services, 700 Camino de Salud NE, Albuquerque, NM 87106).
- Tissue samples (placenta)—send to same test laboratory for animal inoculation.
- Serology—IFA and ELISA methods are available; a fourfold increase in IgG titer over a 4-week period is diagnostic; the use of newer serologic techniques that measure IgM on one sample has not been well documented in small animals.
- PCR—also performed by New Mexico Department of Agriculture laboratory; used to detect organisms in tissue culture or tissue specimens derived from the patient.

THERAPEUTICS

- Alert client of possible zoonotic risk.
- If treat in hospital, wear gloves and mask and maintain in an isolation facility.

TABLE 79-1. Drug Therapy for Q Fever in Dogs and Cats					
Drug	Species	Dose (mg/kg)	Route	Interval (Hours)	Duration (Weeks)
Doxycycline	D	10–20	PO, IV	12–24	2–6
	C	5–10	PO	12–24	2–4
Enrofloxacin	B	3–5	PO	12	2–6
Tetracycline	D	22	PO	8	2–6
	C	10–20	PO	8–12	2–3

D, dogs; C, cats; B, both dogs and cats.

Drugs of Choice

- Tetracycline.
- Doxycycline—use in combination with enrofloxacin for extended periods in chronic infections.
- Enrofloxacin—effective in vitro, but no clinical reports (*Table 79-1*).

Precautions/Interactions

- Tetracycline drugs are associated with yellowing of teeth in young animals; do not use in animals with renal failure.
- Doxycycline—may cause esophagitis and stricture.
- Enrofloxacin—may cause cartilage defects in young animals.
- Enrofloxacin—may cause retinal degeneration when used in cats with concurrent hepatic or renal disease or at high doses.

 COMMENTS

- Difficult to determine success of therapy because many animals spontaneously improve.
- Even asymptomatic cases should be aggressively treated because of the zoonotic potential.
- Utility of predicting success of therapy based on serologic improvement unknown.
- The zoonotic potential cannot be overemphasized.
- By the time the diagnosis is made in a cat or dog, human exposure has occurred.
- Instruct owner and in-contact humans to seek medical advice immediately.
- Humans contract the disease by inhalation of infected aerosols.
- Children commonly infected from ingestion of raw milk, but they are usually asymptomatic.
- Previous urban outbreaks in humans have been related to exposure to infected cats.
- Incubation period from time of contact to illness in humans is 5 to 32 days.
- Person-to-person transmission possible.

Abbreviations

CBC, complete blood count; CNS, central nervous system; ELISA, enzyme-linked immunosorbent assay; FeLV, feline leukemia virus; IFA, immunofluorescence assay; Ig, immunoglobulin; PCR, polymerase chain reaction; RMSF, Rocky Mountain spotted fever.

Suggested Reading

Brouqui P, Badiaga S, Raoult D. Q fever outbreak in homeless shelter. *Emerg Infect Dis* 2004;10:1297–1299.

Komiya T, Sadamasu K, Kang MI, et al. Seroprevalence of *Coxiella burnetii* infections among cats in different living environments. *J Vet Med* Sci 2003;65:1047–1048.

Author: Stephen C. Barr
Consulting Editor: Stephen C. Barr

chapter 80

Rabies

DEFINITION/OVERVIEW

- A severe, invariably fatal viral polioencephalitis of warm-blooded animals, including humans.

ETIOLOGY/PATHOPHYSIOLOGY

- Rabies virus is a single-stranded RNA virus (genus, *Lyssavirus*; family, Rhabdoviridae).
- Virus enters the body through a wound (usually from a bite of rabid animal) or via mucous membranes and replicates in myocytes, then spreads to the neuromuscular junction and neurotendinal spindles; travels to the CNS via intra-axonal fluid within peripheral nerves; spreads throughout the CNS; then finally spreads centrifugally within the peripheral, sensory, and motor neurons.
- Affects nervous system (causing clinical encephalitis—either paralytic or ferocious rabies) and salivary glands (excessive salivation; saliva containing large quantities of virus).
- Once infected, clinical disease is virtually inevitable.
- Prevalence is low, except in enzootic areas, especially in underdeveloped countries, where vaccination rates of cats and dogs are low.
- Distribution is worldwide except in British Isles, Australia, New Zealand, Hawaii, Japan, and parts of Scandinavia.

SIGNALMENT/HISTORY

- All warm-blooded animals can be infected.
- In the United States, four endemic strains within fox, raccoon, skunk, and bat populations exist.
- All endemic strains in the United States can be transmitted to dogs and cats.

CLINICAL FEATURES

- Quite variable—with atypical presentation being the rule rather than exception.
- Classically, three progressive stages of disease—prodromal, ferocious, and paralytic.
- Often first signs are changes in behavior:
  - Seeking solitude.
  - Apprehension.
  - Nervousness.
  - Anxiety.
  - Unusual shyness or aggressiveness.
- Then behavior becomes more erratic:
  - Biting.
  - Snapping.
  - Licking.
  - Chewing at a wound site.
  - Biting at cage.
  - Wandering and roaming.
  - Excitability.
  - Irritability.
  - Viciousness.
  - Changes in tone of bark.
- Progression to more clinical signs of:
  - Disorientation.
  - Incoordination.
  - Seizures.
  - Finally, paralysis.
- Excess salivation or frothing at the mouth—may be exacerbated by mandibular and laryngeal paralysis, with a dropped jaw, and inability to swallow (*Fig. 80-1*).
- Fever—may or may not be present.
- Death—occurs in all infected dogs and cats within 7 to 10 days of onset of clinical signs.

■ **Fig. 80-1** A dog with rabies. Note the slightly dropped jaw, excessive salivation, and manic look. (Courtesy Dr. A. Delahunta, Cornell University.)

DIFFERENTIAL DIAGNOSIS

- Seriously consider rabies—in any unvaccinated (against rabies) dog or cat showing unusual mood or behavioral changes or unaccountable neurologic signs, especially in endemic areas.
- Suspected cases—should be handled with considerable care to limit the number of individuals exposed.
- Any neurologic disease causing diffuse signs—other infectious causes such as canine distemper (no hypersalivation or sudden death; other multisystemic signs present), toxoplasmosis, neosporosis, pseudorabies (no intense pruritus with rabies usually; sudden death is usually not a feature of rabies), toxicity (organophosphate, lead, strychnine, inorganic arsenic), neoplasia, GME, polyradiculoneuropathy, hepatic encephalopathy, and head injury.
- Other causes of laryngeal paralysis, choking, or hypersalivation.

DIAGNOSTICS

- CBC, serum biochemical profile and urinalysis—no characteristic changes.
- CSF—minimally increased protein and leukocyte counts may be seen.

Diagnostic Feature
- **DFA test of nervous tissue—method of choice for definitive diagnosis; rapid and very sensitive test.**
- DFA—brain, head, or entire body can be shipped to rabies-certified laboratory for processing; chill samples immediately, but do not freeze; use extreme care and caution when collecting, handling, and shipping these samples.
- DFA test on dermal tissue—skin biopsy of the sensory vibrissae of the maxillary area, including deeper subcutaneous hair follicles.
- Although skin testing may augment a clinical diagnosis—verification can only be achieved by a DFA test of nervous tissue.

THERAPEUTICS

- Inform client—as to the seriousness of contact with a rabid animal.
- As a veterinarian, you must insist—that clients see a physician immediately to initiate postexposure therapy; local public health officials must be notified as soon as possible.
- Advise clients—to carefully consider any other human exposure.
- If there is doubt regarding the diagnosis—the animal should be quarantined in an approved site with appropriate signage and cage security and only designated people should have access.
- An apparently healthy dog or cat that bites or scratches a person—should be monitored for a period of 10 days; if no signs of illness occur in the animal within 10 days,

the person has had no exposure to the virus; animals do not shed the virus for more than 3 days before development of clinical disease.

- An unvaccinated dog or cat that is bitten or exposed to a known rabid animal—may need to be quarantined for up to 6 months or according to local or state regulations.
- Once a diagnosis is as close to certain as possible—euthanasia with submission of appropriate tissues for a definitive diagnosis is indicated.
- Vaccination—vaccinate according to standard recommendations and state and local requirements; all dogs and cats with any potential exposure to wildlife or other dogs; vaccinate after 12 weeks of age; then 12 months later; then every 3 years (killed vaccines in cats and dogs) or yearly for cats if a nonadjuvanted recombinant vaccine (Purevax Feline Rabies [Merial, Iselin, NJ]) is used.
- Rabies-free countries—entering dogs and cats may be quarantined; contact specific countries for requirements.
- Disinfection—any contaminated area, cage, food dish, or instrument must be thoroughly disinfected; use a 1:32 dilution (4 ounces per gallon of water) of household bleach to quickly inactivate virus; usually virus deposited on a dog or cat hair after a bite from a rabid animal will die after exposure to the air for 1 hour.

Drugs of Choice

- No drug treatment is indicated—once a diagnosis is made, euthanasia is indicated.

Precautions/Interactions

- The seriousness of the zoonotic potential cannot be overemphasized.

 COMMENTS

- Local and state regulations must be adhered to carefully and completely.

Abbreviations

CBC, complete blood count; CNS, central nervous system; CSF, cerebrospinal fluid; DFA, direct fluorescent antibody; GME, granulomatous meningoencephalitis; RNA, ribonucleic acid.

Suggested Reading

Jenkins SR, Auslander M, Conti L, et al. Compedium of animal rabies prevention and control. *J Am Vet Med Assoc* 2004;224:216–222.
Greene CE, Dreesen DW. Rabies. In: Greene CE, ed. *Infectious Diseases of the Dog and Cat.* 2nd ed. Philadelphia: WB Saunders; 1998:114–126.

Author: Fred W. Scott
Consulting Editor: Stephen C. Barr

chapter 81

Reovirus Infection

DEFINITION/OVERVIEW

- A respiratory and intestinal viral infection of cats and dogs resulting in mild upper respiratory signs or diarrhea.

ETIOLOGY/PATHOPHYSIOLOGY

- *Reovirus* (respiratory enteric orphan virus)—nonenveloped, double-stranded RNA virus.
- Easily isolated—from the respiratory and enteric tracts.
- Like rotavirus and coronavirus—affects mature epithelial cells on luminal tips of intestinal villi.
- Damage to villi—villous atrophy and osmotic diarrhea.
- Transmission—fecal/oral (GI) route; also inhalation (respiratory).

SIGNALMENT/HISTORY

- Young animals usually more severely affected.

CLINICAL FEATURES

Dogs

- Conjunctivitis.
- Rhinitis.
- Tracheobronchitis.
- Pneumonia, if secondary bacterial infection involved.
- Diarrhea.

Cats

- Mainly mild respiratory signs (conjunctivitis).
- Diarrhea.

DIFFERENTIAL DIAGNOSIS

Dogs

- Other causes of acute small bowel diarrhea in an otherwise healthy young animal:
  - Infectious; parvovirus, coronavirus, rotavirus, calicivirus, distemper, giardiasis, cryptosporidiosis, hookworms, whipworms, roundworms, GI tract bacterial overgrowth, and clostridia.
  - Toxicity—lead.
  - Dietary indiscretion, allergy.
  - IBD.
  - Foreign body.
  - Intussusception.
- Other causes of canine infectious tracheobronchitis—*Bordetella bronchiseptica*, mycoplasma, CAV, CHV, distemper, and parainfluenza.

Cats

- Other causes of mild upper respiratory disease—rhinotracheitis virus, calicivirus, *Chlamydia* spp., and mycoplasma.

DIAGNOSTICS

- CBC and biochemistry panel—normal.
- Viral isolation—very time consuming, but can be identified on electron microscopy *(Fig. 81-1)*.
- Even if virus is isolated from cat or dog with symptoms—this likely is not the primary pathogen.
- Histopathology—large intracyctoplasmic inclusion bodies.

■ **Fig. 81-1** Electron micrograph of reovirus particles isolated from a dog (bar = 50 nm).

THERAPEUTICS

- Antibiotics may be indicated if fever is present or diarrhea persists.
- Supportive care for osmotic diarrhea as needed.
- Antiviral drugs are not indicated.

Drugs of Choice

- N/A

Precautions/Interactions

- No vaccines are available.

COMMENTS

- If reovirus is demonstrated to be present, search for the presence of other pathogens.

Abbreviations

CAV, canine adenovirus; CBC, complete blood count; CHV, canine herpes virus; GI, gastrointestinal; IBD, inflammatory bowel disease; RNA, ribonucleic acid.

Suggested Reading

Binn LN, Marchwicki RH, Keenan KP, et al. Recovery of reovirus type 2 from an immature dog with respiratory tract disease. *Am J Vet Res* 1977;38:927–929.

Kokubu T, Takahashi T, Takamura K, et al. Isolation of reovirus type 3 from dogs with diarrhea. *J Vet Med Sci* 1993;55:453–454.

Author: J. Paul Woods
Consulting Editor: Stephen C. Barr

Respiratory Capillariasis
(Eucoleus)

chapter 82

DEFINITION/OVERVIEW

- A nematode parasitic infection of both dogs and cats—mainly asymptomatic but can cause a chronic cough and wheezing respiratory sounds.

ETIOLOGY/PATHOPHYSIOLOGY

- *Eucoleus aerophilus* (= previously named *Capillaria aerophila*)—Trichuroidea parasite with bi-operculate eggs.
- Eggs—easily confused with those from other capillarids (*E. boehmi* of the nose and *Pearsonema plica* in the urinary bladder) and whipworms of dogs (*Trichuris vulpis*).
- Adult worms—embed in the mucosal lining of large airways, expelling eggs into the respiratory passages.
- Eggs—coughed up the trachea and swallowed, to be passed in the feces.
- Infection—occurs by ingesting L1 larvae (take about 40 days to mature in eggs).
- Infections—can last as long as a year.
- Direct life cycle—likely, although it is possible that earthworms are paratenic hosts.
- PPP = 3 to 5 weeks.

SIGNALMENT/HISTORY

- Fairly common infection in both cats and dogs.

CLINICAL FEATURES

- Most infections are asymptomatic, rarely causing clinical signs.
- Wheezing.
- Chronic cough.
- Weight loss is rare.
- When complicated with bacterial pneumonia can cause death.

DIFFERENTIAL DIAGNOSIS

- A general differential diagnosis for cough includes such categories as:
    Cardiovascular and congestive heart failure (pulmonary edema; enlarged heart, especially the left atrium; left-sided heart failure; pulmonary emboli; mitral valve insufficiency).
    Allergic (bronchial asthma, eosinophilic pneumonia or granulomatosis, pulmonary infiltrate with eosinophilia).
    Trauma (foreign body, irritating gases, collapsing trachea, hypoplastic trachea).
    Neoplasia (not only of the respiratory tree but also associated structures such as ribs, lymph nodes, muscles).
    Inflammatory (pharyngitis; tonsillitis; kennel cough from such agents as *Bordetella bronchoseptica*, parainfluenza virus, infectious laryngotracheitis virus, and mycoplasma; systemic fungal pneumonia; bacterial bronchopneumonia; aspiration; chronic pulmonary fibrosis; pulmonary abscess or granuloma; chronic obstructive pulmonary disease).
    Parasites (*Oslerus* [*Filaroides*] *osleri*, *Filaroides hirthi*, *F. milksi*, *Paragonimus kellicotti*, *Dirofilaria immitis*—heartworm disease in the dog, and *Aelurostrongylus abstrusus* in the cat).

DIAGNOSTICS

Diagnositic Feature
- **Bi-operculate eggs found in feces or tracheal wash fluids of both cats and dogs** (*Fig. 82-1*).

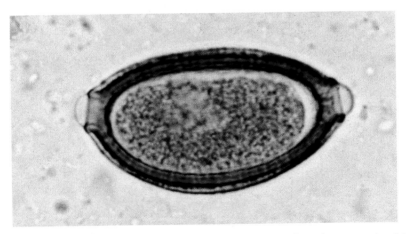

■ **Fig. 82-1** Bi-opurculate egg found in the feces of an infected cat. In dog feces the egg may be distinguished from those of *E. boehmi* by the fine lattice-work lines over the surface as opposed to the fine pitted surface of those of *E. boehmi*.

TABLE 82-1. Drug Therapy for Respiratory Capillariasis in Small Animals				
Drug	Dose (mg/kg)	Route	Interval (Hours)	Duration (Days)
Ivermectin	0.2	PO, SC	Once	—
Fenbendazole	50	PO	24	10–14

- Eggs—very similar to those of *Trichuris vulpis* (whipworms), found in infected dog's feces, and those of *E. boehmi* (nasal capillaria), which also may be found in feces.
- Thoracic radiographs may show diffuse mild bronchoalveolar pattern but are not pathognomonic.

THERAPEUTICS

- Asymptomatic cases do not require treatment.

Drugs of Choice

- Fenbendazole—treatment of choice in dogs; difficult to administer in cats over this time period.
- Ivermectin—efficacy is unknown but is effective against nasal capillariasis and indications are that it is effective against other capillarids as well *(Table 82-1)*.

Precautions/Interactions

- If using ivermectin—ensure dogs do not have microfilaremia before administering ivermectin.
- Ivermectin-sensitive collie breeds or collie-cross dogs—may show neurologic signs with this dose of ivermectin.

COMMENTS

- Pulmonary capillariasis is often found incidentally on routine fecal examinations.
- There is probably not a requirement to treat animals found to be infected with *E. aerophilus* on a routine fecal examination.
- It is the author's impression that the infection has become more uncommon with the advent of the wide use of monthly heartworm preventives.
- Infection is probably acquired from infected earthworms or the environment (eggs can persist for long periods)—one means of preventing reinfection would be to keep pets indoors.

Abbreviation

PPP, prepatent period.

Suggested Reading

Reinemeyer CR. 1995. Parasites of the respiratory system. In: Kirk RW, Bonagura JD, eds. *Current Veterinary Therapy XII*. Philadelphia: WB Saunders; 1995:895–898.

Author: Stephen C. Barr
Consulting Editor: Stephen C. Barr

chapter 83

Rhinosporidium

DEFINITION/OVERVIEW

- A rare chronic fungal infection of the mucous membranes of dogs (reported in one cat).
- Usually forms a cauliflower-like mass that protrudes from the nostril.

ETIOLOGY/PATHOPHYSIOLOGY

- *Rhinosporidium seeberi*—thought to be associated with stagnant water and arid environments.
- Distribution—worldwide.
- Endemic areas—Argentina, Sri Lanka, and India.
- In the United States—most infections reported from the southern states.

SIGNALMENT/HISTORY

- Dogs mainly—no breed or sex predilection.
- Cats—only one case report.

CLINICAL FEATURES

- Cauliflower-like mass in the nasal cavity often seen protruding from the nostril.
- Usually single and polypoid, but may be lobulated or sessile.
- Surface often white or yellowish with superficial flecks, which are fungal sporangia.
- Dog often present with:
  - Sneezing.
  - Epistaxis.
  - Stertorous breathing.

DIFFERENTIAL DIAGNOSIS

- Nasal neoplasia.
- Allergic inflammatory rhinitis.

- Polyps.
- Nasal foreign body.
- Other fungal causes of rhinitis (aspergillosis).
- If epistaxis alone, rule out systemic causes of bleeding (coagulopathy, thrombocytopenia)

 DIAGNOSTICS

- CBC, serum biochemical panel, and urinalysis—usually normal.
- Nasal radiographs—often normal because the mass is usually located in the anterior nasal cavity and does not invade turbinates.
- CT or MRI scans—show a mass effect.

Diagnostic Feature
- **Diagnostic method of choice—cytology of mass aspirate, impression smear, or biopsy of the nasal mass will reveals organisms (periodi acid–Schiff, GMS, and new methylene blue are the best stains) *(Fig. 83-1)*.**

 THERAPEUTICS

- Surgical excision of mass—treatment of choice.
- Approach—through the external nares or by rhinotomy.
- Failure to remove all the mass—usually results in regrowth.

■ **Fig. 83-1** *Rhinosporidium* spores present within a biopsy section of a nasal mass from a dog (GMS stain, 1,000×).

Drugs of Choice

- Dapsone—has been used in one dog with favorable results, but not a complete cure and considerable side effects (dosage: 1.1 mg/kg, PO, q8–12h).
- Ketoconazole—has been used with limited success.

Precautions/Interactions

- Dapsone—can cause hepatotoxicity, anemia, neutropenia, thrombocytopenia, GI signs, and skin reactions.

 COMMENTS

- Careful follow-up is necessary to identify regrowth after surgical removal.
- There is no known risk of direct transmission to humans in contact with infected dogs, but the organism is infectious to humans.

Abbreviations

CBC, complete blood count; CT, computed tomography; GI, gastrointestinal; GMS, Gomori's methamine silver; MRI, magnetic resonance imaging.

Suggested Reading

Caniatti M, Roccabianca R. Scanziani E, et al. Nasal rhinosporidiosis in dogs: four cases from Europe and a review of the literature. *Vet Rec* 1998;142:334–338.

Wallin LL, Coleman GD, Froeling J, et al. Rhinosporidiosis in a domestic cat. *Med Mycol* 2001;39:139–141.

Author: Gary D. Norsworth
Consulting Editor: Stephen C. Barr

chapter 84

Rocky Mountain Spotted Fever

DEFINITION/OVERVIEW

- A tickborne rickettsial disease affecting dogs; considered the most important rickettsial disease in humans.
- Other as yet undefined rickettsial organisms may also cause clinical signs in dogs.

ETIOLOGY/PATHOPHYSIOLOGY

- *Rickettsia rickettsii.*
- Antibodies to *R. akari* (causative agent of rickettsialpox in humans)—have been found in dogs in New York City, but it is not known if it causes disease in dogs.
- Vector—American dog tick (*Dermacentor variabilis*), found east of the Great Plains; wood tick (*Dermacentor andersoni*), found from the Cascade Mountains to the Rocky Mountains.
- Incidence of disease greatest during tick season—late March to end of September.
- Prevalence—overall infection in ticks <2%; varies by geographic location.
- Distribution—mainly in the eastern seaboard states (especially the Carolinas), Mississippi River Valley, and south-central states in the United States; also found in South America.
- Transmission—via the saliva of the vector or blood transfusion.
- Ticks—must attach for 5 to 20 hours to infect a host (humans, dogs, and cats) or reservoir hosts (rodents and dogs).
- Incubation period—2 days to 2 weeks.
- Infection—organism invades and multiplies in vascular endothelium; causes widespread vasculitis in organs with endarterial circulation, leading to microvascular hemorrhage, platelet aggregation (thrombocytopenia), vasoconstriction, increased vascular permeability, increased plasma loss into the interstitial space (organ swelling), hypotension, and eventually DIC and shock.

SIGNALMENT/HISTORY

- Purebred dogs—more prone to developing clinical illness than are mixed-breed dogs.
- German shepherd dogs—more common.

Historical Findings

- Fever—within 2 to 3 days of tick attachment.
- Lethargy.
- Depression.
- Anorexia.
- Swelling (edema)—lips, scrotum, prepuce, ears, and extremities.
- Stiff gait—especially with scrotal or prepucial swelling.
- Spontaneous bleeding—sneezing, epistaxis.
- Respiratory distress.
- Neurologic signs—ataxia, head tilt.
- Ocular pain.

 CLINICAL FEATURES

- Both clinical and subclinical illnesses occur.
- Clinical—variable in severity; lasting 2 to 4 weeks if untreated.
- Ticks may still be present in acute cases.
- Pyrexia.
- Cutaneous lesions—edema of face, limbs, prepuce, and scrotum (*Fig. 84-1*).
- Conjunctivitis.
- Scleral injection (*Fig. 84-2*).
- Respiratory—dyspnea, exercise intolerance, and increased bronchovesicular sounds.
- Generalized lymphadenopathy.
- Neurologic—vestibular dysfunction, altered mental status, and seizures.
- Myalgia/arthralgia.

■ **Fig. 84-1** Severe necrosis of the planum nasale of a dog with Rocky Mountain spotted fever.

■ **Fig. 84-2** Scleral injection in a dog with Rocky Mountain spotted fever (courtesy Dr. R. Riis, Cornell University).

- Petechiae.
- Ecchymoses—ocular (*Fig. 84-3*), oral, and genital regions; in 20% of patients.
- Hemorrhagic diathesis—epistaxis, melena, hematuria in severe cases.
- Cardiac arrhythmias—sudden death.
- DIC and death from shock—in severe acute cases.

■ **Fig. 84-3** Retinal hemorrhage and papilledema in a dog with Rocky Mountain spotted fever (courtesy Dr. R. Riis, Cornell University).

DIFFERENTIAL DIAGNOSIS

- Canine ehrlichiosis—*Erhlichia canis* and other *Anaplasmataceae*; not seasonal; clinically indistinguishable from RMSF (especially acute cases); differentiate with serologic testing; both respond to same treatment.
- Immune-mediated thrombocytopenia—not usually associated with fever or lymphadenopathy; differentiate with serologic testing; may treat for both until results are known.
- SLE—ANA test usually negative in RMSF; serologic testing is diagnostic.
- Brucellosis—scrotal edema; serologic testing is diagnostic.

DIAGNOSTICS

- CBC—thrombocytopenia (~40% of cases) partly due to antiplatelet antibody, megathrombocytosis, mild anemia (normochromic, normocytic), mild leukopenia (early in infection), and leukocytosis (and monocytosis) as disease becomes more chronic.
- Serum biochemical profile—usually nonspecific changes; mild increases in ALT, ALP, BUN, creatinine, total bilirubin (rare); hypercholesterolemia consistently found (cause unknown); hypoalbuminemia (resulting from vascular endothelial damage); azotemia; hyponatremia, hypochloremia, and metabolic acidosis have all been reported.
- Urinalysis—proteinuria, with or without azotemia, from glomerular/tubular damage; hematuria from coagulation defects.
- Serologic tests—several exist, including microscopic immunofluorescence (Micro-IF) test, ELISA, and latex agglutination test:
  - Micro-IF test—most commonly used by diagnostic laboratories; measures IgG; levels may not be elevated when clinical signs first appear; take 2 to 3 weeks to rise; may be negative in very acute cases; perform paired titers 3 weeks apart; fourfold increase between acute and convalescent titers; avoid misdiagnosis because of considerable cross-reactivity with other rickettsial organisms; titers reach peak 3 to 5 months after infection, then decline (some can remain positive for 12 months).
  - ELISA—high sensitivity; can measure both IgG and IgM; therefore detects infection earlier than just measuring IgG alone.
  - Latex agglutination test—high specificity, lower sensitivity than Micro-IF test (false negative results occur); single increased titer is diagnostic.
- Direct immunofluorescence test—skin biopsies obtained by local anesthesia and punch biopsies from affected lesions; detect rickettsial antigens as early as 3 to 4 days postinfection.
- CSF—often normal; may show an increase in protein and nucleated cells.
- PCR—available at some academic institutions (North Carolina State University) for the diagnosis of RMSF.

THERAPEUTICS

- Most cases—treated as inpatient until stable.
- Symptomatic—fluids and electrolyte solutions (dehydration and shock); blood transfusion (anemia); platelet-rich plasma or blood transfusion (hemorrhage from thrombocytopenia).
- Early antibiotic treatment—reduces fever and albumin extravasation and improves patient's attitude with 24 to 48 hours.
- Platelet counts—repeat every 3 days after initiating treatment until within normal range; should return to normal within 2 to 4 days after initiating treatment.
- Serologic titers—lower in treated than in untreated dogs; titers remain positive during convalescence.

Drugs of Choice

- Doxycycline—drug of choice.
- Prednisone—concurrent use; anti-inflammatory or immunosuppressive doses; given early in disease does not seem to be detrimental to the clinical recovery.
- Alternative drugs:
  - Tetracyclines, chloramphenicol, and enrofloxacin—equally efficacious if used early.
  - Oxytetracycline and tetracycline—effective and less expensive.
  - Chloramphenicol—puppies <6 months of age; recommended to avoid yellow discoloration of erupting teeth caused by tetracyclines. (*Table 84-1*).

Precautions/Interactions

- Tetracycline (or derivatives)—do not use in patients <6 months of age because of permanent yellowing of teeth.
- Renal insufficiency—do not use tetracycline; doxycycline may be given (also excreted via the GI tract).
- Enrofloxacin—avoid in young dogs because articular damage can occur; GI upsets (vomiting, anorexia).

Drug	Dose (mg/kg)	Route[a]	Interval (Hours)	Duration (Days)
Doxycycline	10	PO, IV	12	10
Tetracycline	22	PO, IV	8	10
Enrofloxacin	3	PO, SC	12	10
Chloramphenicol	20	PO, IV	12	10

TABLE 84-1. Drug Therapy for Rock Mountain Spotted Fever in Dogs

[a] Begin injectable therapy if patient is vomiting; change over to oral therapy once vomiting stops.

- Chloramphenicol—reduces titers to a greater extent than tetracyclines, so avoid use if serologic confirmation will be conducted after treatment; warn client of public health risk; directly interferes with heme and bone marrow synthesis; avoid use in dogs with thrombocytopenia, pancytopenia, or anemia.

 COMMENTS

- Prognosis—good in acute cases with appropriate and prompt therapy.
- Response—occurs within hours of treatment.
- Recovered dogs—are believed to be permanently immune to reinfection.
- If treatment is not instituted until CNS signs occur or later in the disease process—mortality is high; patients with CNS signs may die within hours.
- Prevention depends on controlling tick infestation on dogs—use dips or sprays containing dichlorvos, chlorfenvinphos, dioxathion, propoxur, or carbaryl.
- Flea and tick collars (e.g., Preventic, Virbac Corp., Fort Worth, TX), weekly insecticide baths (e.g., Ecto-Soothe, Virbac Corp., Fort Worth, TX, or Mycodex, Veterinary Products Lab., Phoenix, AZ) and/or monthly administrations of Revolution (selamectin, Pfizer, Exton, PA), Sentinal, Novartis, Greensboro, NC, (milbemycin/lufenuron), Interceptor, Novartis Greensboro, NC, (milbemycin), Frontline (fiprinol, Merial, Iselin, NJ), or K9Advantix, Bayer, Shawnee Mission, KS (imidacloprid/permithrin) also protect against a number of species of ticks.
- Environment—tick eradication impossible; organism maintained in rodents and other reservoir hosts.
- Avoid—tick-infested areas.
- Removal of ticks by hand—use gloves; ensure tick mouth parts are removed, because a foreign body reaction is likely to result if they are left in place.
- Incidence of RMSF in humans—dropping in the United States; mid-1992 to mid-1993: 300 cases; earlier incidence: up to 1,000 cases/year.
- Source of infection for humans—from ticks that are transferred from dogs; not from dogs directly; when removing ticks from dogs.
- Mainly—causes disease in young adults and children.

Abbreviations

ALP, alkaline phosphate; ALT, alanine aminotransferase; ANA, antinuclear antibody; BUN, blood urea nitrogen; CBC, complete blood count; CNS, central nervous system; CSF, cerebrospinal fluid; DIC, disseminated intravascular coagulation; ELISA, enzyme-linked immunosorbent assay; GI, gastrointestinal; Ig, immunoglobulin; Micro-IF, microscopic immunofluorescence; PCR, polymerase chain reaction; RMSF, Rocky Mountain spotted fever; SLE, systemic lupus erythematosus.

Suggested Reading

Elchos BN, Goddard J. Implications of presumptive fatal Rocky Mountain spotted fever in two dogs and their owner. *J Am Vet Med Assoc* 2003;223:1450–1452.

Warner RD, Marsh WW. Rocky Mountain spotted fever. *J Am Vet Med Assoc* 2002;221:1413–1417.

Author: Stephen C. Barr
Consulting Editor: Stephen C. Barr

chapter **85**

Rotavirus Infection

DEFINITION/OVERVIEW

- A rare intestinal viral infection of mammals, including cats and dogs, causing enteritis and diarrhea.

ETIOLOGY/PATHOPHYSIOLOGY

- Rotavirus (from *rota* meaning wheel)—a nonenveloped, double-stranded RNA virus.
- Relatively resistant—to environmental destruction.
- Resistant to acid—allowing it to pass through the stomach to the intestinal tract.
- Transmission—fecal/oral route.
- Affects mature epithelial cells—on luminal tips of intestinal villi.
- Villus damage—may lead to atrophy and osmotic diarrhea.

SIGNALMENT/HISTORY

- Wide host range (main cause of diarrhea in children <2 years).
- Puppies (often <2 weeks old but usually <12 weeks).
- Kittens (<6 months) more susceptible to infection.
- Animals deprived of colostrum may show more severe disease.

CLINICAL FEATURES

Dogs

- Usually subclinical.
- Mild watery to mucoid diarrhea—occasionally.
- Anorexia and lethargy—rare.
- Fatalities in the very young—very rare.

Cats

- Primarily subclinical or mild diarrhea.
- Diarrhea more severe if concurrent infections or stress environment are present.

DIFFERENTIAL DIAGNOSIS

- Other causes of acute small bowel diarrhea in an otherwise healthy young animal:
  - Infectious; parvovirus, coronavirus, rotavirus, calicivirus, distemper, giardiasis, FeLV, cryptosporidiosis, tritrichomoniasis, hookworms, whipworms, roundworms, GI bacterial overgrowth, and clostridia.
  - Toxicity—lead.
  - Dietary indiscretion, allergy.
  - IBD.
  - Foreign body.
  - Intussusception.

DIAGNOSTICS

- CBC and biochemical panel—usually normal or reflect dehydration and electrolyte abnormalities from diarrhea.
- Viral detection—electron microscopy of negatively stained preparations of diarrheic feces will identify characteristic viral particles (wheel shape, 70 nm diameter) *(Fig. 85-1)*.
- Detection of antigen in feces by ELISA and latex agglutination—commercially available in man (Rotazyme [Abbott Laboratories, Abott Park, IL.) but may be of low sensitivity for dog and cat rotaviruses.

■ **Fig. 85-1** Electron micrograph of rotavirus particles isolated from a dog. Note the wagon-wheel conformation that gives the virus its name (bar = 100 nm).

- Serologic examination (ELISA)—not recommended as most animals (85%) show exposure.
- PCR—very sensitive but not currently commercially available.
- Isolation on cell culture—time consuming, requires considerable expertise, and not all isolates grow.

 # THERAPEUTICS

- Symptomatic for diarrhea (fluids, electrolytes, NPO).
- Antibiotics are not indicated unless fever develops (use broad-spectrum agents).
- Antiviral drugs are not indicated.

Drugs of Choice

- N/A

Precautions/Interactions

- No vaccines are available.

 # COMMENTS

- If outbreaks occur in very young animals in breeding situations, management practices should be scrutinized.
- Pay particular attention to environmental stress (temperature) and ability of animals to receive colostrum.

Abbreviations

CBC, complete blood count; ELISA, enzyme-linked immunosorbent assay; FeLV, feline leukemia virus; GI, gastrointestinal; IBD, inflammatory bowel disease; NPO, nothing per os; PCR, polymerase chain reaction; RNA, ribonucleic acid.

Suggested Reading

Hoskins JD. Canine viral enteritis. In: Greene CE, ed. *Infectious Diseases of the Dog and Cat.* Philadelphia: WB Saunders; 1998:40–49.

Author: J. Paul Woods
Consulting Editor: Stephen C. Barr

chapter 86

Roundworms *(Ascariasis)*

DEFINITION/OVERVIEW

- Large nematode parasites (10 to 12 cm long)—adults live in the small intestine of dogs and cats.
- Infection—can lead to small intestine distention and interference with gut motility and digestion, especially in very young animals.

ETIOLOGY/PATHOPHYSIOLOGY

- *Toxocara canis*—dogs.
- *Toxocara cati*—cats.
- *Toxascaris leonina*—dogs and cats.
- For *T. canis*—dogs may ingest eggs containing larvae, which hatch in the duodenum.
- Larvae—may migrate to the liver and lungs, resulting in pathology in young animals.
- In adult hosts—larvae are widely distributed and become encapsulated in tissues (especially skeletal muscle and kidneys).
- In bitches—encapsulated, sequestered larvae form a source of infection for pups (transplacental and transmammary).
- Larvae—appear in milk as early as day 5 of lactation.
- Transplacental transmission occurs to the fetus—infected animals may be born with a developing worm burden, leading to abdominal distention and pain (can occur before eggs appear in the feces).
- Eggs—can appear in feces as early as 3 weeks of age.
- Older pups and kittens—may become infected by ingesting infective eggs disseminated on the premises by dams with postgestational infections.
- In dogs under 3 months of age (and occasionally adults)—larvae that have migrated to the lungs break out into the airways, migrate up the trachea, and are swallowed, to develop to adults in the GI tract.
- *T. cati* life cycle—similar to that of *T. canis*, except transplacental infection does not occur.
- Transtracheal migration following egg ingestion—probably occurs more commonly in adult cats.
- Paratenic hosts—may be an important reservoir of infection for cats.
- *T. leonina*—infection can occur by ingestion of eggs or by ingesting a paratenic host (rodents) infected with dormant infective larvae.

SIGNALMENT/HISTORY

- Dogs and cats—all ages, although clinical disease most severe in young pups and kittens.

CLINICAL FEATURES

Dogs

- *T. canis*—parasitic pneumonia from tracheal migration of a large burden of prenatally acquired larvae can result in high mortality in pups (first 48 to 72 hours of life).
- Emaciation.
- Digestive disturbances.
- Abdominal distention.
- Mucoid diarrhea and vomiting—sometimes containing adult worms.
- Death—can occur in 2- to 3-week-old pups if burdens are high.
- Less severe burdens.
  - Unthriftiness.
  - Rough hair coat.
  - Pot-bellied appearance (*Fig. 86-1*).
  - Intermittent diarrhea.
  - Anemia.
  - Intestinal loops containing adults easily palpable.
- Aberrant migrations by adults from the GI tract—may cause obstruction or rupture of the common bile duct, gallbladder, and pancreatic duct or migration to distant sites (spinal column).
- Neurologic signs—restlessness, twitching to convulsions (mechanism unknown).
- GI tract—local hypersensitivity response has been reported causing acute vomiting, hemorrhagic enteritis, or chronic eosinophilic enteritis (German shepherd dogs).
- Somatic larval migration—rarely causes clinical signs, but results in nodular lesions in kidneys, liver, lung, and myocardium.
- *T. leonina*—least pathogenic; usually causes no clinical signs other than mild diarrhea and periodic vomiting.

Cats

- *T. cati*—similar to those in dogs, but less severe; potbelly, intermittent diarrhea, unthriftiness.
- Vomiting and coughing (but not neurologic signs).
- Intestinal loops containing adults easily palpable.
- *T. leonina* is the least pathogenic roundworm, usually causing no clinical signs other than mild diarrhea and periodic vomiting.

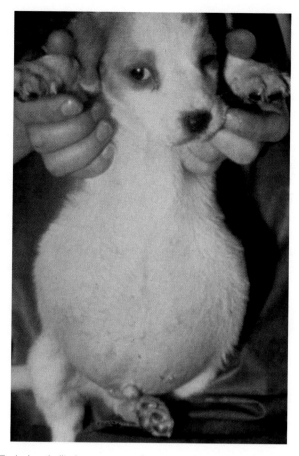

■ **Fig. 86-1** Typical potbellied appearance of a puppy infected with *Toxocara canis* infection.

 DIFFERENTIAL DIAGNOSIS

Dogs

- Causes of potbellied appearance in puppies:
  - Ascites.
  - Hepatomegaly.
  - Splenomegaly.
  - Renomegally.
- Causes of diarrhea in the puppy:
  - Dietary indiscretion.
  - Allergy.
  - Drugs (antibiotics).
  - Toxins—lead.
  - Parasites (*Giardia* spp., cryptosporidiosis, GI parasitism with hookworms or *Strongyloides* spp.).
  - Infectious agents (salmonellosis, enteric calicivirus, reovirus, CPV, coronavirus, canine distemper, CHV, campylobacter, clostridiosis).

- GI tract bacterial overgrowth (coliforms).
- Systemic organ dysfunction (renal, hepatic, pancreas, cardiac).

Cats

- Causes of diarrhea in the kitten:
  - Dietary indiscretion.
  - Allergy.
  - Drugs (antibiotics).
  - Toxins—lead.
  - Parasites (*Giardia* spp., cryptosporidiosis, tritrichomoniasis, GI tract parasitism with hookworms or *Strongyloides* spp.).
  - Infectious agents (panleukopenia, salmonellosis, enteric calici virus, reovirus, FeLV, feline calicivirus).
  - GI tract bacterial overgrowth (coliforms).
  - Systemic organ dysfunction (renal, hepatic, pancreas, cardiac).

DIAGNOSTICS

- *T. canis*—shows marked eosinophilia, mild leukocytosis with eosinophilia, anemia; hepatic enzyme elevations occur in larval migration.
- *T. cati*—eosinophilia with mild leukocytosis; no anemia.
- Fecal flotation (or less sensitive fecal smear)—characteristic eggs of each parasite (Fig. 86-2).

THERAPEUTICS

- Severely debilitated pups—IV fluids and nutritional support while parasiticidal drugs are used.
- Pups with parasite-induced pneumonia—treat severe inflammatory response (due to worm death from parasiticide drug treatment) in the lungs: prednisone (0.25 mg/kg, PO, q12h for 5 days).
- Treat bitch or queen with adulticide/larvacide anthelmintic (fenbendazole)—decreases subsequent litter and mature maternal infections.

Drugs of Choice

Adulticide/Larvacide Anthelmintics

- Fenbendazole (Panacur granules 22.2% [Intervet, Millsboro, DE])—from day 40 of pregnancy to 2 weeks after birth results in ascarid-free pups.
- Unsequestered larvae—treat with fenbendazole for 5 consecutive days (does not kill sequestered larvae).
- Sequestered larvae—treat from day 40 gestation to 2 weeks postgestation to protect pups born in subsequent litters.
- Once larvae are in the fetus (after day 40 of gestation)—probably not killed when fenbendazole is administered to the bitch.

■ **Fig. 86-2** The roundworm eggs of the (**A**) dog (*Toxocara canis*), (**B**) cat (*Toxocara cati*), and (**C**) both dogs and cats (*Toxascaris leonina*). Note that the egg of *T. leonina* is ellipsoid and has a smooth shell that distinguishes it from those of other *Toxocara* spp.

- Ivermectin (Ivomec [Merial, Iselin, NJ])—experimentally, large doses can markedly reduce pup infections (1 mg/kg, PO, q24h on days 20 and 42, or 0.5 mg/kg, PO, on days 38, 41, 44, and 47 of gestation to bitch).

Adulticide Anthelmintics

PUPS <4 WEEKS OF AGE
- Piperazine (Pipfuge and others)—starting in the second week of life, repeat every 3 weeks until pup is 3 months of age).
- Praziquantel/pyrantel/febantel (Drontal Plus [Bayer, Shawnee Mission, KS])—monthly after pups reach 3 weeks of age and weigh over 2 pounds).

PUPS AND DOGS >4 WEEKS OF AGE
- Piperazine (Pipfuge and others).
- Milbemycin oxime (Interceptor or Sentinel [Novartis, Greensboro, NC]).
- Praziquantel/pyrantel/febantel (Drontal Plus [Bayer, Shawnee Mission, KS]).
- Pyrantel (Nemex tablets and suspension [Pfizer, Exton, PA]).
- Ivermectin and pyrantel (Heartguard Plus [Merial, Iselin, NJ])

TABLE 86-1. Drug Therapy of Roundworm Infections in Cats and Dogs

Drug	Species	Dose (mg/kg)	Route	Interval (Hours)	Duration (Days)
Fenbendazole (Panacur)	D	50	PO	24	3[a]
Piperazine (Pipfuge)	B	110	PO	Once	[b]
Praziquantel/pyrantel/febantel (Drontal) Plus	D	[c]	PO	Once	[d]
Milbemycin oxime (Interceptor, Sentinel)	D	0.5	PO	Once	[d]
Selamectin (Revolution)	B	6	Topical	Once	[d]
Pyrantel (Nemex or Drontal)	D	5	PO	Once	[d]
	C	5–10	PO	Once	[d]
Ivermectin/pyrantel (Heartgard Plus)	D	5	PO	Once	[d]
Dichlorvos (Task Tabs)	B	11	PO	Once	[d]
Toluene/dichlorophene (Happy Jack)	B	[e]	PO	Once	[d]
Diethylcarbamazine (Filaribits)	D	6.6	PO	24	Life span[f]

[a] Repeat in 3 weeks in pups >4 wks of age. Give from day 40 of pregnancy to 2 weeks after birth in pregnant bitches for ascarid-free pups.

[b] Pups—start in 2nd week of life, repeat every 3 weeks until pup is 3 months of age. Cats—every 3 weeks.

[c] Dose—praziquantel (5 to 12 mg/kg), pyrantel (5 to 12 mg/kg), and febantel (25 to 62 mg/kg).

[d] Repeat monthly.

[e] Dose—toluene (264 mg/kg), and dichlorophene (220 mg/kg).

[f] Filaribits is primarily given for heartworm prevention so is given daily for the dog's life.

B, cats and dogs; C, cats; D, dogs.

- Fenbendazole (Panacur Granules 22.2% [Intervet, Millsboro, DE]).
- Dichlorvos (Task Tabs [Boehringer Ingelheim, St. Joseph, MO]).
- Toluene and dichlorophene (Happy Jack Trivermicide Worm Capsules, Happy Jack Inc, Snow Hill, NC).
- Diethylcarbamazine (Filaribits [Pfizer, Exton, PA])(*Table 86-1*).

CATS
- Because *T. cati* larvae do not cross the placenta—only necessary to treat cats every 3 weeks for the first 3 to 4 months of life.
- Piperazine (Pipfuge and others).
- Pyrantel (Nemex tablets and suspension [Pfizer, Exton, PA] or Drontal [Bayer, Shawnee Mission, KS.]).
- Dichlorvos, toluene/dichlorophene, milbemycin, and selamectin also work in cats.

Precautions/Interactions

- Piperazine—at low doses (55 mg/kg), worms are not paralyzed long enough to be expelled; use higher doses (110 mg/kg).

- Pay particular attention—to manufacturer's recommendations regarding use of the drugs in pregnant and young animals; for example:
  - Drontal Plus—not for puppies <3 weeks of age or 2 pounds.
  - Heartgard Plus—not for puppies <6 weeks of age.
  - Interceptor—not for puppies <6 weeks of age or 2 pounds.
  - Sentinel—not for puppies <4 weeks of age or 2 pounds.
  - Sentinel Flavor Tabs—not for puppies <4 weeks of age or 11 pounds.
  - Revolution—use in animals >6 weeks of age.
  - Task Tabs—not for puppies <10 days of age or 1 pound.
- Check dogs for microfilaremia before using avermectin products.
- Pups may vomit 30 to 90 minutes after being given Task Tabs—should not affect efficacy.
- Dichlorvos should not be given to animals with GI tract obstruction or liver problems.

 COMMENTS

- *Toxocara* eggs are extremely resistant remaining infective for years—virtually impossible to rid from soils in heavily contaminated situations.
- Entomb eggs—cover runs with a concrete slab or bituminous asphalt.
- Once installed—egg levels can be controlled by at least weekly cleaning of cement or asphalt.
- Contaminated kennel areas—physically clean surfaces using high-pressure washers, followed by 1% sodium hypochlorite (3 cups of bleach/gallon of water), followed by water rinsing. (NOTE: This does not kill the eggs, but merely removes their ability to stick to surfaces).
- Prevent animals (particularly cats) eating potential paratenic hosts (rodents—*Toxocara* infection rates are high).
- Zoonotic potential—visceral and ocular larva migrans may follow ingestion of infective eggs (especially in children).

Abbreviations

CHV, canine herpes virus; CPV, canine parvovirus; FeLV, feline leukemia virus; GI, gastrointestinal.

Suggested Reading

Bowman DD, ed. *Georgis' Parasitology for Veterinarians*, 8th ed. Philadelphia: WB Saunders; 2003:206–211.
Parsons JC. Ascarid infections of cats and dogs. *Vet Clin North Am Small Animal Pract* 1987; 17:1307–1339.

Author: Stephen C. Barr
Consulting Editor: Stephen C. Barr

chapter 87

Salmonellosis

DEFINITION/OVERVIEW

- A bacterial disease that causes enteritis, septicemia, and abortions in both cats and dogs.

ETIOLOGY/PATHOPHYSIOLOGY

- *Salmonella* spp.—gram-negative bacteria of many different serotypes.
- The bacterium colonizes the small intestine (ileum)—invades enterocytes before entering and multiplying in the lamina propria and local mesenteric lymph nodes.
- Cytotoxin and enterotoxin are produced, causing inflammation and prostaglandin synthesis—leads to the development of a secretory diarrhea and mucosal sloughing.
- In uncomplicated enteritis, organisms are prevented from spreading from the mesenteric lymph nodes—patients develop diarrhea, vomiting, and dehydration as a result of secretory diarrhea.
- If organisms spread from the lymph nodes to the circulation to produce bacteremia and septicemia—severe disease occurs.
- Focal extraintestinal infections—can result in abortion, joint disease, or endotoxemia with organ infarction, generalized thrombosis, DIC, and death.
- Some patients recover from the septicemic form—suffer prolonged recovery as a result of their debilitated state.
- The true incidence is unknown—most infections are subclinical.

Dogs

- Most clinical disease seen in young or pregnant animals.
- Fecal swab cultures from clinically normal domestic pets, pets in boarding kennels, and pets in veterinary hospitals showed incidences of 30%, 16.7%, and 21.5%, respectively.
- Common in racing greyhounds and sled dogs.

Cats

- Have a high natural resistance—especially older cats.
- Stressed hospitalized animals—higher risk.

- Fecal swab culture surveys of normal cats and cats from a research colony—incidences of 18% and 10.6%, respectively.
- Shelter cats—more likely to have *Salmonella* spp. in feces.
- Pandemics of salmonellosis in migrating songbirds (usually *S. typhimurium*) in spring—create epidemics in bird-hunting cats.

 SIGNALMENT/HISTORY

- Host factors that increase the likelihood of dogs or cats developing clinical illness:
  - Age (neonatal/young).
  - Overall health status (debilitated older animals; treatment with immunosuppressive drugs or antibiotics for other diseases are used when patient is exposed to virulent drug-resistant *Salmonella* spp. during hospital stay, concurrent GI parasitism).
- Environmental factors:
  - Coprophagia spreads infection.
  - Dehydrated (dry) pet food can harbor organism (semimoist not as likely).
  - Contaminated foods (pig ear dog treats).
  - Dense populations (research colonies, boarding facilities).
- Hunting/stray animals—scavenge for food (exposure to organism in food, dead animals, infected raw meat, song birds).
- Hospitalized animals—increased nosocomial exposure coupled with increased stress of hospitalization and concurrent treatments with antimicrobials and immunosuppressive drugs.
- Historically—patients may have diarrhea, vomiting, fever, and anorexia.
- Vaginal discharge/abortion—may occur in dogs.
- Chronic persistent febrile illness with persistent fever, anorexia, malaise without diarrhea—possible.

Dogs

- Most infections—subclinical (carrier state: *Salmonella* spp. shed in feces).
- Clinical forms—varying from mild, to moderate, to severe are seen in neonatal/immature puppies and pregnant bitches.
- Most adult carrier dogs—clinically normal.

Cats

- Adult cats—highly resistant to clinical disease.
- Neonatal/immature and immunocompromised animals—susceptible to disease.

 CLINICAL FEATURES

Dogs

- Gastroenteritis:
  - Anorexia.
  - Malaise/lethargy.

- Depression.
- Fever.
- Diarrhea containing mucus and blood.

■ As disease progresses—the patient becomes more dehydrated, with:
- Abdominal pain.
- Tenesmus.
- Pale mucous membranes.
- Mesenteric lymphadenopathy.
- Weight loss.

■ Gastroenteritis with bacteremia and septicemia, septic shock, or endotoxemia:
- Pale mucous membranes.
- Weakness.
- Cardiovascular collapse.
- Tachycardia.
- Tachypnea.
- Death preceded by multiple organ failure.

■ Focal extraintestinal infections—conjunctivitis, metritis/abortion, cellulitis, and pyothorax have been reported.

Cats

■ May exhibit a syndrome of a chronic febrile illness (without gastrointestinal signs):
- Persistent fever.
- Prolonged illness with vague, nonspecific clinical signs and leukogram with a left shift.

■ Recovering patients—may exhibit chronic intermittent diarrhea for 3 to 4 weeks; may shed *Salmonella* spp. in stool for 6 weeks or longer.

 DIFFERENTIAL DIAGNOSIS

■ All causes of diarrhea, including systemic or metabolic disease, as well as specific intestinal disorders, should be considered.

■ Other causes of acute enterocolitis—dietary indiscretion, chronic IBD, HGE, neoplasia (especially GI tract lymphoma), drugs (antibiotics), toxins (lead), parasites (cryptosporidiosis, tritrichomoniasis, whipworms), infectious agents (parvovirus; FIP; rickettsia, including salmon poisoning; GI tract bacterial overgrowth; *Campylobacter* spp.; clostridial enterotoxicosis; histoplasmosis; leishmaniasis; other rare infections—pythiosis), systemic organ dysfunction (renal, hepatic, pancreatic), and metabolic (hypoadrenocorticism, hyperthyroidism—cats).

 DIAGNOSTICS

■ CBC—variable; depends on stage of illness.
- Initially neutropenia—often with left shift and toxic neutrophils.

- Nonregenerative anemia.
- Lymphopenia.
- Thrombocytopenia.

■ Serum biochemical profile—hypoalbuminemia and electrolyte abnormalities with secretory diarrhea (metabolic acidosis, hypokalemia).

■ Fecal/rectal culture—positive (requires special media); best performed on fresh feces to maximize culture results.

■ PCR—available but not widely used on a commercial basis.

■ Fecal leukocytes—usually present.

■ Blood cultures (perform if fever is present)—can be positive but not very sensitive.

■ Joint fluid—culture may be positive.

■ Subclinical carrier state—fecal culture intermittently positive often >6 weeks.

■ Use of antimicrobials in patient before sampling—may produce false negative culture results.

 THERAPEUTICS

■ Degree of care—depends largely on severity of diarrhea and whether systemically ill or not.

■ Uncomplicated gastroenteritis cases without bacteremia—treat as outpatients.

■ Bacteremia/septicemia/severe diarrhea—parenteral crystalloid fluid and electrolyte therapy based on degree of dehydration, shock, acid–base status, and ongoing fluid losses.

■ Consider colloid therapy (plasma, hetastarch)—when serum albumin <2 g/dl.

■ Once vomiting and diarrhea abate—consider oral fluids containing hypertonic sugar solutions for secretory diarrhea.

■ Limit movement of patient (isolate)—because patient can excrete large numbers of organisms in stool during acute diarrhea stage.

■ Maintain good hygiene—of associated animal health care workers (including clients).

■ Restrict food until in recovery—then offer highly digestible, low-fat diet.

Drugs of Choice

Asymptomatic Carrier State

■ Antimicrobials—contraindicated because:
  - Increases the risk of resistance developing to the drugs.
  - Prolongs the convalescent excretion period.

■ Quinolone drugs—clear carrier state in humans but unknown in animals.

Uncomplicated Gastroenteritis

■ Antimicrobials—not indicated.

■ Locally acting intestinal absorbents and protectants—mainstay of therapy.

Neonates, Aged, and Debilitated Animals

■ Antimicrobials—indicated, but important to base selection on culture and sensitivity results because *Salmonella* spp. are notoriously resistant to many agents.

■ TMS.

TABLE 87-1. Drug Therapy for Salmonellosis in Dogs and Cats

Drug	Species	Dose (mg/kg)	Route	Interval (Hours)	Duration (Days)
Trimethoprim-sulfadiazine	B	15	PO, IV	12	10
Amoxicillin	B	10–20	PO	8	10
Enrofloxacin	B	5	PO, SC	12	7
Norfloxacin	B	22	PO	12	7
Chloramphenicol	D	15–25	PO, SC	8	7
	C	10–15	PO, SC	12	7

D, dogs; C, cats; B, both dogs and cats.

- Amoxicillin.
- Enrofloxacin.
- Norfloxacin.
- Chloramphenicol (*Table 87-1*).

Precautions/Interactions

- TMS—multiple adverse reactions, including:
  - KCS—monitor tear production weekly throughout treatment.
  - Hepatotoxicity—anorexia, depression, icterus; monitor alanine ALT if prolonged therapy.
  - Megaloblastic–folate acid deficiency anemia—especially in cats after several weeks; supplement with folinic acid (2.5 mg/kg/day).
  - Immune-mediated polyarthritis, retinitis, glomerulonephritis, vasculitis, anemia, thrombocytopenia, urticaria, toxic epidermal necrolysis, erythema multiforme, and conjunctivitis—remove from drug.
  - Renal failure and interference with renal excretion of potassium (leading to hyperkalemia).
  - Salivation, diarrhea, and vomiting (cats).
  - May interfere with thyroid hormone synthesis (dogs)—check T_3 and T_4 after 6 weeks.
- Use chloramphenicol and TMS with caution in neonates and pregnant patients.
- Chloramphenicol—may cause a reversible nonregenerative anemia and myelosuppression.
- Fluoroquinolones—avoid use in pregnant, neonatal, or growing animals (medium-sized dogs <8 months of age; large or giant breeds <12 to 18 months of age) because of cartilage lesions.

COMMENTS

- Repeat a fecal culture monthly for 3 months to detect development of carrier state.
- Monitor for secondary spread to other animals.

- Avoid predisposing factors (host, environmental, etc.) described previously.
- Spread of infection to other animals and humans in the household not uncommon, resulting in chronic bouts of diarrhea, especially during times of stress.
- Prognosis for uncomplicated gastroenteritis is excellent; usually self-limiting, but patients can become chronic shedders of bacteria.
- Prognosis for severe disease is poor if left untreated; aggressive therapy usually produces a cure.

Abbreviations

ALT, alanine aminotransferase; CBC, complete blood count; DIC, disseminated intravascular coagulation; FIP, feline infectious peritonitis; GI, gastrointestinal; HGE, hemorrhagic gastroenteritis; IBD, inflammatory bowel disease; KCS, keratoconjunctivitis sicca; PCR, polymerase chain reaction; TMS, trimethoprim-sulfadiazine.

Suggested Reading

Greene CE. Salmonellosis. In: Greene CE, ed. *Infectious Diseases of the Dog and Cat*. Philadelphia: WB Saunders; 1998:235–240.

McDonough PL, Simpson KW. Diagnosing emerging bacterial infections: salmonellosis, campylobacteriosis, clostridial toxicosis, and helicobacteriosis. *Semin Vet Med Surg (Small Anim)* 1996;11: 187–197.

Author: Patrick L. McDonough
Consulting Editor: Stephen C. Barr

chapter 88

Salmon Poisoning

DEFINITION/OVERVIEW

- A rickettsial infection of dogs living in the Pacific northwest of the United States, causing a systemic illness characterized by vomiting, diarrhea, and fever.

ETIOLOGY/PATHOPHYSIOLOGY

- *Neorickettsia helminthoeca*—a rickettsial organism with a trematode vector, *Nanophyetus salmonincola*.
- Dogs become infected by ingesting raw fish that have eaten the trematode vector or by ingesting the vector or organism directly from water.
- The organism invades the small intestinal epithelium and associated lymphoid tissue.

SIGNALMENT/HISTORY

- Only dogs infected.
- No age, sex, or breed predilection.
- History of ingestion of raw fish caught in an endemic region.

CLINICAL FEATURES

- Fever—initially.
- Anorexia.
- Weight loss.
- Diarrhea and vomiting—may occur.
- Diarrhea—becomes progressively more severe and may consist mainly of blood at the time of death.
- Lymphadenopathy—especially cervical and prescapular.
- Nasal discharge.
- Ocular discharge.

DIFFERENTIAL DIAGNOSIS

- Gastroenteritis from ingestion of garbage, foreign bodies, toxins; infectious (distemper, parvovirus); IBD; systemic organ dysfunction (nephropathy, hepatopathy, pancreatitis); and HGE.
- Diarrhea—can be so severe that sometimes it is misdiagnosed as parvovirus.

DIAGNOSTICS

- CBC, serum biochemical profile, and urinalysis—usually normal.
- Aspirate cytologic specimen of enlarged lymph nodes—may reveal intracytoplasmic rickettsial bodies (Giemsa stain).
- Fecal examination—reveals operculated eggs of the trematode *Nanophyetus salmonincola*.

THERAPEUTICS

- Most require hospitalization for supportive fluid therapy and close monitoring of electrolytes, acid–base status, and body temperature.
- Basic measures to control diarrhea.

Drugs of Choice

- Doxycycline.
- Other tetracyclines are also effective—tetracycline, oxytetracycline, or minocycline.
- If tetracyclines cannot be used—penicillins, chloramphenicol, and sulphonamides are usually also effective.
- Praziquantel—to kill the fluke *Nanophyetus salmonincola* (*Table 88-1*).
- *Nanophyetus salmonincola* does not cause severe clinical disease—treating for it will limit spread of eggs.

TABLE 88-1. Drug Therapy for Salmon Poisoning in Dogs				
Drug	Dose (mg/kg)	Route	Interval (Hours)	Duration (Days)
Doxycycline	10	PO, IV	12	7
Tetracycline	22[a]	PO	8	5
Oxytetracycline	10[a]	PO, IV	8	5
Minocycline	10	PO, IV[b]	12	7
Praziquantel	20–30	PO	Once	—

[a] Reduce dose in renal failure.
[b] Give by slow IV injection; rapid injection can cause hypotension, shock, and urticaria if given too rapidly.

Precautions/Interactions

- In a vomiting dog—best to start therapy with injectable oxytetracycline or doxycycline until the vomiting is controlled; then switch to an orally administered drug.
- Doxycycline—contraindicated in pregnant or lactating bitches.
- Minocycline—give by slow IV injection because too rapid injection can cause hypotension, shock, and urticaria.
- Tetracyclines—can cause discoloration of teeth in young animals; reduce dose in renal failure.

 COMMENTS

- The sooner therapy is instituted after ingestion of raw fish—the better is the prognosis.
- Warn clients—if other dogs may have eaten raw fish from the same area, they should receive a course of doxycycline and praziquantel.
- Prognosis—without treatment, infected dogs usually die within 5 to 10 days.
- Prognosis—with early treatment, prognosis is good.

Abbreviations

CBC, complete blood count; HGE, hemorrhagic gastroenteritis; IBD, inflammatory bowel disease.

Suggested Reading

Gorham JR, Foreyt WJ. Salmon poisoning disease. In:Greene CE, ed. *Infectious Diseases of the Dog and Cat.* 2nd ed. Philadelphia: WB Saunders; 1998:135–139.

Author: Johnny D. Hoskins
Consulting Editor: Stephen C. Barr

chapter **89**

Sarcocystis

 DEFINITION/OVERVIEW

- Enteric protozoa of carnivores causing no disease in the definitive host (carnivores), but the cysts sequestered in the muscle of domestic herbivores (cattle) are of some economic importance.
- The importance of the organism to small animal clinicians (finding *Sarcocystis* oocysts in the feces of dogs and cats)—understanding their significance.

 ETIOLOGY/PATHOPHYSIOLOGY

- *Sarcocystis* spp.—like other coccidia, are obligate intracellular protozoa that infect and reproduce in enterocytes of many carnivores (including cats and dogs).
- Unlike other coccidia—*Sarcocytis* requires a second host (intermediate host) to complete the life cycle.
- Intermediate hosts—domestic (cattle and sheep) and various wild herbivores.
- Intermediate hosts acquire infection—oocysts from contaminated pasture.
- Cysts—develop within muscle (and nervous tissue) of the herbivorous intermediate hosts causing economic downgrade of the carcass at slaughter.
- Dogs and cats—become infected by eating cysts sequestered in the meat of a herbivorous intermediate host.
- *Sarcocystis*—of no pathogenic consequence to definitive hosts (dogs and cats); muscle cyst stages can have a pathogenic effect on some intermediate hosts (cattle).

 SIGNALMENT/HISTORY

- Dogs and cats—eating raw or undercooked meat.
- Prevalence—can be >50% in stray dogs in some countries.

 CLINICAL FEATURES

- None.
- Owners and veterinarians—may be concerned with finding *Sarcocystis* oocysts in feces of a pet.

DIFFERENTIAL DIAGNOSIS

- None.
- Need to differentiate the *Sarcocystis* oocysts from those of other coccidia.

DIAGNOSTICS

- Fecal flotation—small (9 to 16 μm) sporulated oocysts or sporocysts of *Sarcocystis* (Fig. 89-1).
- Individual species—possible to tell apart based on morphology of oocysts.

THERAPEUTICS

- No effective drug treatment known.
- Because the organism is nonpathogenic to dogs and cats, and infection terminates spontaneously, drug therapy is not warranted.

Drugs of Choice

- None.

Precautions/Interactions

- None.

■ **Fig. 89-1** Oocysts of *Sarcocystis* in the feces of a dog (1,000×).

COMMENTS

- Owners should avoid feeding pets raw uncooked meat.
- Fresh meat in retail food stores—can be infected with *Sarcocystis* cysts, which can remain viable for several days under refrigeration.
- Frozen (for longer than 3 days) or well-cooked meat—loses its infectivity to cats and dogs.
- Prevent contact of infected dogs and cats with the feed supply (grain or pasture lands) of herbivores—to reduce the contamination of feed with sporocysts.

Suggested Reading

Kirkpatrick CE, Dubey JP. Enteric coccidial infections. *Vet Clinics North Am Small Anim Pract* 1987;17:1412–1414.

Author: Stephen C. Barr
Consulting Editor: Stephen C. Barr

chapter 90

Spirocerca lupi

DEFINITION/OVERVIEW

- Nematode parasite—adult worms are found in fibrous nodules within the walls of the esophagus and stomach of dogs.
- Cause vomiting or regurgitation, aortic aneurysm (rarely aortic rupture), cervical spondylitis, esophageal osteosarcoma, pulmonary hypertrophic osteoarthropathy, and aberrant migration of adults to unusual sites within the thorax (subcutis, heart).
- Common in Israel (where it seems to be reemerging), South Africa, Greece—rare in North America (mideastern states; Alabama).

ETIOLOGY/PATHOPHYSIOLOGY

- *Spirocerca lupi*—adults (within the esophageal or gastric wall nodules) deposit very small (15 × 30 μm) eggs containing an embryo into the esophageal luminal tract, to be passed in feces.
- Eggs—eaten by intermediate hosts (coprophilic beetles); develop to L3 infective larvae.
- Transmission—dogs infected by ingesting L3 larvae in paratenic hosts (lizards, chickens, mice).
- Dogs—larvae migrate via the adventitia of visceral arteries and aorta to the walls of the stomach and esophagus.
- Aortic aneurysm—develops in about 50% of infected dogs (very rarely, aortic rupture).
- Chronic infections—result in large, calcified fibrous nodules within the esophagus walls.
- Neoplasia of the nodules—occurs occasionally.
- PPP = 5 to 6 months.

SIGNALMENT/HISTORY

- Median age of infection—5 years.
- Infection in dogs under 1 year of age—rare.
- Large hunting-breed dogs—with access to intermediate hosts (mice, uncooked chicken, lizards) are overrepresented.
- Most cases—diagnosed during the colder months (December through April in Israel).

CLINICAL FEATURES

- Vomiting.
- Regurgitation.
- Salivary gland necrosis—resulting in enlarged, hard, painful salivary glands.
- Associated signs—retching; vomiting; regurgitation of saliva.
- Pyrexia.
- Weakness.
- Respiratory abnormalities.
- Anorexia.
- Melena.
- Paraparesis—less common.

DIFFERENTIAL DIAGNOSIS

- Other causes of regurgitation—megaesophagus (idiopathic, myasthenia gravis, polymyositis, hypoadrenocorticism, hypothyroidism, lead toxicity), esophagitis, esophageal diverticulum, vascular ring anomaly, esophageal neoplasia, hiatal hernia, esophageal foreign body, and sialadenitis.
- Other causes of vomiting—dietary; toxins (lead, ethylene glycol), IBD, metabolic (diabetes mellitus, renal disease, hepatic disease, acidosis, heat stroke, hypoadrenocorticism), gastric abnormalities (neoplasia, obstruction, atrophic gastritis, ulcers, dilatation/volvulus), gastroesophageal junction disorders (hiatal hernia), small intestine disorders (IBD, neoplasia, fungal, parasitic, viral, obstruction, paralytic ileus), large intestine disorders (colitis, obstipation, irritable bowel syndrome), abdominal disorders (pancreatitis, gastrinoma, peritonitis, steatitis, prostatitis, pyometra, diaphragmatic hernia, neoplasia), and neurologic disorders (psychogenic, motion sickness, vestibular lesions, head trauma, brain neoplasia).

DIAGNOSTICS

- CBC—anemia (blood loss), 50% of cases.
- Creatine kinase elevations—50% of cases.
- Fecal flotation (sugar best)—identifies eggs in about 80% of infected dogs.
- Thoracic radiology—identifies caudal esophageal masses in about 50% of infected dogs (Fig. 90-1).
- Mid-thoracic vertebral spondylitis—on radiographic examination (33% of cases).

Diagnostic Features
- **Esophageal endoscopy—most sensitive diagnostic procedure (100%).**
- **Endoscopy—may show granulomas in various degrees of severity** (Fig. 90-2) **or tumors** (Fig. 90-3).

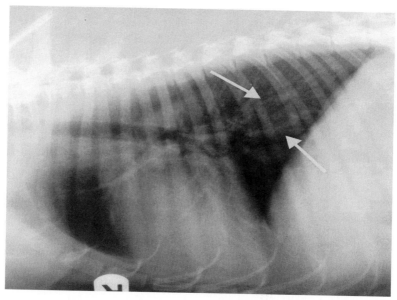

■ **Fig. 90-1** Lateral radiograph of a dog with an esophageal granuloma (*between arrows*) caused by *Spirocerca lupi* (courtesy Dr. Eran Lavy, Israel).

THERAPEUTICS

- Drug therapy—institute quickly.
- If not treated—about 60% of dogs will die or be euthanized within a month of diagnosis if not treated.
- Surgery—to remove nodules has been successful.

Drugs of Choice

- Doramectin (Dectomax Injectable Solution, 10 mg/ml [Pfizer, Exton, PA]).
  - Regimen 1: 0.2 mg/kg, SQ every 14 days for 3 treatments—resolves clinical signs and nodules in most dogs, but further treatment with doramectin (0.5 mg/kg, PO, q24h for 6 weeks) may be required if nodules not fully resolved.
  - Regimen 2: 0.4 mg/kg, SQ every 14 days for 6 treatment and then monthly until all esophageal granulomas are gone—2 years in some cases.

Precautions/Interactions

- Doramectin is not labeled for use in the dog (cattle and pig wormer).

COMMENTS

- Sialidinitis will resolve with long-term treatment with doramectin.

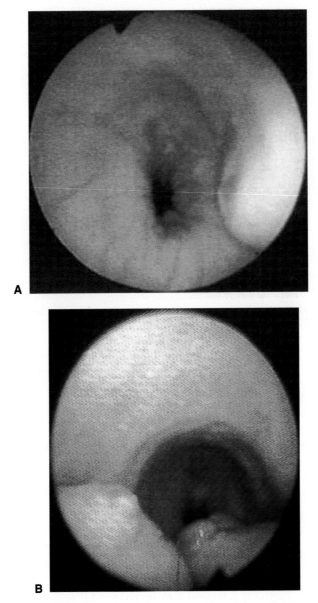

■ **Fig. 90-2** Endoscopic views of esophageal granulomas caused by *Spirocerca lupi* in various forms of development (courtesy Dr. Eran Lavy, Israel).

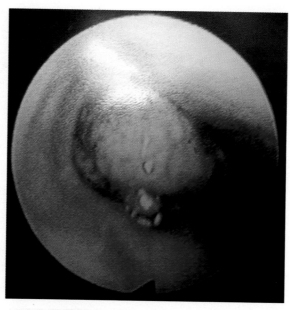

■ **Fig. 90-3** Endoscopic view of esophageal neoplasm caused by *Spirocerca lupi* (courtesy Dr. Eran Lavy, Israel).

Abbreviations

CBC, complete blood count; IBD, inflammatory bowel disease; PPP, prepatent period.

Suggested Reading

Berry WL. *Spirocerca lupi* esophageal granulomas in 7 dogs: resolution after treatment with doramectin. *J Vet Intern Med* 2000;14:609–612.

Lavy E, Aroch I, Bark H, et al. Evaluation of doramectin for the treatment of canine spirocercosis. *Vet Parasitol* 2002;109:65–73.

Mazaki-Tovi M, Baneth G, Aroch I, et al. Canine spirocercosis: clinical, diagnostic, pathologic, and epidemiologic characteristics. *Vet Parasitol* 2002;107:235–250.

Author: Stephen C. Barr

Consulting Editor: Stephen C. Barr

chapter 91

Sporotrichosis

DEFINITION/OVERVIEW

- A zoonotic fungal disease that may affect the integument or lymphatics; may cause systemic disease.

ETIOLOGY/PATHOPHYSIOLOGY

- *Sporothrix schencki*—ubiquitous dimorphic fungus living mainly in soil rich in decaying organic material.
- Infection—occurs typically by direct inoculation such as puncture wounds associated with foreign bodies (dogs mainly), or introduced by scratches (cats).

SIGNALMENT/HISTORY

Dogs

- More commonly seen in hunting breeds because of increased likelihood of puncture wounds associated with thorns or splinters.
- Historically, dogs initially presenting with clinical disease have had a poor response to antibiotic therapy.

Cats

- Intact males that roam outdoors and fight, because of the increased likelihood of puncture wounds and acquiring the disease from their opponents.

CLINICAL FEATURES

Cutaneous Form

Dogs

- Associated with numerous nodules, which may drain or crust, typically affecting the head or trunk but can also be found on the limb *(Fig. 91-1)*.

■ **Fig. 91-1** Sporotrichosis in a dog. Note the crusted excoriated draining tract around the dew claw on the limb.

Cats

■ Lesions often initially appear as wounds or abscesses, mimicking wounds associated with fighting, found on the head, lumbar region, or distal limbs.

Cutaneolymphatic Form

■ Usually an extension of the cutaneous form; spreads via the lymphatics, resulting in new nodules and draining tracts or crusts; lymphadenopathy common.

Disseminated Form

■ Associated with the systemic signs of fever, malaise, and anorexia.
■ Consider underlying immunosuppressive disorder, which is a predisposing factor for systemic form (neoplasia).

 DIFFERENTIAL DIAGNOSIS

■ Various bacterial and fungal diseases—consider when symptoms include a nodular granulomatous disease and draining tracts.
■ Neoplasia.
■ Parasitic infections (*Demodex* or *Pelodera* spp.).

 DIAGNOSTICS

■ CBC, serum biochemical profile, and urinalysis usually normal unless in the systemically ill, in which there can be a leukocytosis with a left shift and monocytosis.
■ REMEMBER: this is a zoonotic disease that can be acquired across intact skin—take particular care when collecting samples from infected patients.

Diagnostic Feature

- **Cytologic examination of the exudate and staining—often the only test necessary to confirm disease (cats)—cigar-shaped to round yeast intracellularly or free in the exudates.**
- Dogs—special fungal stains (periodic acid–Schiff and GMS) may aid in the diagnosis; a negative finding does not rule out the disease.
- Culture of deeply affected tissues—often requires surgery to obtain an adequate sample.
- Important—to alert laboratory that sporotrichosis is on the differential diagnosis list.
- Bacterial contamination of biopsy samples for culture—is common.

THERAPEUTICS

- Warn owner of zoonotic potential of patient under treatment.

Drugs of Choice

SSKI

- Treatment of choice.
  - Dogs—40 mg/kg PO q8h with food.
  - Cats—20 mg/kg PO q12h with food.
- Continue—for 30 days after the resolution of the clinical lesions.
- Dogs—if signs of iodism are noted (see following discussion of signs of iodism), discontinue treatment for 1 week; if symptoms are mild, reinitiate at the same dose; if severe, consider other drugs.
- Cats—iodism is more commonly seen in cats; if develops, discontinue and use other drugs.

Ketoconazole and Itraconazole

- Dogs—ketoconazole: 15 mg/kg, PO, q12h, preferably with an acidic meal (e.g., tomato juice), until 1 month after clinical resolution, which should occur within about 3 months.
- Cats—ketoconazole: 5 to 10 mg/kg, PO, q12-24h, or itraconazole 10 mg/kg/day until 1 month after clinical resolution.

Precautions/Interactions

Signs of Iodism

- Dogs—dry hair coat, excessive scales, nasal or ocular discharge, vomiting, depression, or collapse.
- Cats—depression, vomiting, anorexia, twitching, hypothermia, and cardiovascular collapse.

Side Effects of Azole Therapy

- Dogs—anorexia, acute hepatopathy (follow hepatic enzymes to monitor), pruritus, alopecia, and lightening of the hair color reported.

- Cats—GI disturbances, depression, fever, jaundice, and neurologic signs; may be necessary to alternate drugs.

 COMMENTS

- Reevaluate—every 2 to 4 weeks for clinical signs and side effects associated with treatment.
- Although difficult—try to determine the source of the original infection to prevent repeat infections.
- Consider—having male cats neutered to stop fighting behavior.
- Unresponsive therapy—not unexpected; consider alternative treatment or combined regimens (SSKI and ketoconazole).
- Zoonotic—proper precautions and client education can not be over emphasized.

Abbreviations

CBC, complete blood count; GI, gastrointestinal; GMS, Gomori's methamine silver (stain); SSKI, supersaturated potassium iodide.

Suggested Reading

Scott DW, Miller WH, Griffin CE. *Muller and Kirk's Small Animal Dermatology*, 5th ed. Philadelphia: WB Saunders; 1995.

chapter 92

Streptococcal Infections

DEFINITION/OVERVIEW

- A bacterial infection causing a wide range of clinical entities depending on which organ is infected.

ETIOLOGY/PATHOPHYSIOLOGY

- *Streptococcus* spp. is a gram-positive, nonmoltile coccal or spherical bacteria.
- Normal flora of the upper respiratory tract, oropharynx, lower genital tract, and skin.
- Under appropriate conditions, capable of infecting all areas of the body, but primary infections involve the respiratory, circulatory, integumentary, urogenital, or central nervous systems.
- Frequently a secondary invader of body tissues.
- Classified by ability to RBCs and produce a zone around the bacterial colony on blood agar plates.
- Hemolytic strains subdivide further by antigenic differences in cell wall carbohydrates into Lancefield serogroups A to H and K to T.
- Some groups more likely to be associated with disease, depending on species (e.g., group G associated with cats and dogs; group A with humans).
- Produce exotoxins, streptolysins (hemolysins), streptokinase, deoxyribonucleases, and hyaluronidases.

SIGNALMENT/HISTORY

- Very young—more prone to infection because of immature immune system, especially kittens born to primiparous queens.
- Severity of disease—dependent on age, exposure, and immune response; virulence.
- Opportunistic circumstances—wounds, trauma, surgical procedures, and concurrent viral infections.
- Maternal antibodies—generally protect puppies and kittens against clinical disease.
- Carrier states—do occur.

CLINICAL FEATURES

- Vary—with site of infection and host immunocompetence.
- Respiratory tract—weakness, cough, dyspnea, fever, and hemoptysis.
- Urinary tract—hematuria, stranguria, and pollakiuria.
- Local wound—purulent exudates with lymphadenopathy.

Dogs

- Septicemia, endometritis, vaginitis, mastitis (*Fig. 92-1*), fading puppies, abortion, urinary tract infection, pneumonia, necrotizing fasciitis, and streptococcal shock syndrome.

Cats

- Septicemia, peritonitis, cervical lymphadenitis, pharyngitis, tonsillitis, and fading kitten.

 ## DIFFERENTIAL DIAGNOSIS

- Other systemic infectious diseases causing fever, lymphadenopathy, and pneumonia, including viral, bacterial, fungal, rickettsial, and protozoal infections.

 ## DIAGNOSTICS

- CBC—usually leukocytosis with neutrophilia and left shift (degenerative or regenerative).
- Cocci—may be found in circulating neutrophils in overwhelming sepsis.
- Serum biochemical profile—may suggest a predisposing condition.

■ **Fig. 92-1** The mammary gland of a rottweiler bitch with streptococcal mastitis, showing swelling, discoloration, and sinus development within the mammary gland.

- Urinalysis—pyuria, bacteruria.
- Diagnosis—best made with culture of affected tissue, exudate, urine, blood, or needle aspirate to confirm causative organism.
- Direct microscopy with Gram stain of exudates—reveals single gram-positive cocci or chains of organisms.
- Thoracic radiographs—interstitial or alveolar pulmonary pattern with pneumonia.
- UTI—radiodense uroliths (struvite) often present with streptococcal cystitis.

 THERAPEUTICS

- Drain and flush abscesses, débride necrotic tissue.
- Septic shock or deep infections (pneumonia, mastitis) causing systemic illness—fluid therapy support with intravenous antibiotic therapy.

Drugs of Choice

- Base on culture and sensitivity results.
- First choice—penicillin G or penicillin V.
- Ampicillin.
- Erythromycin.
- Cephalexin (*Table 92-1*).
- Prophylactic treatment—all kittens born to a primiparous queen indicated by neonatal infections.

Precautions/Interactions

- Erythromycin—may cause vomiting, abdominal discomfort, anorexia, and diarrhea; if occurs, stop medicating until symptoms abate, then restart at half the initial dose, giving medication with food, then raise to required dose if tolerates drug.
- Cephalexin—may cause anorexia, vomiting, diarrhea, and hypersalivation.

Drug	Species	Dose (mg/kg)	Route	Interval (Hours)	Duration (Days)
Penicillin G	B	10,000–20,000 U/kg	IM, SC	12–24	7
Penicillin V	B	10–30	PO	8	7
Ampicillin	B	10–40	PO, IV, SC	8	7–14
Erythromycin	D	5–20	PO	12–24	7
Cephalexin	B	10–40	PO	12	7

TABLE 92-1. Drug Therapy for Streptococcal Infections in Dogs and Cats

D, dogs; B, both dogs and cats.

COMMENTS

- Avoid—overcrowding and poor environmental sanitation.
- Prevention in newborns—dip navel and umbilical cord in 2% tincture of iodine.
- Prevention in colonies—avoid overcrowding, maintain clean feeders, and segregate infected animals.
- *Streptococci* isolated from humans—usually of human (group A) and not animal origin.
- Dogs and cats—can develop pharyngeal colonization with group A *Streptococcus* (with no clinical signs) acquired from an infected human; the pet may serve as a source of reinfection of humans; important to treat all family members, including the pets, in a household to break the reinfection cycle.

Abbreviations

CBC, complete blood count; RBCs, red blood cells; UTI, urinary tract infection.

Suggested Reading

Greene CE, Prescott JF. Streptococcal and other gram-positive bacterial infections. In: Greene CE, ed. *Infectious Diseases of the Dog and Cat*. Philadelphia: WB Saunders; 1998:205–214.

Author: J. Paul Woods
Consulting Editor: Stephen C. Barr

chapter 93

Strongyloides

DEFINITION/OVERVIEW

- Nematode parasite—adult worms infect the paramucosa of the small intestine of dogs and cats, causing diarrhea.
- Larval migration—may cause respiratory signs.

ETIOLOGY/PATHOPHYSIOLOGY

- *Strongyloides stercoralis*—parasitizes humans, dogs, and cats.
- Neonates—infected from larvae in colostrums.
- Larvae migrate via lungs (possibly causing bronchopneumonia)—to small intestinal tract.
- Female worms only—inhabit dogs and cats and lay eggs that hatch into L1 larvae.
- Some L1 larvae molt to infective L3 larvae—can infect the host (autoinfection) before leaving in feces.
- Transmission—infective L1 larvae via skin penetration and ingestion (usually in colostrum).
- Relatively host specific—with possible transmission to humans.
- *Strongyloides tumefaciens*—adenomatous mass in colon of cats.
- PPP = 2 weeks.

SIGNALMENT/HISTORY

- Most disease—neonatal puppies and kittens after transcolostral transmission.
- Most infections—occur in hot humid summer conditions.
- Dogs and cats in kennel and cattery situations—higher prevalence.

CLINICAL FEATURES

- Asymptomatic to watery diarrhea—main sign.
- Severe debilitation—especially in neonates.
- Dermatitis—intense pruritus and erythema at site of larvae skin penetration.
- Cough—may develop a few days after skin penetration as larvae migrate through lungs (*Fig. 93-1*).

■ **Fig. 93-1** Hemorrhagic lesions on the surface of a puppy's lungs infected with *Strongyloides* organisms.

■ Watery diarrhea (but may contain blood and mucus)—develops a few days after cough as parasites reach small intestine.

 DIFFERENTIAL DIAGNOSIS

Dogs

■ Causes of diarrhea in the puppy:
  - Dietary indiscretion.
  - Allergy.
  - Drugs (antibiotics).
  - Toxins—lead.
  - Parasites (*Giardia* spp., cryptosporidiosis, GI parasitism with hookworms or *Strongyloides* spp.).
  - Infectious agents (salmonellosis, enteric calici virus, reovirus, CPV, coronavirus, canine distemper, CHV, *Campylobacter* spp., clostridiosis).
  - GI tract bacterial overgrowth (coliforms).
  - Systemic organ dysfunction (renal, hepatic, pancreas, cardiac).

Cats

■ Causes of diarrhea in the kitten:
  - Dietary indiscretion.
  - Allergic.
  - Drugs (antibiotics).

- Toxins—lead.
- Parasites (*Giardia* spp., cryptosporidiosis, tritrichomoniasis, GI tract parasitism with hookworms or *Strongyloides* spp.).
- Infectious agents (panleukopenia, salmonellosis, enteric calici virus, reovirus, FeLV, and feline calicivirus).
- GI tract bacterial overgrowth (coliforms).
- Systemic organ dysfunction (renal, hepatic, pancreas, cardiac).

 # DIAGNOSTICS

- CBC—normal; may see mild nonregenerative anemia, and stress leukogram.
- Biochemistry profile—normal.
- Fecal flotation or direct smear—eggs (50 to 60 μm by 30 to 35 μm)—must use very fresh feces because eggs usually hatch before examination can occur.

Diagnostic Feature
- **L1 larvae—most common diagnostic form in feces either by fecal flotation or Baermann's technique** (*Fig. 93-2*).
- L1 larvae—380 μm long, large genital rudiment, esophagus with three distinct sections, and a long, straight tail.
- Differentiate *Strongyloides* spp. L1 larvae from *Ancylostoma* spp. L1 larvae—incubate fecal specimen in Baermann's apparatus for 48 hours—*Strongyloides* larvae will develop into unique filariform infective larvae (long, cylindrical esophagus, split tail).

 # THERAPEUTICS

- Isolate infected animals from noninfected animals and avoid human contact.
- After treatment, examine feces monthly for at least 6 months to ensure treatment success.
- One post-treatment fecal examination is not enough to ensure treatment success because of the intermittent nature of fecal larvae shedding.
- Treat not only affected pups, but dams also.

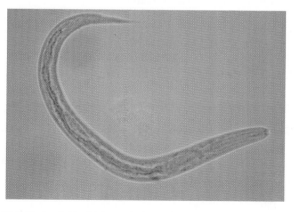

■ **Fig. 93-2** *Strongyloides* L1 larvae is the main diagnostic form found in feces.

TABLE 93-1. Drug Therapy for Strongyloidiasis in Dogs					
Drug	Dose (mg/kg)	Route	Interval (Hours)	Duration (Days)	Repeat Interval (Weeks)
Ivermectin (Ivomec)	0.2	SC, PO	Once	—	4
Fenbendazole (Panacur)	50	PO	24	5	4

Drugs of Choice

- Ivermectin (Ivomec 1% Injectable or Ivomec 0.27% Sterile Solution [Merial, Iselin, NJ]).
- Fenbendazole (Panacur Granules 22.2% [Intervet, Millsboro, DE]—use in adults and bitches (*Table 93-1*).

Precautions/Interactions

- This dose of ivermectin is extralabel use—ensure heartworm negative before treatment.
- Do not use this dose of ivermectin in collie dogs or collie-like breeds.

 COMMENTS

- Warn owners of zoonotic nature of *Strongyloides* spp.
- *Strongyloides stercoralis*—may produce dermatitis, severe abdominal discomfort and diarrhea in humans.
- May cause death in immunosuppressed individuals.
- Frequent cleaning of cages (every 24 hours) and monthly administration of ivermectin—needed to clear kennels of infection.
- Alternate anthelmintic—between ivermectin and fenbendazole to prevent resistance from developing.
- Using wire-bottom cages in colony situations—no guarantee of preventing infection.
- Cage cleaning—high-pressure washers followed by 1% sodium hypochlorite (3 cups of bleach/gallon of water) followed by water rinsing.

Abbreviations

CBC, complete blood count; CHV, canine herpes virus; CPV, canine parvovirus; FeLV, feline leukemia virus; GI, gastrointestinal; PPP, prepatent period.

Suggested Reading

Bowman DD, ed. *Georgi's Parasitology for Veterinarians*, 8th ed. Philadelphia: WB Saunders; 2003:197–201.
Hendrix CM, Blagburn BL, Lindsay DS. Whipworms and intestinal threadworms. *Vet Clin North Am Small Anim Pract*. 1987;17:1355–1375.

Author: Stephen C. Barr
Consulting Editor: Stephen C. Barr

chapter 94

Tapeworms *(Cestodiasis)*

DEFINITION/OVERVIEW

- Helminth parasites in the class Cestodes—infect the small intestine of cats and dogs but cause few clinical signs.

ETIOLOGY/PATHOPHYSIOLOGY

- *Taenia pisiformis*—dogs.
- *T. taeniaeformis*—cats.
- *Dipylidium caninum*—cats and dogs.
- Transmission—predation of rabbits and rodents.
- *D. caninum*—flea vectored, with flea maggots ingesting tapeworm eggs in dog or cat feces.
- Transmission—occurs when dogs and cats ingest the adult flea.
- Tapeworms—attach to the small intestinal mucosa, causing virtually no pathological condition or clinical signs, other than mild perianal pruritus.
- The sight of tapeworm segments crawling from the anus or around the perianal fur of a pet, or in its feces, is often repugnant to owners (*Fig. 94-1*).

SIGNALMENT/HISTORY

- Cats and dogs of all ages—exposure to fleas or ingesting the viscera of rodents or rabbits.

CLINICAL FEATURES

- Chains or segments in feces or attached to perianal fur.
- Perianal pruritus (*D. caninum*) manifested by dragging anus on ground.

DIFFERENTIAL DIAGNOSIS

- Anal sac impaction, sacculitis or abscess, perianal fistulas, and anal sac neoplasia.
- Perianal pruritus—food hypersensitivity, flea allergy dermatitis, atopy, tail-fold pyoderma, and seborrheic skin disorders affecting the perineum.

■ **Fig. 94-1** Tapeworm segment on the perianal region of a cat.

 DIAGNOSTICS

- *D. caninum*—Scotch tape pressed to the perianal skin for egg capsules containing eggs (*Fig. 94-2*) ~50 μm in diameter, pale yellow, hexacanth embryo.
- Even if owners report or you see tapeworm segments on the perianal fur—eggs may not be found using this method.
- *Taenia*—eggs spherical, brown, ~30 μm, hexacanth embryo (*Fig. 94-3*); segments are square with a single lateral pole (*Fig. 94-4*).

■ **Fig. 94-2** Egg packet of *Dipylidium caninum* containing several eggs.

■ **Fig. 94-3** Egg of *Taenia pisiformis*; brown spheroid egg containing hexocanth embryo with hooks.

■ **Fig. 94-4** The square segment of *Taenia pisiformis* with a single lateral pore.

THERAPEUTICS

- Outpatient.
- Discuss flea control (*D. caninum*).

Drugs of Choice

Dogs
- Fenbendazole (Panacur Granules 22.2% [Intervet, Millsboro, DE]).
- Praziquantel (Droncit [Bayer, Shawnee Mission, KS]).
- Praziquantel/pyrantel/febantel (Drontal Plus [Bayer, Shawnee Mission, KS]).
- Epsiprantel (Cestex [Pfizer, Exton, PA]).

Cats
- Praziquantel (Droncit [Bayer, Shawnee Mission, KS]).
- Praziquantel/pyrantel (Drontal [Bayer, Shawnee Mission, KS]).
- Epsiprantel (Cestex [Pfizer, Exton, PA] (*Table 94-1*).

Precautions/Interactions

- Praziquantel or epsiprantel—do not use in puppies or kittens <4 weeks old.

 COMMENTS

- Careful attention to flea control using monthly preparations, including:
  - Selamectin (Revolution [Pfizer, Exton, PA]).
  - Lufenuron (Program [Novartis, Greensboro, NC]).
  - Imidacloprid (Advantage [Bayer, Shawnee Mission, KS]).
  - Fipronil (Frontline [Merial, Iselin, NJ]).
- *D. caninum* may be infective to children.

Drug	Species	Dose (mg/kg)	Route	Interval (Hours)	Duration (Days)
TABLE 94-1. Drug Therapy for Tapeworm Infections in Dogs and Cats					
Fenbendazole (Panacur)	D	50	PO	24	3
Praziquantel (Droncit)	B	5–7.5	PO, SC, IM	Once	—
Praziquantel/pyrantel/febantel (Drontal Plus)	D	a	PO	Once	—
Epsiprantel (Cestex)	B	5.5	PO	Once	—
Praziquantel/pyrantel (Drontal)	C	b	PO	Once	—

a Praziquantel (22.7), pyrantel (22.7), febantel (113.6).
b Praziquantel (18.2), pyrantel (72.6).
B, both dogs and cats; C, cats; D, dogs.

Suggested Reading

Bowman DD. In: *Georgis' Parasitology for Veterinarians*, 8th ed. Philadelphia: WB Saunders; 2003:138–148.

Georgi JR. Tapeworms. *Vet Clin North Am Small Anim Pract* 1987;17:1285–1306.

Author: Stephen C. Barr
Consulting Editor: Stephen C. Barr

Tetanus

DEFINITION/OVERVIEW

- Disease caused by a bacterium found in soil and as part of the normal bacterial flora of mammalian intestinal tracts.
- When it contaminates necrotic anaerobic wounds, germinating spores in the wound produce a potent exotoxin (tetanospasmin).

ETIOLOGY/PATHOPHYSIOLOGY

- *Clostridium tetani*—obligate anaerobic spore-forming gram-positive rod.
- Distribution—worldwide.
- Very resistant—to disinfectants and environmental exposure.
- Tetanospasmin—blocks release of neurotransmitters by entering the axon of the nearest motor nerves at the neuromuscular end plate, migrates up axon to neuronal cell body within spinal cord, and then ascends to the brain.
- Hematogenous tetanospasmin—can enter the brain through an intact blood–brain barrier to cause intracranial signs before development of generalized limb rigidity.
- Early involvement of facial musculature after hematogenous spread—due to shortness of cranial nerve motor axons (relative to those of limbs).
- Tetanospasmin—inhibits glycine and GABA release (neurotransmitters of inhibitory interneurons of the brain and spinal nerves).
- May also cause autonomic dysfunction—resulting in increased vagal tone.
- Tetanospasmin binding to inhibitory neuron presynaptic sites—irreversible.
- Recovery—depends on growth of new axon terminals.

SIGNALMENT/HISTORY

- Dogs—small wounds, often unseen.
- Association—with foreign bodies.
- Hunting breeds—higher prevalence near horse farms, where *C. tetani* reaches high levels.
- Cats—very resistant; large obvious wounds with extensive contamination.

CLINICAL FEATURES

Localized
- Rigidity—of muscle(s) or entire limb closest to wound site.
- Thoracic limb—often fixed extended elbow; carpus flexed or extended; spreads to include opposite extremity and eventually involves entire CNS.
- Pelvic limb—held rigidly extended out behind; often associated with infection in female reproductive tract.
- Localized—may spontaneously resolve if infection source removed and partial immunity to tetanospasmin present.

Generalized
- Initially, stiff gait with outstretched or dorsally curved (cats) tail.
- Difficulty walking progressing to stretched out "sawhorse" appearance *(Fig. 95-1)*.
- Difficulty lying down.
- Difficulty opening jaw and eating.
- Eventually, difficulty breathing.
- Eyelids retract, enophthalmos and prolapsed third eyelids *(Fig. 95-2)*.
- Forehead skin wrinkles *(Fig. 95-3)*.
- Ears erect or pulled back, grinning (commissure of lips retracted).
- Hypersalivation.
- Tachycardia, laryngeal spasm.
- Fever (from muscle rigidity).
- Dysuria.
- Constipation.
- Tetanic muscle spasms, especially when stimulated by noise or touch.

■ **Fig. 95-1** Dog with generalized tetanus showing classical "sawhorse" stance (courtesy Dr. A. Delahunta, Cornell University).

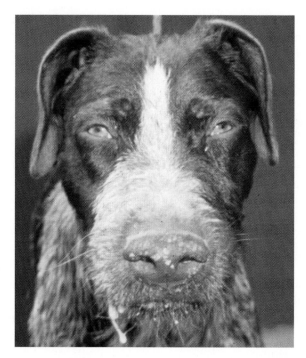

■ **Fig. 95-2** Facial features of a dog with tetanus can show prolapse of the third eyelid and retraction of the ears (courtesy Dr. A. Delahunta, Cornell University).

■ **Fig. 95-3** This dog shows the wrinkling of the forehead to give the apprehensive appearance of dogs with tetanus. Note the nasal oxygen tube, which may be helpful in dogs with respiratory depression from tetanus.

- Clonic seizures; opisthotonus initially (animals often vocalize as muscle contraction painful), progressing to seizure and loss of consciousness.
- Death usually due to respiratory system compromise from laryngeal and respiratory muscle spasm.

DIFFERENTIAL DIAGNOSIS

- Intoxications—lead, strychnine, organophosphate, carbamate, and 1080 poison usually show GI signs and less severe muscle spasm.

DIAGNOSTICS

- Diagnosis—made mainly on history, presence of wound and clinical appearance.
- CBC—mild leukopenia initially then leukocytosis.
- Serum biochemistry panel—AST and CK elevations (muscle spasms).
- Anti-tetanus antibody—often provides false negative results but a positive result helps confirm diagnosis.
- Wound culture for *C. tetani*—unrewarding as high contamination risk.

THERAPEUTICS

- Warn owners—of lengthy hospital stay (and subsequent costs), complications in generalized cases.
- Localized or mild cases—good survival if treated aggressively.

Drugs of Choice

- Therapy involves a combination of—anti-toxin, local wound treatment, antibiotics, sedation, nursing care, and autonomic agents.

Anti-toxin
- ATS—binds circulating tetanospasmin (will not eliminate bound toxin to neuroreceptors).
- Anaphylaxis reactions—possible (see Precautions/Interactions).
- No need to repeat injection—therapeutic levels of anti-tetanus serum persist for 14 days.
- Risk for anaphylaxis—increases on subsequent injections.

Local Wound Treatment
- Administer ATS before surgical manipulation of wound to counteract toxin release into circulation.
- Remove any foreign material and necrotic tissue.
- Irrigate wound with hydrogen peroxide (increases oxygen tension in tissue, inhibits growth of obligate anaerobes).

Antibiotics

- Penicillin G.
- Tetracycline.
- Metronidazole and clindamycin are also effective.

Sedation

- A combination of phenothiazine and barbiturates controls reflex spasm and convulsions but maintains consciousness.
- Chlorpromazine.
- Pentobarbital.

Nursing Care

- Dark, quiet environment—with minimal stimulation.
- Soft bedding or air/water bed—protects against decubital ulcers.
- Encourage to eat, drink unassisted—homogenize food so it can be sucked in through clenched teeth.
- Maintain hydration—parenteral balanced isotonic fluids.
- PEG tube—if megaesophagus or hiatal hernia develop, or severely debilitated.
- Urinary catheterization (sterile system essential) and periodic enemas—may be required.
- Tracheostomy—if laryngeal obstruction from laryngeal spasm develops.
- Hyperthermia—control with parenteral fluids, fans, alcohol on footpads.

Autonomic Agents

- Bradycardia—may occur when chlorpromazine and pentobarbital are used together.
- If heart rate drops below 60 beats/minute—give glycopyrrolate or atropine.

Precautions/Interactions

- To test for anaphylaxis from ATS administration—0.1 to 0.2 ml given SC or ID, 30 minutes before IV dose; wheal at injection site indicates anaphylactic reaction may occur.
- Treat anaphylaxis—epinephrine *(Table 95-1)*.
- Use glucocorticoids and antihistamine—only if necessary.

    COMMENTS

- Careful nursing care and attention to details—most generalized tetanus cases show improvement after 1 week and fully recover after 3 to 4 weeks.
- Tetanus toxoid—not recommended for dogs and cats.

Abbreviations

AST, aspartate aminotransferease; ATS, anti-tetanus equine serum; CBC, complete blood count; CK, creatine kinase; CNS, central nervous system; GABA, gamma-aminobutyric acid; GI, gastrointestinal; PEG, percutaneous endoscopic gastrostomy.

TABLE 95-1. Drug Therapy for Tetanus in Dogs				
Drug	Dose (mg/kg)	Route	Interval (Hours)	Duration (Days)
Anti-tetanus equine serum	100–1,000[a]	IV	Once	—
Penicillin G	20,000–100,000[b]	IV	8	10–14
Tetracycline	22	PO, IV	8	10–14
Chlorpromazine	0.5–2	PO, IV, IM	8	As needed
Pentobarbital	3–15	IV	3–4	To effect
Glycopyrrolate	0.005	SC, IV	—	To effect
Atropine	0.05	SC	—	To effect
Epinephrine	0.1[c]	IV	Once	To effect

[a] Units per kilogram to a maximum dose of 20,000 U given slowly over 10 minutes.
[b] Units per kilogram.
[c] Milliliters per kilogram of 1:10,000 dilution.

Suggested Reading

Greene CE. Tetanus. In: Greene CE, ed. *Infectious Diseases of the Dog and Cat.* Philadelphia: WB Saunders; 1998:267–273.

Author: Patrick L. McDonough
Consulting Editor: Stephen C. Barr

chapter 96

Tick Bite Paralysis

DEFINITION/OVERVIEW

- Flaccid lower motor neuron paralysis caused by salivary neurotoxins from certain species of female ticks.

SIGNALMENT/HISTORY

- In North America, ticks include:
    - *Dermacentor variabilis* (common wood tick—distributed over eastern two thirds of country and into California and Oregon).
    - *D. andersoni* (Rocky Mountain wood tick—distributed from the Cascade Mountains to the Rocky Mountains).
    - *Amblyomma americanum* (lone star tick—distributed from Texas and Missouri to the Atlantic Coast).
    - *A. maculatum* (Gulf Coast tick—found in the high temperatures and humidity of the Atlantic and Gulf of Mexico seaboards).
- In Australia—*Ixodes holocyclus* secretes a far more potent neurotoxin than the North American ticks; incidence of disease is much more common in Australia.
- *I. holocyclus*—injects salivary neurotoxins.
- Neurotoxin—probably interferes with the depolarization/acetylcholine release mechanism in the presynaptic nerve terminal, leading to reduction in the release of acetylcholine.
- One adult tick is sufficient to cause neurologic signs—a large larval or nymphal tick infestation can also induce signs.
- Signs—occur 6 to 9 days after tick attachment.
- Not all adult female ticks produce neurotoxin—not all tick-infected animals develop signs.
- Overall incidence is low in the United States—occurs mainly in the warmer months and regions of the southern states.
- Incidence—higher in Queensland, Australia (only other country where the disease exits) than in United States.

SIGNALMENT/HISTORY

- Australia—dogs and cats.
- United States—dogs; cats appear to be resistant.
- History—exposure of animal while walking in woods a week or so before the onset of signs.
- Onset of signs is gradual—initial unsteadiness and weakness in pelvic limbs.

CLINICAL FEATURES

Non-*Ixodes* Tick (American Ticks)

- Once neurologic signs appear—rapidly ascending lower motor neuron paresis progressing to paralysis occurs.
- Recumbency occurs 1 to 3 days after onset—hyporeflexia to areflexia and hypotonia to atonia.
- Pain sensation preserved.
- Cranial nerve dysfunction—not a prominent feature.
- May note facial weakness and reduced jaw tone—sometimes dysphonia and dysphagia early in course.
- Respiratory paralysis—uncommon in the United States.
- Urination and defecation—usually normal.

Ixodes Tick (Australian)

- Neurologic signs—much more severe and rapidly progressive.
- Ascending motor weakness—can progress to paralysis within a few hours.
- Signs—ptyalism, megaesophagus, and vomiting or regurgitation characteristic.
- Sympathetic nervous system affected—mydriatic and poorly responsive pupils; hypertension; tachyarrhythmias; high pulmonary capillary hydrostatic pressure; and pulmonary edema.
- Caudal medullary respiratory center affected—additive to the peripheral pulmonary changes, causing progressive fall in respiratory rate without a change in the tidal volume, resulting in hypoxia, hypercapnia, and respiratory acidosis.
- Respiratory muscle paralysis—much more prevalent.
- Progression to dyspnea, cyanosis, and respiratory paralysis within 1 to 2 days if not treated.

DIFFERENTIAL DIAGNOSIS

- Botulism—history of ingestion of toxin source (dead birds); more cranial nerve involvement and autonomic signs than tick bite paralysis in the United States.
- Coonhound paralysis—may follow a raccoon bite, systemic illness, or vaccination; cranial nerve involvement usually limited to facial and pharyngeal/laryngeal paresis; no autonomic signs; often shows diffuse hyperesthesia.

- Acute polyneuropathy—no ticks present or history of exposure.
- Distal denervating disease—tick bite paralysis usually more diffuse.
- Myelopathy—generalized or multifocal.
- Rabies—no ticks present or history of exposure; no vaccination against rabies; other behavioral signs.

DIAGNOSTICS

- CBC and other laboratory parameters—usually within normal range, except arterial blood gases in severely affected patients —low PaO_2, high $PaCO_2$, and low blood pH.

Diagnostic Feature
- **Most important diagnostic procedure is to search for ticks—remove immediately.**
- Electrodiagnostics—normal insertion activity and an absence of spontaneous myofiber activity (no fibrillation potentials or positive sharp waves); lack of motor unit action potentials; motor nerve stimulation is followed by either a dramatic decrease in amplitude or a complete absence of compound muscle action potentials.

THERAPEUTICS

- Hospitalize—until tick is found and removed or administer treatment to kill hidden ticks.
- Supportive care—until patient begins to show signs of recovery.
- Oxygen therapy if hypoventilation and hypoxia present—may require artificial ventilation if respiratory failure ensues.

Drugs of Choice

- United States—if ticks not found, dip patients in insecticidal bath; often only treatment needed.
- Australia—able to obtain hyperimmune serum (0.5 to 1 mg/kg, IV); given depending on severity of signs; if severe, can also give phenoxybenzamine, an α-adrenergic antagonist (1 mg/kg, IV, diluted in saline, given slowly over 20 min), which appears to be beneficial in relieving the sympathetic effects of the tick toxin; acepromazine (0.1 to 0.2 mg/kg, IV, up to 2 mg total dose) can be used as an alternative because it also has α-adrenergic antagonist effects.

Precautions/Interactions

- Drugs that interfere with neuromuscular transmission—contraindicated (e.g., tetracyclines, aminoglycosides, and procaine penicillin).
- Atropine—contraindicated in advanced stages of disease or with marked bradycardia from *Ixodes* tick bite.

COMMENTS

- Non-*Ixodes* tick—once tick is removed, recovery is rapid with minimal nursing care required; recovery usually complete within 1 to 3 days.
- *Ixodes* ticks—signs will often progress despite tick removal; thus aggressive treatment to neutralize toxin is indicated; prognosis often guarded and recovery can be prolonged.
- To reduce risk of disease—owners should check for ticks within 2 to 3 days of possible exposure.
- Treatment—weekly insecticide baths (Ecto-Soothe Shampoo [Virbac, Fort Worth, TX]; Adams Flea and Tick Shampoo and Mycodex products [Veterinary Products Laboratories, Phoenix, AZ]) or the use of insecticide-impregnated collars (Preventic [Virbac, Fort Worth, TX]) help.
- Some monthly topical parasiticides (Frontline [Merial, Iselin, NJ]; K9Advantix [Bayer, Shawnee Mission, KS]; Revolution [Pfizer, Exton, PA]) also protect against a number of species of ticks.
- Zoonosis—ticks are not transmitted from dogs to humans, although humans can suffer tick bite paralysis (especially in Australia).
- Be aware—tick species that can cause tick bite paralysis are also capable of transmitting certain rickettsial diseases RMSF, *Erhlichia* spp.).

Abbreviations

CBC, complete blood count; RMSF, Rocky Mountain spotted fever.

Suggested Reading

Malik R, Farrow BRH. Tick paralysis in North America and Australia. *Vet Clin North Am* 1991;21:157–171.

Author: Paul A. Cuddon
Consulting Editor: Stephen C. Barr

Ticks and Tick Control

DEFINITION/OVERVIEW

- Dogs and cats may be parasitized by hard ticks of the family Ixodidae.
- Ectoparasites that feed only on the blood of their hosts; arthropods; closely related to scorpions, spiders, and mites.
- Transmitted microbial pathogens: protozoa, helminths, fungi, bacteria, rickettsiae, and viruses.
- May cause toxicosis, hypersensitivity, paralysis, and blood loss anemia.

ETIOLOGY/PATHOPHYSIOLOGY

- Hard ticks—four life stages: egg, larva, nymph, and adult; larvae and nymphs must feed to repletion before detaching and molting; as adult female ixodid ticks engorge, they may increase their weight by more than 100-fold; after detachment females may lay thousands of eggs.
- Blood loss anemia—from heavy infestations.
- Damage to the integument—tick mouth parts cut through the host's skin; bites are generally painless; local irritation and infection may occur.
- Salivary secretion of neurotoxins—may lead to systemic signs (tick paralysis); local action may cause impaired hemostasis and immune suppression.
- Pathogens—acquired when ticks feed on infected reservoir hosts (often rodents and small feral mammals); sometimes transovarial transmission occurs and infected eggs hatch and produce infected larvae; greatest potential for systemic disease occurs when infections acquired in early life stages are transmitted to new hosts when the next stage feeds; may affect virtually any organ system.
- Transmission of pathogens and toxins—often requires periods of attachment from hours to days; the essentially painless bite allows adequate feeding times.

SIGNALMENT/HISTORY

Geographic Distribution

- Strong geographic specificities exist for some tick species; thus geographic prevalence of associated diseases.

- *Ixodes scapularis*—Lyme disease; midwest, northeast, and parts of the southeast United States.
- *Ixodes pacificus*—western coastal states of the United States.
- *Rhipicephalus sanguineus*—found throughout the continental United States; but canine ehrlichiosis and babesiosis most common in the southeast.

Species

- Dogs and cats.
- Cats are thought to be quite efficient at removing ticks, but tick attachment and subsequent tick-vectored diseases are routinely diagnosed.

Risk Factors

- Large hunting breeds (dogs)—considered to be at high risk because they are likely to come in contact with environments harboring questing ticks.
- Domestic animals—can be in close contact with ticks owing to encroachment of ticks into suburban environments and expansion of suburban environment into surrounding forests, prairies, and coastline areas.

 CLINICAL FEATURES

- Attached ticks or tick-feeding cavities from which ticks have detached may be seen on the skin.
- Associated tickborne diseases (borreliosis, ehrlichiosis, babesiosis, RMSF, and others)—vary with the organ system(s) affected.
- Irritation caused by ticks and subsequent self-trauma—may lead to pyotraumatic dermatitis ("hot spots") in dogs.

 DIAGNOSTICS

- Ticks—examine the skin for attached ticks or tick feeding cavities.
- Tickborne diseases—evaluate epidemiologic considerations for each disease, history of tick parasitism, and complete clinical examination.

 THERAPEUTICS

- Outpatient—after removal of ticks.
- Removal—do as soon as possible to limit time available for neurotoxin or pathogen transmission; grasp ticks close to the skin with fine-pointed tweezers and gently pull free; species with short, strong mouth parts (e.g., *Dermacentor* spp.) usually pull free with host skin attached; species with long, fragile mouth parts (e.g., *Ixodes* spp.) often leave fragments of mouth parts embedded in the feeding cavity.
- Wash feeding cavity with soap and water—generally sufficient to prevent local inflammation or secondary infection.

- Inform client—that application of hot matches, Vaseline, or other materials not only fails to cause tick detachment but allows for longer periods of attachment and feeding.

Prevention/Avoidance

- Avoid environments that harbor ticks—may be difficult except for pets kept strictly indoors.
- Tick control—essential to realize that this does not always equal control of tickborne diseases; often the goal is the perceived absence of ticks on the host animal.
- Pets—owners report complete tick control, even though there may be some period of attachment and tick feeding or live ticks may spend some time crawling on the animal after they have been exposed to lethal levels of an acaricide; immature ticks of some species (*R. sanguineus* and *I. scapularis*) may be undetected because of their minute size.
- Tickborne pathogens—may be transmitted very rapidly (viruses) or may require several hours (*Rickettsia rickettsii*) or days (*Borrelia burgdorferi*).

Insecticides and Acaricides

- In the United States—the EPA licenses agents as effective against various species of pests.
- Control—inferred as providing control of diseases carried by that species; although this may be correct in some or all cases, veterinarians should be sophisticated enough to require demonstration of efficacy in prevention of disease transmission before accepting a disease-control claim at face value; challenging because ticks are widely dispersed in the environment, spend a relatively short time on their hosts, possess great reproductive capacities, and have long lifetimes.
- Acaricidal collars (Preventic, Virbac, Fort Worth, TX) and spot treatment (Frontline, Merial, Iselin, NJ)—have gained wide use; ease of application is as important as efficacy; direct marketing to pet owners of veterinarian-dispensed products has been a major factor in shifting tick control away from OTC formulations.
- Bathing, spraying, or powdering with appropriate organophosphate or pyrethrin-containing products has become far less common with the advent of new convenient and effective products.

 COMMENTS

Conditions

- Canine babesiosis—vectored by *R. sanguineus*, caused by protozoan parasite *Babesia canis*, infects canine RBCs, leading to sludging in capillaries and destruction in the spleen.
- RMSF—vectored by *Dermacentor variabilis*, caused by *R. rickettsii*, invades vascular endothelial tissues, leading to necrotizing vasculitis.
- Canine ehrlichiosis—vectored by *R. sanguineus*, caused by *Ehrlichia canis*, infects mononuclear cells and platelets.
- Granulocytic ehrlichiosis—emerging disease; caused by *E. equi* (also called *E. phagocytophila*); infects granulocytes, leading to nonspecific signs and fever.

- Lyme disease—vectored by *I. scapularis* and *I. pacificus*, caused by *B. burgdorferi*; dogs may develop fevers associated with arthritis or syndromes leading to complete heart block, protein-losing nephropathy, and neurologic abnormalities.
- Canine hepatozoonosis—caused by protozoal organism *Hepatozoon canis* after the dog ingests an infected *R. sanguineus*; cysts and pyogranulomas in the muscles and other tissues associated with myositis and renal failure, often leading to death in chronic cases.
- Tick paralysis—caused by a neurotoxin; affects acetylcholine synthesis and/or liberation at the neuromuscular junction of the host animal; signs (typified by ascending flaccid paralysis often initially affecting the pelvic limbs) develop 5 to 9 days after tick attachment.

Vaccines

- Currently for "prevention" of only Lyme disease; two types for dogs: whole-cell, killed bacterin (since 1990) and Osp A (since 1996).
- Safety and efficacy—peer-reviewed published data for dogs naturally exposed to *B. burgdorferi* available only for bacterin; 1969 dogs received a total of 4,033 doses of bacterin during a 20-month period; 4,498 control dogs were not vaccinated; immunization was found to be safe regardless of previous history of Lyme disease or exposure to *B. burgdorferi*, 38 (1.9%) of vaccinated dogs had minor reactions that resolved without complications immediately or within 72 hours after vaccination; cumulative incidence of Lyme disease was 1.0% in vaccinated dogs and 4.7% in control dogs; 40% of vaccinated dogs had serologic evidence of infection with *B. burgdorferi* before vaccination but the incidence of Lyme disease was only 2%; incidence of Lyme disease in infected control dogs was 4.8%; thus vaccination of infected dogs was associated with about a 50% decrease in the incidence of Lyme disease; some clinical experiences have not shown this high degree of efficacy and have reported potentially harmful side effects (e.g., immune-mediated phenomena).

Zoonotic Potential

- Ticks may parasitize many different species of mammals, birds, and reptiles at different stages in their developmental cycles; infections acquired in early life stages may be transmitted when ticks feed again in the next stage.
- Humans, if parasitized, may be exposed to babesiosis, RMSF, ehrlichiosis, borreliosis, or tick paralysis.

Abbreviations

EPA, Environmental Protection Agency; OTC, over-the-counter; RBCs, red blood cells; RMSF, Rocky Mountain spotted fever.

Suggested Reading

Hoskins JD. Tick-borne zoonoses: Lyme disease, ehrlichiosis, and Rocky Mountain spotted fever. *Vet Clin North America* 1991:6;236–243.

Levy SA, Barthold SW, Dombach DM, et al. Canine borreliosis. *Compend Contin Educ* 1993;15:833–848.

Levy SA, Lissman BA, Ficke CM. Performance of a *Borrelia burgdorferi* bacterin in borreliosis endemic areas. *J Am Vet Med Assoc* 1993;202:1834–1838.

Author: Steven A. Levy

Consulting Editor: Karen Helton Rhodes

chapter 98

Toxoplasmosis

DEFINITION/OVERVIEW

- A multisystemic protozoal disease affecting both cats and dogs; affects nearly all mammals, with Felidae being the definitive host.

ETIOLOGY/PATHOPHYSIOLOGY

- *Toxoplasma gondii*—an obligate intracellular coccidian protozoan parasite.
- Infection—acquired by ingestion of tissue cysts or oocysts.
- After infection—organism spreads to extraintestinal organs via blood or lymph, resulting in focal necrosis of many organs (heart, eye, central nervous system).
- Acute disseminated infection—rarely fatal.
- Chronically—tissue cysts form to produce low-grade disease that usually is not clinically apparent unless immunosuppression or concomitant illness allows *T. gondii* to proliferate and cause an acute inflammatory response.
- Clinical toxoplasmosis—often associated with other infections causing severe immunosuppression (e.g., canine distemper, FIP, FIV, FeLV).
- Severity and manifestations of disease—depend on location and degree of tissue injury caused by tissue cysts.
- Distribution—worldwide.
- Approximately 30% of cats and up to 50% of humans in some countries are serologically positive for *T. gondii*.
- Clinical disease—uncommon; most animals with toxoplasmosis are asymptomatic.

SIGNALMENT/HISTORY

- Cats (particularly males)—more commonly clinically affected than dogs.
- Historically—initially get nonspecific signs of lethargy, depression, and anorexia.
- Weight loss.
- Fever.
- Ocular discharge, photophobia, and miotic pupils (cats).
- Respiratory distress.
- Neurologic signs—ataxia, seizures, tremors, paresis/paralysis, and cranial nerve deficits.

- Digestive tract signs—vomiting, diarrhea, abdominal pain, and jaundice.
- Stillborn kittens.
- Abortion.

CLINICAL FEATURES

Cats

- Disease is most severe in transplacentally infected kittens—may be stillborn or die before weaning.
- Surviving kittens:
  - Anorexia.
  - Lethargy.
  - High fevers unresponsive to antibiotics.
  - Signs reflecting necrosis/inflammation of lungs (dyspnea, increased respiratory noises), liver (icterus, abdominal enlargement from ascites), and CNS (encephalopathic) (Fig. 98-1).
- Respiratory and gastrointestinal signs (postnatal):
  - Anorexia.
  - Lethargy.
  - High fevers unresponsive to antibiotics.
  - Dyspnea.
  - Weight loss.
  - Icterus.
  - Vomiting.
  - Diarrhea.
  - Abdominal effusion.
  - Neurologic signs—seen in <10% of patients, blindness, stupor, incoordination, circling, torticollis, anisocoria, and seizures.

■ **Fig. 98-1** A young kitten with toxoplasmosis showing ventral flexion of the neck due to muscle weakness from neurologic and muscular involvement.

■ **Fig. 98-2** Eye of a cat with ocular toxoplasmosis, showing nodular iritis and a fibrin clot within the anterior chamber, as a result of severe uveitis (courtesy Dr. R. Riis, Cornell University).

- • Ocular signs—common (approximately 80% of affected cats show intraocular inflammation); uveitis (aqueous flare, hyphema, mydriasis), iritis, detached retina, iridocyclitis, and keratic precipitates (*Fig. 98-2*).
- ■ Rapid course—acutely affected patients with CNS and/or respiratory involvement.
- ■ Slow course—patients with reactivation of chronic infection.

Dogs

- ■ Young—usually generalized infection:
  - • Fever.
  - • Weight loss.
  - • Anorexia.
  - • Tonsillitis.
  - • Dyspnea.
  - • Diarrhea.
  - • Vomiting.
- ■ Older—usually localized infections; mainly associated with neural and muscular systems.
- ■ Neurologic—quite variable; usually reflecting diffuse neurologic inflammation; seizures, tremors, ataxia, paresis, paralysis, muscle weakness, and tetraparesis.
- ■ Ocular—rare; similar to those found in the cat.
- ■ Cardiac involvement—occurs; usually is not clinically apparent.

 DIFFERENTIAL DIAGNOSIS

Cats

- ■ Intraocular disease (anterior uveitis)—FIP, FeLV, FIV, immune-mediated, trauma, lens-induced, and corneal ulceration with reflex uveitis.
- ■ Dyspnea (respiratory signs)—asthma, cardiogenic, pneumonia (bacterial, fungal, parasitic), neoplasia, heartworm disease, pleural disease (effusions), diaphragmatic hernia, and chest wall injury.

- Neurologic signs (causes of meningoencephalitis)—viral (FIP, rabies, pseudorabies), fungal (cryptococcosis, blastomycosis, histoplasmosis), parasitic (cuterebriasis, coenurosis, aberrant heartworm migration), bacterial, and idiopathic disease (feline polioencephalomyelitis).

Dogs

- Often associated with other immunosuppressive diseases—for example, signs of distemper may be seen.
- Neurologic—usually in very young dogs; differentiate from *Neospora caninum* (both produce CNS and neuromuscular disease) using serology or PCR.
- Consider other conditions causing multifocal neurologic signs—infectious/inflammatory toxicity, metabolic diseases, neoplasia, GME, and hereditary and congenital defects.

 DIAGNOSTICS

- CBC—mild normocytic normochromic anemia.
- Approximately 50% of infected cats have leukopenia (severe disease)—mainly as a result of lymphopenia; some have neutropenia alone, lymphopenia, and/or a degenerative left shift; leukocytosis may occur during recovery.
- Serum biochemical profile—ALT and AST increased in most patients; approximately 25% of cats have icterus; most have hypoalbuminemia.
- Cats that develop pancreatitis as a result of toxoplasmosis—mildly low serum calcium concentrations.
- Urinalysis—mild proteinuria in a small proportion of cats; bilirubinuria (in icteric cats).
- Serology (ELISA)—IgM, IgG, and antigen serum titers give the most definitive information from one sample; a follow-up sample 3 weeks after the first will provide more complete information as to the type of infection (active, recent, or chronic).
- IgM—single serologic titer of choice for diagnosis of active infection; elevated 2 weeks postinfection (usually coincides with onset of clinical signs), persists for a maximum of 3 months, then falls; a prolonged titer may indicate reactivation or delay in antibody class shift from IgM to IgG (a result of immunosuppression from FeLV or FIV infection or steroid therapy).
- IgG—rises 2 to 4 weeks postinfection and persist beyond a year.
- A single high IgG titer is not diagnostic for active infection—a 4× increase in IgG titer over a 3-week period suggests active infection; most cats remain IgG positive for life.
- Antigen—positive 1 to 4 weeks postinfection; however, as it remains positive during active or chronically persistent infection, measurement does not give much more information than antibody titers.
- PCR—on CSF, aqueous humor, or infected tissues can differentiate toxoplasmosis from neosporosis; not commercially available.

■ **Fig. 98-3** Lateral thoracic radiograph of a cat with pulmonary toxoplasmosis. Note the patchy alveolar and interstitial pulmonary infiltrates.

- Radiographic examination—mixed pattern of patchy alveolar and interstitial pulmonary infiltrates (*Fig. 98-3*), with occasional pleural effusion; abdominal effusions and hepatomegaly.
- CSF—elevated leukocyte count (both mononuclear cells and neutrophils) and protein in encephalopathic animals.
- Cytologic examinaiton—tachyzoites, although rare, in body fluids (CSF, pleural or peritoneal effusions) during acute infection; BAL (pulmonary involvement) can reveal tachyzoites (*Fig. 98-4*).

■ **Fig. 98-4** Transtracheal wash from a cat with pulmonary toxoplasmosis. Note the banana-shaped tachyzoites in the process of rupturing out of the cell. (Wright-Giemsa stain, 1,000×).

■ **Fig. 98-5** A fecal preparation from a cat showing the relative sizes of *Toxoplasma gondii* (*T*), *Isospora rivolta* (*R*), *Isospora felis* (*F*), and *Toxocara cati* (*C*) (courtesy Dr. J.P. Dubey, U. S. Department of Agriculture, Beltsville, Md).

- Fecal examination (Sheather's sugar solution)—oocysts may be detected on routine fecal examinations in asymptomatic cats but are morphologically indistinguishable from *Hammondia* spp. and *Besnoitia* spp. (*Fig. 98-5*); PCR or mouse inoculation may distinguish species; oocysts are rarely shed during clinical disease.

  THERAPEUTICS

- Patients with severe disease will require hospitalization and fluid and nutritional support while receiving antiprotozoal therapy.

Drugs of Choice

- Clindamycin—for at least 2 weeks after clinical signs clear.
- Uveitis—1% prednisolone drops.
- Alternative to clindamycin—sulfadiazine in combination with pyrimethamine; TMS; azithromycin.
- Folinic acid (2.5 mg/kg/day) or brewer's yeast (100 mg/kg/day)—correct bone marrow suppression caused by sulfadiazine/pyrimethamine therapy (*Table 98-1*).

Precautions/Interactions

- Clindamycin and azithromycin—can cause GI signs (vomiting, anorexia, transient diarrhea); dose should be reduced or temporarily discontinued; reinitiate when signs stopped; give with food.
- Sulfonamide and pyrimethamine—can cause vomiting, leukopenia, myelosuppression, fetal teratogenesis, myelodysplasia; reduce dose with hepatic insufficiency.
- TMS—multiple adverse reactions including:
  - KCS—monitor tear production weekly throughout treatment.

TABLE 98-1. Drug Therapy for Toxoplasmosis

Drug	Species	Dose (mg/kg)	Route	Interval (Hours)	Duration (Weeks)
Clindamycin	D	10–20	PO, IM	12	2–4
	C	10–12.5	PO, IM	12	2–4
Sulfadiazine[a]	B	30	PO	12	2
Pyrimethamine	B	0.5	PO	12	2
Trimethoprim-sulfadiazine	B	15	PO, IV	12	2
Azithromycin	B	7.5	PO	12	2–4
Prednisilone (1% ophthalmic drops)	B	[b]	Topically	8	2
Folinic acid[c]	B[d]	2.5	PO	24	2

[a] Use in combination with pyrimethamine.
[b] 2 to 3 drops in affected eye(s).
[c] If giving sulfonamide drugs.
[d] Especially cats.
D, dogs; C, cats; B, both dogs and cats.

- Hepatotoxicity—anorexia, depression, icterus; monitor ALT if prolonged therapy.
- Megaloblastic–folate acid deficiency anemia—especially in cats after several weeks; supplement with folinic acid (2.5 mg/kg/day).
- Immune-mediated polyarthritis, retinitis, glomerulonephritis, vasculitis, anemia, thrombocytopenia, urticaria, toxic epidermal necrolysis, erythema multiforme, conjunctivitis—remove from drug.
- Renal failure and interference with renal excretion of potassium (leading to hyperkalemia).
- Salivation, diarrhea, and vomiting (cats).
- May interfere with thyroid hormone synthesis (dogs)—check T_3 and T_4 after 6 weeks.

COMMENTS

- Examine 2 days after initiating clindamycin treatment—clinical signs (fever, hyperesthesia, anorexia, uveitis) should begin to resolve; uveitis should resolve completely within 1 week.
- Examine 2 weeks after initiating treatment—assess neuromuscular deficits; should partially resolve (some deficits permanent owing to CNS or peripheral neuromuscular damage) (Fig. 98-6).
- Examine 2 weeks after owner-reported resolution of signs—consider discontinuing treatment; some neuromuscular deficits permanent.
- Prognosis—guarded in cats needing therapy because response is inconsistent.
- Worse prognosis in neonates and the severely immunocompromised.

■ **Fig. 98-6** A cat that has survived treatment for toxoplasmosis, displaying residual hind limb atrophy and rigid contracture.

- Prevent cats from eating raw meat, bones, viscera, or unpasteurized milk (especially goat milk) or from eating mechanical vectors (flies, cockroaches)—meat may be eaten if well cooked.
- Prevent—cats from free roaming to hunt prey (birds, rodents) or from entering buildings where food-producing animals are housed.

Zoonotic Potential

- Healthy cat with a positive *T. gondii* antibody titer—poses little danger to its owner.
- Cats with no antibody titer—are at more risk of becoming infected, shedding oocysts in the feces, and constituting a source of infection to humans.
- To avoid contact with oocysts or tissue cysts:
  - Do not feed raw meat.
  - Wash hands and surfaces (cutting boards) after preparing raw meat.
  - Boil drinking water if the source is unreliable.
  - Keep sandboxes covered to prevent cats defecating in them.
  - Wear gloves when gardening.
  - Wash hands and vegetables before eating to avoid contact with oocyst soil contamination.
  - Empty cat litterboxes daily (oocysts need at least 24 hours to become infective).
  - Disinfect litterboxes with boiling water.
  - Control stray cat population to avoid oocyst contamination of environment.
  - Pregnant women should avoid contact with cats excreting oocysts in feces, soil, cat litter, and raw meat (meat cooked to 150° F will kill *T. gondii*).
- Parasitemia during pregnancy—can cause spread of tachyzoites to the fetus; probably does not happen unless first-time infection of dam occurs during pregnancy (as with humans).
- Placental transmission—rare.

Abbreviations

ALT, alanine aminotransferase; AST, aspartate aminotransferase; BAL, bronchoalveolar lavage; CBC, complete blood count; CNS, central nervous system; CSF, cerebrospinal fluid; ELISA, enzyme-linked immunosorbent assay; FeLV, feline leukemia virus; FIP, feline infectious peritonitis; FIV, feline immunodeficiency virus; GI, gastrointestinal; GME, granulomatous meningoencephalopathy; Ig, immunoglobulin; KCS, keratoconjunctivitis sicca; PCR, polymerase chain reaction; TMS, trimethoprim-sulfadiazine.

Suggested Reading

Dubey JP, Lappin MR. Toxoplasmosis and neosporosis. In: Greene CE, ed. *Infectious Diseases of the Dog and Cat*. Philadelphia: WB Saunders; 1998:493–509.

Author: Stephen C. Barr

Consulting Editor: Stephen C. Barr

chapter 99

Trichinosis

DEFINITION/OVERVIEW

- Nematode infection—adults infect the small intestine of a wide range of carnivores (including dogs and humans) and omnivores (pigs), causing little GI disease.
- Larvae—sequest in skeletal muscle throughout the body.
- Of major zoonotic importance—humans obtain infection by eating poorly cooked meat containing sequestered larvae from a wide range of animals (pigs, bears, seals, horses).
- Zoonosis—causes severe myositis and sometimes death in humans.
- In China—eating dog meat is an important source of trichinosis in humans.
- Distribution—worldwide.

ETIOLOGY/PATHOPHYSIOLOGY

- *Trichinella spiralis*—dogs and cats become infected by eating L1 larvae sequestered in the muscle of other animals.
- Sources of infection—wild caught rodents or the carcasses of carnivores (mainly cats), or foxes, opossum, raccoons, and wild pigs (dogs).
- L1 larvae—molt to adults in the small intestine.
- Adult worms—produce large numbers of "prelarvae," which are injected into the intestinal mucosa.
- Prelarvae—migrate via lymphatics initially, then the blood stream to skeletal muscles, where they coil up and develop to L1 in cyst-like structures.
- L1 larvae—remain infective in the muscle for months to years.
- Dogs—only a very few larvae are needed for infection.
- Ingestion of large numbers of larvae—results in same degree of muscle sequestration as very small infections because most infecting larvae in large infections pass right through the GI tract without developing to adults.
- Infection rate in dogs—higher than in pigs in some studies.

SIGNALMENT/HISTORY

- Hunting dogs (including those that foxhunt)—high rate of infection.
- Puppies—more susceptible to infection than older dogs.

CLINICAL FEATURES

- Mild GI upset—vomiting, diarrhea.
- Myalgia, muscle stiffness—mild and rarely observed.

DIFFERENTIAL DIAGNOSIS

- Other causes of mild transient gastroenteritis—dietary indiscretion, early IBD, drugs (antibiotics), parasites (giardiasis, trichomoniasis, whipworms), infectious agents, partial foreign body (hairballs in cats).

DIAGNOSTICS

- CBC—eosinophilia during acute stage of infection; may persist for several weeks in severe infections.
- Identification of the small adults (female: 3 mm, male 1.5 mm) in the feces—may require examination of feces collected over time (*Fig. 99-1*).
- Adults and larvae in feces—distinguished from the larvae of *Crenosoma*, *Angiostrongylus*, and *Filaroides* spp. by the stichosome esophagus (both adults and larvae), copulatory lobes (male), and presence of prelarvae within the uterus (female).
- May identify prelarvae in blood (100 μm as opposed to the ~300 μm of larvae of *Dirofilaria immitis* and *Dipetalonema reconditum*)—by modified Knott's technique.
- Muscle biopsy—L1 larvae with characteristic stichosome esophagus in "cysts" (*Fig. 99-2*).

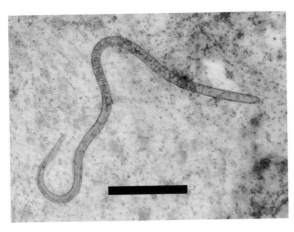

■ **Fig. 99-1** A male adult *Trichinella spiralis* organism in the feces of a dog (bar = 300 μm).

■ **Fig. 99-2** A cyst containing a *Trichinella spiralis* larvae in the muscle of a dog (bar = 100 μm).

 THERAPEUTICS

- No specific treatment required—for GI tract signs or myalgia.
- Albendazole—shown to significantly reduce muscle larval forms.
- Because of the efficacy of albendazole—fenbendazole is likely to be efficacious with no side effects.

Drugs of Choice

- Fenbendazole (Panacur Granules 22.2% [Intervet, Millsboro, DE]).
- Albendazole (Valbazen suspension 11.36% [Pfizer, Exton, PA]) (*Table 99-1*).

Precautions/Interactions

- Albendazole—has been shown to cause myelosuppression in cats and dogs at these doses.
- If use albendazole—monitor CBC for signs of pancytopenia.

 COMMENTS

- Although not a serious health problem in dogs or cats—may act as a source of infection to other species (pigs) that are eaten by humans.
- Humans could become infected directly—from the feces of infected dogs and cats (in theory).

TABLE 99-1. Drug Therapy for Trichinosis in Dogs and Cats				
Drug	Dose (mg/kg)	Route	Interval (Hours)	Duration (Days)
Fenbendazole (Panacur)	50	PO	24	10
Albendazole (Valbazen)	50ª	PO	12	7

ª May cause myelosuppression at this dose in dogs and cats.

Abbreviations

CBC, complete blood count; GI, gastrointestinal tract; IBD, inflammatory bowel disease.

Suggested Reading

Bowman DD, Frongillo MF, Johnston KB, et al. Signs, larval burdens, and serological responses of dogs experimentally infected with *Trichinella spiralis* Owen, 1835. *Folia Parasitol (Praha)* 1991;38:245–253.

Darrigrand RA, Bowman DD, Frongillo M, et al. Treatment of experimentally induced trichinosis in dogs and cats. *Am J Vet Res* 1993;54:1303–1305.

Author: Stephen C. Barr
Consulting Editor: Stephen C. Barr

chapter 100

Trichomoniasis

DEFINITION/OVERVIEW

- Enteric pear-shaped motile flagellated protozoa similar to *Giardia* organisms that inhabits the large intestine of cats, dogs, and humans.
- One species causes diarrhea in cats.

ETIOLOGY/PATHOPHYSIOLOGY

- *Pentatrichomonas hominis* (family: trichomonads)—inhabits the large intestine of cats, dogs, and humans.
- Nonpathogenic in dogs and cats—except very rarely, when it may become an opportunistic pathogen.
- *Tritrichomonas foetus* (etiologic agent of infertility and abortion in cattle)—causes diarrhea in cats.
- *T. foetus* prevalence in cats—~30% in show cats but very low in feral or indoor cats.
- Pathogenic factors leading to infected cats developing diarrhea—endogenous bacterial flora, adherence of parasite to host epithelium, and cytotoxin and enzyme elaboration.
- Parasites colonize the terminal ileum, cecum, and colon—leads to large bowel diarrhea.

SIGNALMENT/HISTORY

- High population density (catteries, shelters)—may be a risk factor for infection.
- Coinfection with *Giardia* spp.—common.
- Young cats—usually under 1 year (range: 3 months to 13 years).

CLINICAL FEATURES

Cats

- Intermittent large bowel diarrhea.
- Diarrhea occasionally contains blood and mucus.
- Anus may become edematous, erythematous, and painful in very young cats.
- Rectal prolapse if anal irritation becomes severe.
- Diarrhea improves with antibiotic treatment but reoccurs when treatment stops.

DIFFERENTIAL DIAGNOSIS

Cats

- Dietary indiscretion, IBD, neoplasia (especially GI lymphoma), drugs (antibiotics), toxins (lead), parasites (cryptosporidiosis, *Giardia* spp., hookworms, roundworms), infectious agents (FIP, salmonellosis, GI bacterial overgrowth, clostridia), systemic organ dysfunction (renal, hepatic, pancreatic, cardiac), and metabolic (hyperthyroidism).

DIAGNOSTICS

- Direct fecal smear—low sensitivity.
- Method—dilute fresh feces 50:50 in saline, coverslip, examine at 40× objective with condenser lowered to increase contrast.

Diagnostic Feature
- **Distinguish from *Giardia* spp. (concave ventral disc, spiral forward motion)— *T. foetus* has jerky forward motion, is spindle-shaped, and has undulating membranes** (*Fig. 100-1*).
- *T. foetus* trophozoites—are not seen on fecal flotation.
- *T. foetus* trophozoites—will not survive refrigeration.

■ **Fig. 100-1** *Tritrichomonas foetus* tachyzoites in the feces from a kitten. Note the undulating membrane protruding from the posterior of the tachyzoite which partly distinguishes it from *Giardia* spp.

- Fecal protozoal culture—use in-house culture system (In Pouch TF, Biomed Diagnostics, San Jose, CA).
- Method—inoculate with 0.05 g of fresh feces, incubate at room temperature, examine for motile trophozoites daily for 12 days.
- *Giardia* spp. and *P. hominis*—do not grow after 24 hours in In Pouch culture system.
- PCR—more sensitive than fecal culture above but not commercially available.

 THERAPEUTICS

- Essential to rule out coexisting disease (cryptosporidiosis, giardiasis), especially if diarrhea persists after specific treatment.

Drugs of Choice

- *P. hominis*—metronidazole (20 mg/kg, PO, q12h for 7 days).
- *T. foetus*—failed all attempted drug treatment protocols to date.
- Most cats spontaneously resolve their diarrhea—but may take years.

Precautions/Interactions

- Glucocorticoids may exacerbate clinical disease.

 COMMENTS

- Possible zoonotic transmission should be discussed with owner.

Abbreviations

CBC, Complete blood count; FIP, feline infectious peritonitis; GI, gastrointestinal; IBD, inflammatory bowel disease; PCR, polymerase chain reaction.

Suggested Reading

Gookin JL, Breitschwerdt EB, Levy MG, et al. Diarrhea associated with trichomonosis in cats. *J Am Vet Med Assoc* 1999;215:1450–1455.

Gookin JL, Levy MG, Law JM, et al. Experimental infection of cats with *Tritrichomonas foetus*. *Am J Vet Res* 2001;62:1690–1697.

Gookin JL, Birkenheuer AJ, Breitschwerdt EB, et al. Single-tube nested PCR for diagnosis of *Tritrichomonas foetus* in feline feces. *J Clin Microbiol* 2002;40:4126–4130.

Gookin JL, Foster DM, Poore MF, et al. Use of a commercially available culture system for diagnosis of *Tritrichomonas foetus* infection in cats. *J Am Vet Med Assoc* 2003;222:1376–1379.

Levy MG, Gookin JL, Poore M, et al. *Tritrichomonas foetus* and not *Pentatrichomonas hominis* is the etiologic agent of feline trichomonal diarrhea. *J Parasitol* 2003;89:99–104.

Author: Stephen C. Barr
Consulting Editor: Stephen C. Barr

chapter 101

Trichosporonosis

DEFINITION/OVERVIEW

- A systemic or localized fungal infection causing granulomas usually on the nose; also can cause systemic infections in cats.

ETIOLOGY/PATHOPHYSIOLOGY

- *Trichosporon* spp.—yeastlike saprophytic fungi of the family Cryptococcaceae.
- Not considered to be primary pathogens—infect animals that are immunosuppressed, are receiving multiple broad-spectrum antibiotics, or have neoplasia.
- In severely immunosuppressed host—fungus invades mucosal surfaces of the GI, urinary, and respiratory tracts, with subsequent dissemination.
- Cats—infections are characterized by pyogranulomatous inflammation of the mucosa, submucosa, and subcutaneous tissue.

SIGNALMENT/HISTORY

- Usually older cats.
- Although immunosuppression has not been documented in most feline cases, it has been suspected.

CLINICAL FEATURES

- Nasal mass *(Fig. 101-1)*.
- Mass sometimes protrudes from the nostril (similar to that with *Cryptococcus neoformans*).
- Fever.
- Inspiratory stridor.
- Regional lymphadenopathy—uncommon.
- Subcutaneous lesions—secondary to a cat bite (one reported case).
- Chronic cystitis—hematuria and dysuria.

■ **Fig. 101-1** Nasal mass in a cat caused by *Trichosporon* sp.

DIFFERENTIAL DIAGNOSIS

- Other causes of nasal masses:
  - Other fungal infections—*C. neoformans*, *Aspergillus*, and *Penicillium*.
  - Neoplasia.
  - Nasal polyps.

DIAGNOSTICS

Diagnostic Feature
- **Requires—histologic confirmation on biopsied tissue.**
- Culture of mucosal surfaces not adequate—normal microflora of these areas may include *Trichosporon*.
- Culture biopsy material—Sabouraud's or Mycosel agar at 25°C for several days.
- Culture—cream-colored yeastlike colonies with blastoconidia that do not have a capsule when stained with mucin stains (unlike *C. neoformans*).

THERAPEUTICS

- Benzimidazoles—drugs of choice.
- *Trichospora* spp.—demonstrate resistance to amphotericin B.

Drugs of Choice

- Itraconazole (Sporanox [Janssen, Titusville, NJ]).
- Fluconazole (Diflucan [Pfizer, Exton, PA]) (*Table 101-1*).

TABLE 101-1. Drug Therapy for Trichosporonosis in Cats				
Drug	Dose (mg/kg)	Route	Interval (Hours)	Duration (Weeks)
Itraconazole (Soranox)	10	PO	12	4
Fluconazole (Diflucan)	10–25[a]	PO	12	4

[a] Up to a maximum dose of 200 mg/cat/day.

Precautions/Interactions

- Itraconazole—can cause vomiting, diarrhea, inappetence, elevations in hepatic enzymes, peripheral edema, fever, hypertension, and skin rash.
- Monitor ALT—if rises, stop drug for 2 weeks and restart at 50% original dose.
- Fluconazole—can cause similar side effects to itraconazole but less hepatotoxic in cats.

 # COMMENTS

- It is essential to examine the cat for underlying immunosuppressive conditions and direct therapy toward these if found.

Abbreviations

ALT, alanine aminotransferase; GI, gastrointestinal.

Suggested Reading

Doster AR, Erickson ED, Chandler FW. Feline trichosporonosis. *J Am Vet Med Assoc* 1987; 190:1184–1186.

Greene CE, Chandler FW. Trichosporosis. In: CE Greene, ed. *Infectious Diseases of the Dog and Cat.* Philadelphia: WB Saunders; 1998:418–420.

Author: Stephen C. Barr
Consulting Editor: Stephen C. Barr

chapter 102

Tularemia

DEFINITION/OVERVIEW

- An acute systemic bacterial infection of cats (rarely dogs) that can result in septicemia, generalized lymphadenopathy, splenomegaly, hepatomegaly, lingual ulcers, and icterus.

ETIOLOGY/PATHOPHYSIOLOGY

- *Francisella tularensis*—small gram-negative facultative intracellular coccobacilli found mainly in wild rabbits and rodents.
- North America—most cases described from Missouri, Alaska, Oklahoma, Illinois, Utah, Maine, South Dakota, Tennessee, Kansas, and Colorado.
- Peak occurrence—June to August.
- Infection—occurs by ingestion of tissue or body fluids of infected animal or contaminated water or by bite of a blood-sucking insect (ticks, flies, mites, midges, fleas, and mosquitoes).
- Dogs resistant.
- Only a few bacteria needed to infect cats through skin, airways, or conjunctiva.
- Large number of bacteria needed to infect—via GI tract.
- Once inoculated—organisms spread via lymphatics to regional lymph nodes, then blood stream (septicemia), causing acute disease 2 to 7 days after infection.

SIGNALMENT/HISTORY

- Cats mainly; dogs relatively resistant.
- Higher prevalence in outdoor/hunting cats.
- Exposure to infected lagomorphs and rodents.
- Contact with biting insects.

CLINICAL FEATURES

- Serologic surveys—suggest many animals exposed but few develop clinical disease.
- In acute disease:
  - Fever.
  - Anorexia.

- Lethargy.
- Lymphadenopathy (especially cervical and submandibular).
■ Later—hepatomegaly with icterus.
■ Splenomegaly.
■ Multifocal ulcers—sometimes with white pseudomembrane along glossopalantine arches and tongue.

DIFFERENTIAL DIAGNOSIS

■ Any acute systemic disease causing fever, lymphadenopathy, malaise, oral ulceration, and often a fatal outcome, including:
- Lymphoma.
- Bubonic plague (*Yersinia pestis*).
- FIP.
- FeLV.
- FPV.
- Bacterial sepsis.
- Endotoxemia.

DIAGNOSTICS

■ CBC—initially panleukopenia followed by leukocytosis, left shift, toxic neutrophils, and thrombocytopenia as DIC develops.
■ Biochemical panel—elevated bilirubin, ALT.
■ Decreased glucose—late in infection.
■ Coagulation parameters—reflect DIC.
■ Serologic examination—animal may die before antibody titer rises.
■ Gram stain of lesions—difficult to see organism as they are small gram-negative organisms (*Fig. 102-1*).

Diagnostic Features
■ Culture—use blood, pleural fluid, lymph node aspirate into special medium (containing cysteine, usually on chocolate agar), because not recoverable on routine laboratory media.
■ DFA assay—of clinical material and tissues provides the most rapid and accurate assay for infection.

THERAPEUTICS

■ Aggressive treatment for septicemia and DIC—indicated with IV fluids, plasma, and heparin.

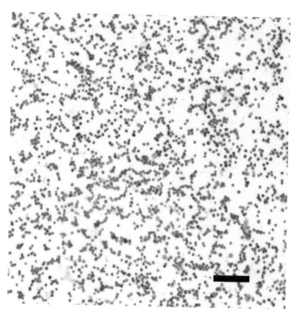

■ **Fig. 102-1** *Francisella tularensis* are very small gram-negative coccobacilli that are difficult to find in lesions because they stain poorly (bar = 10 μm).

Drugs of Choice

■ Little information available on efficacy of antimicrobials, because usually fatal before treatment can begin.
■ Amoxicillin (20 mg/kg, IM or SC, q12h) combined with gentamicin (4.4 mg/kg, IM or SC, q24h) until a clinical response is achieved (*Table 102-1*).
■ Fluoroquinolones may show some efficacy.

Precautions/Interactions

■ The organism is infectious to humans (only 100 organisms inhaled or splashed on a conjunctiva will cause infection).
■ Extreme care must be taken on handling infected animals/tissues; send tissues out for culture, or body out for autopsy; do not perform these in the veterinary clinic.
■ Monitor renal function, mainly by examining urine sediments, while administering gentamicin especially in dehydrated animals.

TABLE 102-1. Drug Therapy for Tularemia in Dogs and Cats				
Drug	Dose (mg/kg)	Route	Interval (Hours)	Duration
Amoxicillin	20	IM, SC	12	a
Gentamicin[b]	4.4	IM, SC	24	a
Enrofloxacin	10–15	PO, IM, IV, SC	12	a

[a] Until a clinical response is achieved.
[b] Give in combination with amoxicillin.

COMMENTS

- Prognosis poor—if not treated very early or if lymph nodes are palpable.
- Most human cases of tularemia—result from tick-borne infections rather than contact with infected rodents or rabbits.
- Some human cases—develop from cat scratches and bites, with initial lesion developing at the site of the injury.
- Human cases acquired from dogs—rarely include injury but have been reported from dogs licking humans (an excellent reason not to let dogs lick the mouths of humans).
- In endemic areas—cats should be neutered to prevent roaming, limit hunting behavior, prevent exposure to contaminated water, and treated for ectoparasites.

IMPORTANT: Zoonosis potential is high—gloves, gowns, face masks should be worn when handling a suspected case, which should be isolated from others in the hospital.

Abbreviations

ALT, alanine aminotransferase; CBC, complete blood count; DFA, direct fluorescent antibody; DIC, disseminated intravascular coagulation; FeLV, feline leukemia virus; FIP, feline infectious peritonitis; FPV, feline panleukopenia virus; GI, gastrointestinal.

Suggested Reading

Feldman KA. Tularemia. *J Am Vet Med Assoc* 2003;222:725–730.

Kaufmann AF. Tularemia. In: Greene CE, ed. *Infectious Disease of the Dog and Cat*. Philadelphia: WB Saunders; 1998:300–302.

Woods JP, Crystal MA, Morton RJ, et al. Tularemia in two cats. *J Am Vet Med Assoc* 1998;212:81–83.

Author: Patrick L. McDonough
Consulting Editor: Stephen C. Barr

chapter 103

Tyzzer's Disease

DEFINITION/OVERVIEW

- Bacterial infection of dogs and cats initially proliferating within the GI tract, then spreading via hepatic portal vein to the liver to cause hepatic colonization with multifocal periportal hepatic necrosis.

ETIOLOGY/PATHOPHYSIOLOGY

- *Clostridium piliformis* (formally *Bacillus piliformis*)—gram-negative obligate intracellular bacterium.
- Organisms—initially proliferate in intestinal epithelial cells before spreading to liver.
- In liver—multifocal hepatic necrosis.
- Sudden death—occurs after a short (24 to 48 hours) illness.
- Occasional spread to other organs—focal myocarditis and enteric lymphadenitis.

SIGNALMENT/HISTORY

- Dogs and cats—any age, although young at higher risk.
- Other risk factors—contact with rodents, immunosuppression.

CLINICAL FEATURES

- Rapid onset.
- Lethargy.
- Depression.
- Anorexia.
- Abdominal discomfort.
- Hepatomegaly.
- Terminally—hypothermia.
- Death within 24 to 48 hours.
- Small amounts of pasty feces—diarrhea infrequent.

DIFFERENTIAL DIAGNOSIS

- Other causes of acute hepatitis:
  - Infectious canine hepatitis.
  - FIP.
  - Toxoplasmosis.
  - Suppurative cholangitis.
  - DIC.
  - RMSF.
  - Acute hemorrhagic necrotizing pancreatitis.
  - Leptospirosis.
  - Idiosyncratic hepatotoxin (drugs and chemicals).

DIAGNOSTICS

- Diagnosis usually made at necropsy—hepatic necrosis with filamentous organisms within cytoplasm of hepatocytes (Fig. 103-1).
- ALT—markedly elevated if taken shortly before death.
- Serologic examination—to identify latent infections in rodent colonies.
- Serology—could be used to investigate illness in dogs and cats.
- Organism isolation—requires mice, embryonating eggs, or cell culture inoculation.

■ **Fig. 103-1** Filamentous organisms of *Clostridium piliformis* (the etiologic agent of Tyzzer's disease) in the cytoplasm of hepatocytes (Giemsa stain; bar = 5 μm).

THERAPEUTICS

- None effective.

Drugs of Choice

- None.

Precautions/Interactions

- None.

COMMENTS

- Avoid contact of cats and dogs with rodents.
- Examine causes of immunosuppression.

Abbreviations

ALT, alanine aminotransferase; DIC, disseminated intravascular coagulation; FIP, feline infectious peritonitis; GI, gastrointestinal tract; RMSF, Rocky Mountain spotted fever.

Suggested Reading

Jones BR, Greene CE. Tyzzer's disease. In: Greene CE, ed. *Infectious Diseases of the Dog and Cat.* Philadelphia: WB Saunders; 1998:242–243.

Author: Kenneth W. Simpson
Consulting Editor: Stephen C. Barr

chapter 104

Urinary Capillariasis
(*Pearsonema*)

DEFINITION/OVERVIEW

- A parasitic infection of the bladder and occasionally the renal pelvis of dogs and cats.

ETIOLOGY/PATHOPHYSIOLOGY

- *Pearsonema* (previously *Capillaria*) *plica* (dogs and cats) and *P. feliscati* (cats)—capillarid parasite that invades the mucosa and submucosa of the urinary bladder, renal pelvis, and ureters (rarely), causing a mild inflammatory response.
- *P. plica*—produces ova with bipolar plugs in urine; after earthworms ingest embryonated ova, the parasite develops into the infective stage.
- Ingestion of infective earthworms—result in a patent infection in dogs.
- PPP = 58 to 88 days.
- *P. feliscati*—life cycle poorly understood.
- Infection of cats—thought to occur by ingestion of eggs or possibly some undetermined paratenic host.

SIGNALMENT/HISTORY

Dogs

- No predilection reported.
- High prevalence (up to 50%) in natural hosts (foxes and raccoons) in southeastern United States may predispose to infection in dogs in this region.
- In kennels—dirt surfaces may predispose to high infection rates.

Cats

- Affected cats >8 months of age.
- In the United States, infection is rare.
- In Australia, prevalence is up to 35%.

CLINICAL FEATURES

- Usually asymptomatic, except in heavy infections.
- Pollakiuria.
- Hematuria.
- Stranguria.
- Dysuria.

DIFFERENTIAL DIAGNOSIS

- Consider—other causes of lower urinary tract disease (calculi, bacterial infection, trauma, and neoplasia).
- Differentiated from other conditions—finding parasite eggs in urine.

DIAGNOSTICS

- CBC, serum biochemical profile—normal.
- Urinalysis—ova with bipolar plugs (60 μm to slightly smaller than those of *Trichuris vulpis*) in urine sediment are diagnostic (*Fig. 104-1*).
- Consider the possibility of fecal contamination of urine with *T. vulpis* (dogs) or other *Capillaria* spp. ova if the urine was free-catch.
- Note also that a false diagnosis of trichuriasis may be made if feces are contaminated with urine containing *P. plica* ova.

THERAPEUTICS

- Infection is usually self-limiting in both cats and dogs.
- Ova are no longer detectable in the urine sediment of infected dogs after 10 to 12 weeks if dogs are isolated from reinfection.

■ **Fig. 104-1** The ova of *Pearsonema plica* from the urine of an infected dog.

TABLE 104-1. Drug Therapy for *Pearsonema plica* Infection in Dogs and Cats				
Drug	Dose (mg/kg)	Route	Interval (Hours)	Duration (Days)
Fenbendazole	50	PO	24	5
Ivermectin (1% injectable)	0.2	SC, PO	Once[a]	—

[a] Repeat in 2 weeks.

- Consider anthelmintic therapy if clinical signs are present.
- Monitor success of therapy by clinical signs and examining urine sediment for ova.

Drugs of Choice

- Fenbendazole—not approved but is effective.
- Ivermectin—1% injectable; has been suggested also but is not approved (*Table 104-1*).

Precautions/Interactions

- If using ivermectin, check for presence of circulating *Dirofilaria* microfilaria before administration to avoid complications.

 COMMENTS

- Prevalence of infection in kennels can be reduced by replacing soil surfaces with sand, gravel, or cement.

Abbreviations

CBC, complete blood count; PPP, prepatent period.

Suggested Reading

Brown SA, Prestwood KA. Parasites of the urinary tract. In: Kirk RW, ed. *Current Veterinary Therapy IX*. Philadelphia: WB Saunders; 1986:1153–1155.

Author: Susan E. Little and Scott A. Brown
Consulting Editor: Stephen C. Barr

chapter 105

Whipworms *(Trichuriasis)*

DEFINITION/OVERVIEW

- A nematode parasite of dogs and cats; adult worms live in the cecum and may cause large bowel diarrhea and pseudohypoadrenocorticism in dogs.
- Asymptomatic in cats.

ETIOLOGY/PATHOPHYSIOLOGY

- *Trichuris vulpi*—dogs.
- *T. campanula* and *T. serrata*—cats.
- *T. vulpis*—widely distributed throughout North America.
- *T. campanula* and *T. serrata*—occur sporadically in North America, Caribbean Islands, and Australia.
- Adult *T. vulpis* worms—embed within the large intestinal and cecal mucosa, causing inflammation.
- Cecal mucosal damage—can be severe enough to result in severe bloody mucoid diarrhea and electrolyte abnormalities similar to Addison's disease.
- Female worms—lay large numbers (about 2,000 per day) of bi-opurculated eggs, which are passed in feces.
- Eggs—extremely resistant to environmental conditions (can remain viable for years).
- Eggs—susceptible to desiccation, extreme temperatures, and ultraviolet radiation.
- Infection—dogs ingesting eggs containing mature L1 larvae.
- Larvae hatch in the small intestine—migrate to large intestine, molt, and become adults.
- *T. vulpis* PPP = 11 weeks.
- *T. campanula* PPP = 9 weeks.

SIGNALMENT/HISTORY

- No sex, breed, or age predilection.
- Pseudohypoadrenocorticism syndrome due to trichuriasis—middle-aged to older dogs.
- Housing—dogs in outside runs, housed on dirt floors, under constant exposure to high build-up of fecal material, and seldom cleaned are predisposed to infection.

CLINICAL FEATURES

Dogs

- Many infections—asymptomatic.
- Large bowel diarrhea—hematochezia; mucus; straining; increased frequency.
- Vomiting—secondary to large bowel inflammation.
- Weakness—from dehydration.
- Metabolic acidosis.
- Electrolyte abnormalities—hyponatremia, hyperkalemia may be present.
- Pseudohypoadrenocorticism syndrome—severe diarrhea caused by the parasite results in isotonic GI fluid loss.
    - When GI fluid loss replaced by water intake—hyponatremia develops.
    - Diarrhea—also leads to dehydration and bicarbonate loss, resulting in metabolic acidosis.
    - Metabolic acidosis—causes the translocation of potassium from the intracellular to extracellular fluid, resulting in hyperkalemia.
    - If hyponatremia and hyperkalemia severe enough—Na:K ratio falls below 27, resembling Addison's disease.

Cats

- Asymptomatic.

DIFFERENTIAL DIAGNOSIS

Dogs

- Other causes of large bowel diarrhea, including idiopathic chronic IBD, immune-mediated eosinophilic colitis, histiocytic colitis, parasites (giardiasis, trichomoniasis, amebiasis, balantidiasis, leishmaniasis), fungal (histoplasmosis, prototheca), bacterial, irritable bowel syndrome, ileocolic and cecocolic intussusception, and neoplasia.
- Other causes of reduced Na:K ratio, including hypoadrenocorticism (Addison's disease), renal failure, chylothorax, other GI tract disorders (salmonellosis, perforated duodenal ulcer), pregnancy with diarrhea, and peritoneal effusions.

DIAGNOSTICS

- CBC and serum biochemical profile—no abnormalities if diarrhea is not severe.
- If diarrhea is severe (resulting in pseudohypoadrenocorticism)—hyponatremia, hyperkalemia with a reduced Na:K ratio (<27), normal ACTH response test.
- Fecal flotation; trichurid eggs (*Fig. 105-1*).
- Endoscopy—may view adult parasites in the colonic mucosa (should a clinician be unfortunate enough to miss a diagnosis by fecal flotation or by treatment trial).

■ **Fig. 105-1** *Trichuris vulpis* egg in dog feces. Note the prominent bipolar plugs, brown color, single cell (zygote) within the egg shell membrane, and size, ~90 × 45 μ.

 THERAPEUTICS

- A dog with severe diarrhea, dehydration, metabolic acidosis, and a reduced Na:K ratio—IV isotonic fluid support (initially isotonic saline).
- Perform ACTH response test—to rule out Addison's disease.
- Dogs with trichuriasis-induced pseudohypoadrenocorticism—will not be harmed by treatment with physiologic mineralcorticoid or glucocorticoid supplementation.

Drugs of Choice

- Fenbendazole (Panacur Granules 22.2% [Intervet, Millsboro, DE]).
- Praziquantel/pyrantel/febantel (Drontal Plus [Bayer, Shawnee Mission, KS]).
- Diethylcarbamazine/oxibendazole (Filaribits Plus [Pfizer, Exton, PA]).
- Milbemycin (Interceptor [Novartis, Greensboro, NC]) *(Table 105-1)*.

TABLE 105-1. **Drug Therapy for Whipworms (Trichuriasis) in Dogs**				
Drug	Dose (mg/kg)	Route	Interval (Hours)	Duration (Days)
Fenbendazole (Panacur)	50	PO	24	3[a]
Praziquantel/pyrantel/febantel (Drontal Plus)	[b]	PO	24	3[a]
Diethylcarbamazine/oxibendazole (Filaribits Plus)	[c]	PO	Daily[d]	—
Milbemycin (Interceptor)	0.5	PO	Monthly[e]	—

[a] Retreat in 3 to 4 weeks time.
[b] Praziquantel (5 to 12), pyrantel (5 to 12), and febantel (25 to 65).
[c] Diethylcarbamazine (6.6), and oxibendazole (5).
[d] Given as daily heartworm preventive.
[e] Given as monthly heartworm preventive.

Precautions/Interactions

- Fenbendazole—can be used in pregnant animals, but praziquantel/pyrantel/febantel should not be.
- Diethylcarbamazine/oxibendazole—has been associated with hepatic injury (sometimes fatal) in dogs and should not be used when there is evidence of concurrent hepatic injury.

 COMMENTS

- Dogs living in chronically infected environment—initially treat with fenbendazole; then place the dog on monthly milbemycin.
- Cats—have been successfully treated with fenbendazole.

Abbreviations

ACTH, adrenocorticotropic hormone; CBC, complete blood count; GI, gastrointestinal; IBD, inflammatory bowel disease; PPP, prepatent period.

Suggested Reading

Bowman DD, ed. *Georgi's Parasitology for Veterinarians*, 8th ed. Philadelphia: WB Saunders; 2003: 228–229.
DiBartola SP, Johnson SE, Davenport DJ, et al. Clinicopathologic findings resembling hypoadrenocorticism in dogs with primary gastrointestinal disease. *J Am Vet Med Assoc* 1985;187:60–63.

Author: Stephen C. Barr
Consulting Editor: Stephen C. Barr

Vaccination Schedule

NOTE: Tailor vaccination schedule for each individual animal based on:

1. Age of presentation for the animal's first vaccination.
2. Risk of exposure to diseases.
3. Risk of developing disease if exposed.
4. Likelihood of the owner complying with instructions for revaccination (booster yearly versus every 3 years).
5. Risk of complications developing as a consequence of vaccination (adjuvanted versus nonadjuvanted recombinant vaccines).
6. Modified live vaccine not recommended for pregnant or immunocompromised animals.

FELINE

| Vaccine Antigen | Age of Initial Vaccination[a] | | Booster Interval |
	6 to 12 Weeks	>12 Weeks	
FVRCP[b]	Every 3 weeks until >12 weeks	1 dose	1 year later, then every 3 years
FeLV[c]	2 doses 3 to 4 weeks apart >9 weeks	2 doses 3 to 4 weeks	1 year later, then annually
Rabies[d]		1 dose	1 year later, then annually or every 3 years[d]

[a] Vaccination of kittens 4 to 6 weeks of age may be indicated in high-risk environments (catteries, shelters); FVRC recommended in kittens >2 weeks (IN) or >4 weeks (MLV parenteral) if enzootic viral respiratory infections are present.

[b] FVRC: MLV and inactivated for SC administration, and MLV and IN products are available; IN provides more rapid (protection within 48 hours) protection than parenteral dosing but has a high incidence of mild contagious respiratory illness. P: MLV and inactivated for SC administration available; maternal antibody may last to 12 weeks; give last vaccine in initial series at or after 12 weeks of age; if MLV vaccine is used, only one vaccine needed if given after 12 weeks of age until first year booster; booster at 1 year of age, then every 3 years; use inactivated vaccine in the pregnant or immunocompromised.

[c] Recommended for cats at risk (cats that are outdoor, indoor/outdoor, stray/feral, open multicat households, FeLV-positive households, households of unknown FeLV status). All (except Merial's Purevax recombinant leukemia vaccine) products contain inactivated noninfectious viral antigens with an adjuvant, and are given SC distally on the hind limb due to possibility of producing a vaccine-induced sarcoma; Purevax is adjuvant-free in a canarypox vector (reducing risk of tumor formation) and administered in a small volume (0.25 ml) using a transdermal (Vetjet) vaccination system; pretest before considering vaccination (if positive on an ELISA, retest in 4 to 8 weeks; if negative, start vaccine series).

[d] Inactivated adjuvanted products and one nonadjuvanted recombinant product (Merial) available; adjuvanted products require booster every 3 years; nonadjuvanted recombinant product requires yearly booster (follow manufactures and local law specifications).

ELISA, enzyme-linked immunosorbent assay; FeLV, feline leukemia virus; FVRCP, feline viral rhinotracheitis/calici virus; IN, intranasal; MLV, modified live virus; P, panleukopenia; SC, subcutaneous.

CANINE

| Vaccine Antigen | Age of Initial Vaccination[a] | | Booster Interval |
	6 to 12 Weeks	12 to 18 Weeks	
M/DA2Pi[b]	Every 3 weeks until 12 weeks	2 doses 3 to 4 weeks apart	1 year later, then every 3 years[c]
p[d]	2 doses, 3 to 4 weeks apart until 18 weeks	3 doses 3 to 4 weeks apart	1 year later, then every 3 years[e]
Rabies[f]		1 dose	1 year later, then annually or triennially

[a] Vaccination of puppies 4 to 6 weeks of age may be indicated in high-risk environments (shelters).

[b] M: can be given up to 12 weeks of age, but should be reserved for 6-week-old pups as first vaccine, 3 weeks later by D. D: MLV vaccines and one recombinant in a canary virus vector available; risk of postvaccinal disease for MLV but not for recombinant vaccine; yearly boosters required with recombinant product and every 3 years with MLV. A2: use A-2 MLV vaccines to avoid blue eye (anterior uveitis) seen with A-1 products. Pi: MLV and inactivated for SC administration, and MLV and IN products are available; IN provides more rapid (protection within 48 hours) protection than parenteral dosing but has a high incidence of mild contagious respiratory illness.

[c] Can check titers and booster if titer to D <1:32, Pi <1:16, A2 <1:16.

[d] P: killed, MLV, and potentiated MLV vaccines available; use MLV or potentiated in most pups (killed in pregnant animals, immunosuppressed pups, or pups under 5 weeks of age); can begin MLV at 6 weeks, booster every 3 weeks until 16 to 18 weeks of age; dogs vaccinated with MLV will excrete virus in feces for up to 2 weeks postvaccination.

[e] Can check titer and booster if titer to P <1:80.

[f] Inactivated adjuvanted products available for IM and/or SC administration; require booster 1 year after the first dose at 12 weeks, then annually or triennially (follow manufacturer's and local law specifications).

A, adenovirus type 1 (hepatitis) or type 2 (respiratory); D, distemper; IM, intramuscular; IN, intranasal; M, measles; MLV, modified live virus; P, parvovirus; Pi, parainfluenzap; SC, subcutaneous.

Products for Treatment of Canine Intestinal Parasites

APPENDIX B. Products for Treatment of Canine Intestinal Parasites

Trade Name®	Active Ingredient(s) and Dosage	Toxocara canis	Toxascaris leonina	Ancylostoma caninum	Ancylostoma braziliense	Uncinaria stenocephala	Trichuris vulpis	Taenia pisiformis	Dipylidium caninum	Echinococcus granulosus	Echinococcus multilocularis
Sergeant's Vetscription Worm-Away for Dogs	Piperazine (62 to 300 mg/kg)	+	+								
Nemex-2 Suspension	Pyrantel pamoate (5 mg/kg >2.25 kg; 10 mg/kg <2.25 kg)	+	+	+		+					
Panacur Granules 22.2%	Fenbendazole (50 mg/kg × 3 days)	+	+	+		+	+	+			
Cestex	Epsiprantel (2.75 mg/kg cats and 5.5 mg/kg for dogs)							+	+		
Droncit	Praziquantel (2.5 to 7.5 mg/kg)							+	+	+	+
Drontal Plus	Praziquantel/pyrantel/febantel (5–7 mg, 5–7 mg, 25–35 mg/kg)	+	+	+		+	+	+	+	+	+

Parasiticides for Cats

APPENDIX C. Parasiticides for Cats

Trade Name®	Active Ingredient(s) and Dosage	Age at First Administration	Toxocara cati	Toxascaris leonina	Ancylostoma tubaeformis	Dirofilaria immitis (prevention)	Taenia taeniaeformis	Dipylidium caninum	Cteno-cephalides felis	Ticks	Otodectes cynotis
D-Worm Liquid Wormer for Cats and Dogs (sample of several OTC products)	Piperazine (45 to 65 mg/kg)	No age restriction	+	+							
Cestex	Epsiprantel (2.8 mg/kg)	7 weeks					+	+			
Droncit Feline Cestocide Tablets	Praziquantel (2.5 to 7.5 mg/kg)	6 weeks					+	+			
Tape Worm Tabs for Cats and Kittens	Praziquantel (2.5 to 7.5 mg/kg)	6 weeks					+	+			
Droncit Injectable Cestocide for Dogs and Cats	Praziquantel (5 to 7 mg/kg)	6 weeks					+	+			
Drontal	Praziquantel/pyrantel (5 mg + 20 mg, resp./kg)	4 weeks >1.5 lb	+	+	+		+	+			

Product	Drug (dose)	Minimum age					
Program Suspension	Lufenuron (30 mg/kg) monthly	6 weeks				+	
Program Flavor Tabs	Lufenuron (30 mg/kg) monthly	6 weeks				+	
Program 6 Month Injectable for Cats	Lufenuron (10 mg/kg) every 6 months	6 weeks				+	
Capstar	Nitenpyram (1 mg/kg) daily as needed	4 weeks, >2 lb				+	
Heartgard Chewables for Cats	Ivermectin (0.024 mg/kg) monthly	6 weeks		+	+		
Interceptor Flavor Tabs	Milbemycin oxime (2 mg/kg) monthly	8 weeks	+	+	+		
Revolution	Selamectin (6 mg/kg) monthly	8 weeks	+	+	+	+	+
Acarexx	0.5 ml of 0.01% ivermectin per ear	4 weeks					+

(continues)

APPENDIX C. Parasiticides for Cats (continued)

Trade Name®	Active Ingredient(s) and Dosage	Age at First Administration	Toxocara cati	Toxascaris leonina	Ancylostoma tubaeformis	Dirofilaria immitis (prevention)	Taenia taeinaeformis	Dipylidium caninum	Cteno-cephalides felis	Ticks	Otodectes cynotis
MilbeMite Otic Solution	0.25 ml of 0.1% milbemycin oxime per ear	4 weeks									+
Frontline Plus	Fipronil and (S)-methoprene	8 weeks							+	+	
Advantage	Imidacloprid	8 weeks							+		

Canine Heartworm Preventatives

APPENDIX D. Canine Heartworm Preventatives

Trade Name®	Active Ingredient(s) and Dosage	Application	Earliest Administration as per Label	Toxocara canis	Toxascaris leonina	Ancylostoma caninum	Ancylostoma braziliense	Uncinaria stenocephala	Trichuris vulpis
Filaribits	Diethylcarmazine (6.6 mg/kg daily)	Oral/daily	8 weeks						
Heartgard Tablets for dogs	Ivermectin (0.006 mg/kg)	Oral/monthly	6 weeks						
Heartgard Chewables for dogs	Ivermectin (0.006 mg/kg)	Oral/monthly	6 weeks						
Heartgard Plus Chewables for dogs	Ivermectin + pyrantel (0.006 + 5 mg/kg, respectively)	Oral/monthly	6 weeks	T	T	T	T	T	
Iverhard Plus Flavored Chewables	Generic form of Heartgard Plus Chewables for dogs	Oral/monthly	6 weeks	T	T	T	T	T	
Interceptor Flavor Tabs	Milbemycin (0.5 mg/kg)	Oral/monthly >2 lb	4 weeks or	T	T	C			T
Revolution	Selamectin (6 mg/kg)	Topical/monthly	6 weeks						
Sentinel Flavor Tabs	Milbemycin + Lufenuron (0.5 mg + 10 mg/kg, respectively)	Oral/monthly >2 lb	4 weeks or	T	T	C			T

T, treatment or removal—removes >90% of worms from dogs at the time of dosing.
C, control—removes >90% of existing worms from dogs after two to several treatments.

Canine Products with Efficacies Against Arthropods

APPENDIX E. Canine Products with Efficacies Against Arthropods

Trade Name®	Active Ingredient(s) and Dosage	FDA or EPA Registered	Application	Age at First Administration	Adult Fleas	Flea Eggs or Larvae	Ticks	Sarcoptes	Otodectes	Mosquitoes
Sentinel Flavor Tabs	Milbemycin/Lufenuron (0.5 mg + 10 mg/kg, respectively)	FDA	Oral/daily	>2 lb	+					
Program Flavor Tabs	Lufenuron (10 mg/kg)	FDA	Oral/monthly	6 weeks		+				
Revolution	Selamectin (6 mg/kg)	FDA	Oral/monthly	6 weeks	+	+	+	+	+	
Capstar	Nitempyram (1 mg/kg)	FDA as needed	Oral/daily and >2 lb	4 weeks	+	+				
Frontline Top Spot for dogs and puppies	Fipronil	EPA	Topical/monthly	10 weeks	+					
Frontline Spray Treatment for cats and dogs	Fipronil	EPA	Topical/monthly	8 weeks	+					
Frontline Plus for dogs and puppies	Fipronil and (S)-methoprene	EPA	Topical/monthly	8 weeks	+	+	+			

Advantage	Imidacloprid	EPA monthly	Topical/	7 weeks	+		
K9 Advantix	Imidacloprid and permethrin	EPA	Topical/ monthly	7 weeks	+	+	+
Acarexx	IvermectinFDA	Topical to ear	4 weeks		+	+	
MilbeMite Otic Solution	Milbemycin oxime	FDA to ear	Topical	4 weeks		+	

EPA, Environmental Protection Agency; FDA, Food and Drug Administration.

Drug Formulary

APPENDIX F. Drug Formulary

Drug Name (Trade or Other Names)	Pharmacology and Indications	Adverse Effects and Precautions	Dosing Information and Comments	Formulations	Dosage
Acemannan	Immunostimulant. A polysaccharide acetylated mannan extract from aloe. Proposed to stimulate T-cell activity in animals. It has been used to treat tumors in dogs and cats. It may stimulate tumor necrosis factor (TNF) and other cytokine release.	No reported side effects.	After reconstitution, shake well to dissolve. Use within 4 hr after preparation. Beneficial effect is controversial. There has been a lack of demonstrated effect on lymphocyte blastogenic response in cats.	10-mg vials reconstituted to 1 mg/ml.	Intraperitoneal (1 mg/kg) and intralesional injection (2 mg) every week for 6 treatments.
Albendazole (Valbazen)	Benzimidazole antiparasitic drug. Inhibits glucose uptake in parasites.	At approved doses, there is a wide margin of safety. Adverse effects can include anorexia, lethargy, and bone marrow toxicity. At high doses, has been associated with bone marrow toxicity (*J Am Vet Med Assoc* 213: 44–46, 1998). Adverse effects are possible when administered for longer than 5 days.	Used primarily as antihelmintic, but also has demonstrated efficacy for giardiasis.	113.6 mg/ml suspension and 300 mg/ml paste.	25–50 mg/kg q12h PO × 3 days. For giardia, use 25 mg/kg q12h × 2 days.
Allopurinol (Lopurin, Zyloprim)	Decreases production of uric acid by inhibiting enzymes responsible for uric acid.	May cause skin reactions (hypersensitivity).	Used in humans primarily for treating gout. In animals, used to decrease formation of uric acid uroliths.	100, 300 mg tablets	10 mg/kg q8h, then reduce to 10 mg/kg q24h, PO. For leishmaniasis, use 10 mg/kg q12h PO for at least 4 months.

Drug	Description	Adverse Effects/Cautions	Instructions for Use	Formulations	Dosage
Amikacin (Amiglyde-V [veterinary] and Amikin [human])	Aminoglycoside antibacterial drug (inhibits protein synthesis). Mechanism is similar to that of other aminoglycosides (see Gentamicin sulfate), but may be more active than gentamicin.	May cause nephrotoxicosis with high doses or prolonged therapy. May also cause ototoxicity and vestibulotoxicity. (See Gentamicin sulfate.)	Once-daily doses are designed to maximize peak minimum inhibitory concentration (MIC) ratio. Consider therapeutic drug monitoring for chronic therapy. (See also Gentamicin sulfate.)	50, 250 mg/ml injection	Dog and cat: 6.5 mg/kg q8h IV, IM, SC. Dog: 15–30 mg/kg q24h IV, IM, SC. Cat: 10–14 mg/kg q24h IV, IM, SC.
Amitraz (Mitaban)	Antiparasitic drug for ectoparasites. Used for treatment of mites, including *Demodex*. Inhibits monoamine oxidase in mites.	Causes sedation in dogs (α_2-agonist), which may be reversed by yohimbine or atipamezole. When high doses are used, other side effects reported include pruritus, polyuria and polydipsia (PU/PD), bradycardia, hypothermia, hyperglycemia, and (rarely) seizures.	Manufacturer's dose should be used initially. But, for refractory cases, this dose has been exceeded to produce increased efficacy. Doses that have been used include: 0.025, 0.05, and 0.1% concentration applied 2× week and 0.125% solution applied to half of body every day for 4 weeks to 5 months.	10.6 ml concentrated dip (19.9%).	10.6 ml per 7.5 L water (0.025% solution). Apply 3 to 6 topical treatments q14d. For refractory cases, this dose has been exceeded to produce increased efficacy. Doses that have been used include: 0.025, 0.05, and 0.1% concentration applied 2× week and 0.125% solution applied to half of body every day for 4 weeks to 5 months.
Amoxicillin (Amoxi-Tabs, Biomox, and other brands. [Omnipen, Principen, Totacillin are human forms])	β-Lactam antibiotic. Inhibits bacterial cell wall synthesis. Generally broad-spectrum activity. Used for a variety of infections in all species.	Usually well tolerated. Allergic reactions are possible. Diarrhea is common with oral doses.	Dose recommendations vary depending on the susceptibility of bacteria and location of infection. Generally, more frequent or higher doses needed for gram-negative infections.	50, 100, 150, 200, 400 mg tablets. 250 and 500 mg capsules (human forms).	6.6–20 mg/kg q8–12h PO

(continues)

APPENDIX F. Drug Formulary (continued)

Drug Name (Trade or Other Names)	Pharmacology and Indications	Adverse Effects and Precautions	Dosing Information and Comments	Formulations	Dosage
Amoxicillin trihydrate (Amoxi-Tabs, Amoxi-Drops, Amoxil, and others)	β-Lactam antibiotic. Inhibits bacterial cell wall synthesis. Generally broad-spectrum activity, but resistance is common.	Use cautiously in animals allergic to penicillin-like drugs.	Dose requirements vary depending on susceptibility of bacteria.	50, 100, 200, 400 mg tablets. 50 mg/ml oral suspension.	6–20 mg/kg q8–12h PO.
Amoxicillin + clavulanate potassium (Clavamox)	β-Lactam antibiotic + β-lactamase inhibitor (clavulanate/clavuanic acid).	Same as for amoxicillin.	Same as for amoxicillin.	62.5, 125, 250, 375 mg tablets and 62.5 mg/ml suspension.	Dog: 12.5–25 mg/kg q12h PO. Cat: 62.5 mg/cat q12h PO. Consider administering these doses q8h for gram-negative infections.
Amphotericin B (Fungizone)	Antifungal drug. Fungicidal for systemic fungi, by damaging fungal membranes.	Produces a dose-related nephrotoxicosis. Also produces fever, phlebitis, and tremors.	Administer IV via slow infusion diluted in fluids, and monitor renal function closely. When preparing IV solution, do not mix with electrolyte solutions (use D_5W, for example); administer NaCl fluid loading before therapy. (One study administered this drug subcutaneously: Aust Vet J 73:124, 1996.)	50 mg injectable vial.	0.5 mg/kg IV (slow infusion) q48h to a cumulative dose of 4–8 mg/kg.

Drug	Mechanism/Indications	Precautions	Comments	How Supplied	Dosage
Amphotericin B, liposomal formulation (ABLC, Abelcet)	Same indications as for conventional amphotericin B. Liposomal formulations may be used at higher doses, and safety margin is increased. Expense is much higher than for conventional formulations.	Renal toxicity is the most dose-limiting effect.	Higher doses can be used compared to conventional formulation of amphotericin B. Dilute in 5% dextrose in water to 1 mg/ml and administer IV over 1–2 hr.	100 mg/20 ml in lipid formulation.	Dog: 2–3 mg/kg IV 3 x/week for 9–12 treatments to a cumulative dose of 24–27 mg/kg. Cat: 1 mg/kg IV 3 x/week for 12 treatments.
Ampicillin (Omnipen, Principen, others [human forms])	β-Lactam antibiotic. Inhibits bacterial cell wall synthesis.	Use cautiously in animals allergic to penicillin-like drugs.	Dose requirements vary depending on susceptibility of bacteria. Absorbed approximately 50% less, compared with amoxicillin, when administered orally. Generally, more frequent or higher doses needed for gram-negative infections.	250, 500 mg capsules; 125, 250, 500 mg vials of ampicillin sodium. Ampicillin trihydrate: 10 and 25 g vials for injection.	Ampicillin sodium: 10–20 mg/kg q6–8h IV, IM, SC or 20–40 mg/kg q8h PO. Ampicillin trihydrate: Dog: 10–50 mg/kg q12–24h IM, SC. Cat: 10–20 mg/kg q12–24h IM, SC. Dogs and cats: doses as high as 100 mg/kg have been used for some resistant infections, such as those caused by enterococci.
Ampicillin + sulbactam (Unasyn)	Ampicillin plus a β-lactamase inhibitor (sulbactam). Sulbactam has similar activity as clavulanate.	Same as for ampicillin.	Same as for amoxicillin + clavulanate.	2:1 combination for injection. 1.5 and 3 g vials.	10–20 mg/kg IV, IM q8h.
Ampicillin trihydrate (Polyflex)	β-Lactam antibiotic. Inhibits bacterial cell wall synthesis.	Use cautiously in animals allergic to penicillin-like drugs.	Absorption is slow and may not be sufficient for acute serious infection.	10, 25 mg vials for injection	Dog: 10–50 mg/kg q12–24h IM, SC. Cat: 10–20 mg/kg q12–24h IM, SC.

(continues)

APPENDIX F. Drug Formulary (continued)

Drug Name (Trade or Other Names)	Pharmacology and Indications	Adverse Effects and Precautions	Dosing Information and Comments	Formulations	Dosage
Amprolium (Amprol, Corid)	Antiprotozoal drug. Antagonizes thiamine in parasites. Used for treatment of coccidiosis, especially in puppies.	Toxicity observed only at high doses (CNS signs due to thiamine deficiency). Eye irritation—flush with water.	Usually administered as feed additive to livestock. For dogs, 30 ml 9.6% amprolium has been added to 3.8 L of drinking water for control of coccidiosis.	9.6% (9.6 g/100 ml) oral solution; 20% soluble powder.	1.25 g of 20% amprolium powder to daily feed, or 30 ml of 9.6% amprolium solution to 3.8 L of drinking water for 7 days.
Azithromycin (Zithromax)	Azalide antibiotic. Similar mechanism of action as macrolides (erythromycin), which is to inhibit bacteria protein synthesis via inhibition of ribosome. Spectrum is primarily gram-positive.	Has not been in common use in veterinary medicine to establish adverse effects. Vomiting is likely with high doses. Diarrhea may occur in some patients.	Azithromycin may be better tolerated than erythromycin. Primary difference from other antibiotics is the high intracellular concentrations achieved.	250 mg capsules, 250 and 600 mg tablets, 100 or 200 mg/5 ml oral suspension, and 500 mg vials for injection.	Dog: 10 mg/kg PO once every 5 days or 3.3 mg/kg q24h for 3 days. Cat: 5 mg/kg PO q48h.
AZT (Azidothymidine)	See Zidovudine.				
Bactrim (sulfamethoxazole + trimethoprim) (See Trimethoprim-sulfonamide combinations.)					

Drug	Action	Precautions	Comments	Supply	Dosage
Benznidazole (Ragonil)	Antiprotozoal drug with activity against *Trypanosoma cruzi*. Thought to inhibit protein and RNA synthesis in the parasite.	Vomiting is the main side effect. May cause hepatic and renal toxicity; monitor organ function while treating.	Available in United States only from the CDC. Best efficacy in acute cases; little effect on outcome of chronic disease.	100 mg tablet	5–10 mg/kg q24h PO for 2 months.
Carbenicillin (Geopen, Pyopen)	β-Lactam antibiotic. Inhibits bacterial cell wall synthesis. Active against *Pseudomonas* and other gram-negative bacteria.	Use cautiously in patients sensitive to penicillins (e.g., allergy).	Carbenicillin injection often is administered with an aminoglycoside. Do not mix with aminoglycosides before administration, or inactivation will result.	1, 2, 5, 10, and 30 g vials for injection.	40–50 mg/kg and up to 100 mg/kg q6–8h IV, IM, SC.
Carbenicillin indanyl sodium (Geocillin)	Same as for carbenicillin. Primary use is for treating infections of lower urinary tract.	Same as for carbenicillin.	Oral formulation of carbenicillin, but attains concentrations that are only sufficient for treating urinary tract infections. Do not use for systemic infections.	500 mg tablets.	10 mg/kg q8h PO.
Cefaclor (Ceclor)	Cephalosporin antibiotic. Action is similar to that of other β-lactam antibiotics, inhibiting synthesis of bacterial cell wall, leading to cell death. Cephalosporins are divided into 1st, 2nd, or 3rd generation, depending on spectrum of activity. Consult package insert or specific reference for spectrum of activity of individual cephalosporin. Cefaclor is a 2nd-generation cephalosporin.	All cephalosporins are generally safe; however, sensitivity can occur in individuals (allergy). Rare bleeding disorders have been known to occur with some cephalosporins.	Used primarily when resistance has been demonstrated to 1st-generation cephalosporins.	250, 500 capsules and 25 mg/ml oral suspension.	15 mg/kg q8h PO.

(continues)

APPENDIX F. Drug Formulary (continued)

Drug Name (Trade or Other Names)	Pharmacology and Indications	Adverse Effects and Precautions	Dosing Information and Comments	Formulations	Dosage
Cefadroxil (Cefa-Tabs, Cefa-Drops)	See Cefaclor. Cefadroxil is a 1st-generation cephalosporin.	See Cefaclor. Cefadroxil has been known to cause vomiting after oral administration in dogs.	Spectrum of cefadroxil is similar to that of other 1st-generation cephalosporins. For susceptibility test, use cephalothin as test drug.	50 mg/ml oral suspension; 50, 100, 200, 1000 mg tablet.	Dog: 22 mg/kg q12h, up to 30 mg/kg q12h PO. Cat: 22 mg/kg q24h PO.
Cefazolin sodium (Ancef, Kefzol, and generic)	See Cefadroxil. Cefazolin is a 1st-generation cephalosporin.	See Cefaclor. For cefazolin, use cephalothin to test susceptibility.	Commonly used 1st-generation cephalosporin as injectable drug for prophylaxis for surgery, as well as for acute therapy for serious infections.	50 and 100 mg/50 ml for injection	20–35 mg/kg q8h IV, IM. For perisurgical use: 22 mg/kg q2h during surgery.
Cefdinir (Omnicef)	Oral 3rd-generation cephalosporin. Activity includes staphylococci and many gram-negative bacilli. Other characteristics are similar to those of other drugs in this class.	Similar to those of other oral cephalosporins.	Use in veterinary medicine has not been reported. Use and doses are extrapolated from human medicine.	300 mg capsules, 25 mg/ml oral suspension	Dose not established. Human dose is 7 mg/kg q12h PO.
Cefixime (Suprax)	See Cefaclor. Cefixime is a 3rd-generation cephalosporin.	See Cefaclor.	Although not approved for veterinary use, pharmacokinetic studies in dogs have provided recommended dosages.	20 mg/ml oral suspension and 200 and 400 mg tablets	10 mg/kg q12h PO. For cystitis: 5 mg/kg q12–24h PO.

Drug		Description	Formulation	Dosage
Cefotaxime sodium (Claforan)	See Cefaclor.	See Cefaclor. Cefotaxime is a 3rd-generation cephalosporin. Cefotaxime is used when resistance to other antibiotics is encountered or when infection is in CNS.	3rd-generation cephalosporin used when resistance encountered to 1st- and 2nd-generation cephalosporins.	500 mg; 1, 2, and 10 g vials for injection.	Dog: 50 mg/kg IV, IM, SC q12h. Cat: 20–80 mg/kg q6h IV, IM.
Cefotetan disodium (Cefotan)	See Cefaclor.	See Cefaclor. Cefotetan is a 2nd-generation cephalosporin.	2nd-generation cephalosporin similar to cefoxitin, but may have longer half-life in dogs	1, 2, and 10 g vials for injection.	30 mg/kg q8h IV, SC.
Cefoxitin sodium (Mefoxin)	See Cefaclor.	See Cefaclor. Cefoxitin is a 2nd-generation cephalosporin. May have increased activity against anaerobic bacteria.	2nd-generation cephalosporin, which is often used when activity against anaerobic bacteria is desired.	1, 2, and 10 g vials for injection	30 mg/kg q6–8h IV
Cefpodoxime proxetil (Vantin)	No adverse effects reported for animals, but be aware of possibility of reactions seen with other oral cephalosporins (e.g., vomiting, diarrhea, allergy).	Oral 3rd-generation cephalosporin. Activity includes gram-negative bacilli resistant to 1st-generation cephalosporins. Activity also includes staphylococcus.	Use for infections (e.g., UTI) resistant to other oral drugs.	100, 200 mg tablets; 10 or 20 mg/ml oral suspension.	Systemic infections: 10 mg/kg q8h PO. Urinary tract infections: 10 mg/kg q12h PO.
Ceftazidime (Fortaz, Ceptaz, Tazicef)	See Cefaclor.	3rd-generation cephalosporin. Ceftazidime has more activity than other cephalosporins against *Pseudomonas aeruginosa*.	3rd-generation cephalosporin. May be reconstituted with 1% lidocaine for IM injection.	Vials (0.5, 1, 2, 6 g) reconstituted to 280 mg/ml.	Dog and cat: 30 mg/kg q6h IV, IM. Dog: 30 mg/kg q4–6h SC.

(continues)

APPENDIX F. Drug Formulary (continued)

Drug Name (Trade or Other Names)	Pharmacology and Indications	Adverse Effects and Precautions	Dosing Information and Comments	Formulations	Dosage
Ceftiofur (Naxcel [ceftiofur sodium]; Excenel [ceftiofur HCl]).	See Cefaclor. Ceftiofur is a unique cephalosporin that does not fit into a distinct class; however, its spectrum resembles that of many of the 3rd-generation cephalosporins.	See Cefaclor. Ceftiofur is primarily used only for urinary tract infections.	Available as powder for reconstitution before injection. After reconstitution, stable for 7 days when refrigerated or 12 hr at room temperature, or frozen for 8 weeks. Excenel is not approved for use in dogs.	50 mg/ml injection.	2.2–4.4 mg/kg SC q24h (for urinary tract infections).
Cephalexin (Keflex and generic forms)	See Cefaclor. Cephalexin is a 1st-generation cephalosporin.	See Cefaclor. For cephalexin, use cephalothin to test susceptibility.	Although not approved for veterinary use, trials in dogs with pyoderma show similar efficacy.	250, 500 mg capsules; 250, 500 mg tablets; 100 mg/ml or 125, 250 mg/5 ml oral suspension.	10–30 mg/kg q6–12h PO; for pyoderma, 22–35 mg/kg q12h PO.
Cephalothin sodium (Keflin)	See Cefaclor.	See Cefaclor.	1st-generation cephalosporin. Used as test drug for susceptibility tests of other 1st-generation cephalosporins.	1 and 2 g vials for injection	10–30 mg/kg q4–8h IV, IM
Cephapirin (Cefadyl)	See Cefaclor. Cephapirin is a 1st-generation cephalosporin.	See Cefaclor.		500 mg, 1, 2, 4 g vials for injection.	10–30 mg/kg q4–8h IV, IM.
Cephradine (Velosef)	See Cefaclor. Cephradine is a 1st-generation cephalosporin.	See Cefaclor.		250, 500 mg capsules, and 250, 500 mg, 1 and 2 g vials for injection.	10–25 mg/kg q6–8h PO.

Drug	Description	Precautions	Notes	How Supplied	Dosage
Chloramphenicol and chloramphenicol palmitate (Chloromycetin, generic forms)	Antibacterial drug. Mechanism of action is via inhibition of protein synthesis via binding to ribosome. Broad spectrum of activity. Florfenicol acts via similar mechanism and has been substituted in some animals. (See Florfenicol.)	Bone marrow suppression is possible with high doses or prolonged treatment (especially in cats). Avoid use in pregnant or neonatal animals. Drug interactions with other drugs (e.g., barbiturates) possible because chloramphenicol will inhibit hepatic microsomal enzymes.	Chloramphenicol use based on susceptibility data. Chloramphenicol palmitate requires active enzymes and should not be administered to fasted (or anorectic) animals. NOTE: Some forms of chloramphenicol are no longer available in the United States.	30 mg/ml oral suspension (palmitate), 250 mg capsules, and 100, 250, and 500 mg tablets	Dog: 40–50 mg/kg q8h PO. Cat: 12.5–20 mg/kg q12h PO.
Chloramphenicol sodium succinate (Chloromycetin, generic)	Injection form of chloramphenicol. Converted by liver to parent drug.	Same as for chloramphenicol.	Injectable solution converted to chloramphenicol by hepatic metabolism.	100 mg/ml injection.	Dog: 40–50 mg/kg q6–8h IV, IM. Cat: 12.5–20 mg/cat q12h IV, IM.
Chlortetracycline (generic)	Tetracycline antibacterial drug. Inhibits bacterial protein synthesis by interfering with peptide elongation by ribosome. Bacteriostatic agent with broad spectrum of activity.	Avoid use in young animals; may bind to bone and developing teeth. High doses have caused renal injury.	Broad-spectrum antibiotic. Used for routine infections and intracellular pathogens.	Powdered feed additive.	25 mg/kg q6–8h PO.
Ciprofloxacin (Cipro)	Fluoroquinolone antibacterial. Acts to inhibit DNA gyrase and inhibit cell DNA and RNA synthesis. Bactericidal. Broad antimicrobial activity.	Avoid use in dogs 4 weeks to 7 months of age. High concentrations may cause CNS toxicity, especially in animals with renal failure. Use cautiously in epileptic patients. Causes occasional vomiting. IV solution should be given slowly (over 30 min).	Doses are based on plasma concentrations needed to achieve sufficient plasma concentration above MIC. Efficacy studies have not been performed in dogs or cats. Ciprofloxacin is not absorbed orally as well as enrofloxacin.	250, 500, 750 mg tablets; 2 mg/ml injection.	10–20 mg/kg q24h PO, IV.

(continues)

APPENDIX F. Drug Formulary (continued)

Drug Name (Trade or Other Names)	Pharmacology and Indications	Adverse Effects and Precautions	Dosing Information and Comments	Formulations	Dosage
Clarithromycin (Biaxin)	Macrolide antibiotic with bacteriostatic activity. Spectrum includes primarily gram-positive bacteria. Resistance is expected for most gram-negative bacteria. Efficacy is not established for animals. Most common use in humans is for treatment of *Helicobacter* gastritis, and respiratory infections.	Well tolerated in animals. Most common side side effects are vomiting, nausea, and diarrhea.	Doses are not established for animals because of lack of clinical trials. Dose recommendations are extrapolated from human or empirical use.	250, 500 mg tablets; 25 and 50 mg/ml oral suspension.	7.5 mg/kg q12h PO.
Clavamox	See Amoxicillin/ clavulanate potassium.				
Clavulanic acid	See Amoxicillin/ clavulanate potassium.				
Clindamycin (Antirobe [veterinary], Cleocin [human])	Antibacterial drug of the lincosamide class (similar in action to macrolides). Inhibits bacterial protein synthesis via inhibition of bacterial ribosome. Primarily bacteriostatic, with spectrum of activity primarily against gram-positive bacteria and anaerobes.	Generally well tolerated in dogs and cats. Oral liquid product may be unpalatable to cats. Lincomycin and clindamycin may alter bacterial population in intestine and cause diarrhea; for this reason, do not administer to rodents or rabbits.	Most doses are based on manufacturer's drug approval data and efficacy trials. See dosing column for specific guidelines for different infections.	Oral liquid 25 mg/ml; 25, 75, and 150 mg capsules; and 150 mg/ml injection (Cleocin).	Dog: 11–33 mg/kg q12h PO; for periodontal and soft tissue infection, 5.5–33 mg/kg q12h PO. Cat: 11–33 mg/kg q24h PO; for skin and anaerobic infections, 11 mg/kg q12h PO; for toxoplasmosis, 12.5–25 mg/kg PO q12h.

Clofazimine (Lamprene)	Antimicrobial agent used to treat feline leprosy. Slow bactericidal effect on *Mycobacterium leprae*.	Adverse effects have not been reported in cats. In humans, the most serious adverse effects are GI.	Doses based on empiricism or extrapolation of human studies.	50 and 100 mg capsules.	Cat: 1 mg/kg up to a maximum of 4 mg/kg/day PO.
Clotrimazole (Lotrimin)	Azole antifungal agent for topical (dermal candiasis) or infusion use (nasal for aspergillosis, urinary bladder for candiasis). Inhibits ergosterol formation in fungal cell wall.	Propylene glycol or isopropyl alcohol carrier in infusion solution can cause irritation of mucous membranes and esophagitis if swallowed. May prolong barbiturate anesthesia.	Topical solutions contain propylene glycol and isopropyl alcohol carrier. Various creams and lotion also. All products available from most pharmacies.	1% topical solution in 10 ml and 30 ml, creams, lotion, and vaginal tablets.	Nasal infusion (aspergillosis): 60 ml (2 × 30 ml bottles of 1% solution) usually sufficient to infuse into each nasal cavity (120 ml total) of a large-breed dog; maintain infusion over 60 min while animal is under general anesthesia. Drain out drug completely once completed. Topical: apply q12h for 3–4 weeks.
Cloxacillin sodium (Cloxapen, Orbenin, Tegopen)	β-lactam antibiotic. Inhibits bacterial cell wall synthesis. Spectrum is limited to gram-positive bacteria, especially staphylococci.	Use cautiously in animals allergic to penicillin-like drugs.	Doses based on empiricism or extrapolation from human studies. No clinical efficacy studies available for dogs or cats. Oral absorption is poor; if possible, administer on empty stomach.	250, 500 mg capsules, 25 mg/mL oral solution	20–40 mg/kg q8h PO

(continues)

APPENDIX F. Drug Formulary (continued)

Drug Name (Trade or Other Names)	Pharmacology and Indications	Adverse Effects and Precautions	Dosing Information and Comments	Formulations	Dosage
Dapsone (generic)	Antimicrobial drug used primarily for treatment of mycobacterium infection. May have some immunosuppressive properties or inhibit function of inflammatory cells. Used primarily for dermatologic diseases in dogs and cats.	Hepatitis and blood dyscrasias may occur. Toxic dermatologic reactions have been seen in humans. *Drug interactions:* Do not administer with trimethoprim (may increase blood concentrations).	Doses are derived from extrapolation of human doses or empiricism. No well-controlled clinical studies have been performed in veterinary medicine.	25 and 100 mg tablets.	1.1 mg/kg q8–12h PO.
Decoquinate (Deccox)	Coccidiostat with activity against *Hepatozoon* spp. Disrupts electron transport in mitochondrial cytochrome system.	Should not be given to pregnant animals.	Efficacy against *Hepatozoon* spp. unknown.	0.8% medicated powder, 6% medicated feed.	Long-term treatment of *Hepatozoon* infection: 10–20 mg/kg q12h PO for 33 months (1/4 oz of the 6% feed additive preparation will medicate 20–40 kg body weight of dog).
Dichlorvos (Task)	Antiparasitic drug, used primarily to treat hookworms, roundworms, and whipworms. Kills parasites by anticholinesterase action.	Do not use in heartworm-positive patients. Overdoses can cause organophosphate intoxication. (treat with 2-PAM, atropine).	Doses based on manufacturer's recommendations.	10, 25 mg tablets.	Dog: 26.4–33 mg/kg PO. Cat: 11 mg/kg PO.

Drug	Action/Use	Precautions/Adverse effects	Comments	How supplied	Dosage
Dicloxacillin sodium (Dynapen)	β-Lactam antibiotic. Inhibits bacterial cell wall synthesis. Spectrum is limited to gram-positive bacteria, especially staphylococci.	Use cautiously in animals allergic to penicillin-like drugs.	No clinical efficacy studies available for dogs or cats. In dogs, oral absorption is very low and may not be suitable for therapy (J Vet Pharmacol Ther 21:414–417, 1998). Administer, if possible, on empty stomach.	125, 250, 500 mg capsules, 12.5 mg/ml oral suspension.	11–55 mg/kg q8h PO.
Diethylcarbamazine (DEC) (Caricide, Filaribits)	Heartworm preventive. For action, see Piperazine.	Safe in all species. Reactions can occur in animals with positive microfilaria.	Doses based on manufacturer's recommendations. Specific protocols for heartworm administration may be based on region of country.	50, 60, 180, 200, 400 mg chewable tablets.	Heartworm prophylaxis: 6.6 mg/kg q24h PO.
Difloxacin hydrochloride (Dicural)	Fluoroquinolone antibacterial drug. Acts via inhibition of DNA gyrase in bacteria to inhibit DNA and RNA synthesis. Bactericidal, with broad spectrum of activity. Used for variety of infections, including skin infections, wound infections, and pneumonia.	Adverse effects include seizures in epileptic animals, arthropathy in young animals, vomiting at high doses. Drug interactions: May increase concentrations of theophylline if used concurrently. Coadministration with di- and trivalent cations (e.g., sucralfate) may decrease absorption. Ocular safety not established in cats.	Dose range can be used to adjust dose, depending on severity of infection and susceptibility of bacteria. Bacteria with low MIC can be treated with low dose; susceptible bacteria with higher MIC should be treated with higher dose. Difloxacin is primarily eliminated in feces rather than urine (urine is 5% of clearance). Sarafloxacin is an active desmethyl metabolite.	11.4, 45.4, and 136 mg tablets.	Dog: 5–10 mg/kg q24h PO (see dosing information guidelines).

(continues)

APPENDIX F. Drug Formulary (continued)

Drug Name (Trade or Other Names)	Pharmacology and Indications	Adverse Effects and Precautions	Dosing Information and Comments	Formulations	Dosage
Doramectin (Dectomax)	Macrocyclic antiparasitic agent (similar to ivermectin) active against *Spirocerca* spp. Neurotoxic to parasites by potentiating effects of inhibitory neurotransmitter GABA.	See Ivermectin.	Not approved for use in dogs. Cattle or swine injectable product effective in treating spirocercosis if used early in disease. Can administer PO or SC in dogs.	1% (10 mg/ml) injectable solution.	Regimen 1: 0.2 mg/kg SC every 14 days for 3 treatments—resolves clinical signs and nodules in most dogs. If not fully resolved, use 0.5 mg/kg q24h PO for 6 wk. Regimen 2: 0.4 mg/kg SC every 14 days for 6 treatments and then monthly until all esophageal granulomas are gone (2 years in some cases).
Doxycycline (Vibramycin and generic forms)	Tetracycline antibiotic. Mechanism of action of tetracyclines is to bind to 30S ribosomal subunit and inhibit protein synthesis. Usually bacteriostatic. Broad spectrum of activity, including bacteria, some protozoa, *Rickettsia*, and *Ehrlichia*.	Severe adverse reactions not reported with doxycycline. Tetracyclines in general may cause renal tubular necrosis at high doses. Tetracyclines can affect bone and teeth formation in young animals. *Drug interactions:* Tetracyclines bind to calcium-containing compounds, which decreases oral absorption.	Many pharmacokinetic and experimental studies have been conducted in small animals, but no clinical studies. Ordinarily considered the drug of choice for *Rickettsia* and *Ehrlichia* infections in dogs. Doxycycline IV infusion is stable for only 12 hr at room temperature and 72 hr if refrigerated.	10 mg/ml oral suspension; 100 mg tablets; 100 mg injection vial.	3–5 mg/kg q12h PO IV or 10 mg/kg q24h PO. For *Rickettsia* in dogs: 5 mg/kg q12h.

Drug	Description	Formulation	Dosage
Enilconazole (Imaverol, Clinafarm EC)	Azole antifungal agent for topical use only. Like other azoles, inhibits membrane synthesis (ergosterol) in fungus. Highly effective for dermatophytes.	Administered topically. Adverse effects have not been reported.	Imaverol is available only in Canada as 10% emulsion. In the United States, Clinafarm EC is available for use in poultry units as 13.8% solution. Dilute solution to at least 50:1, and apply topically every 3–4 days for 2–3 wk. Enilconazole also has been instilled as 1:1 dilution into nasal sinus for nasal aspergillosis.	10% or 13.8% emulsion.	Nasal aspergillosis: 10 mg/kg q12h instilled into nasal sinus for 14 days (10% solution diluted 50/50 with water). Dermatophytes: dilute 10% solution to 0.2%, and wash lesion with solution 4 times at 3- to 4-day intervals.
Enrofloxacin (Baytril)	Fluoroquinolone antibacterial drug. Acts via inhibition of DNA gyrase in bacteria to inhibit DNA and RNA synthesis. Bactericidal. Broad spectrum of activity.	Adverse effects include seizures in epileptic animals, arthropathy in dogs aged 4–28 wk, vomiting in dogs and cats at high doses. Blindness in cats has been reported. *Drug interactions:* May increase concentrations of theophylline if used concurrently. Coadministration with di- and trivalent cations (e.g., sucralfate) may decrease absorption.	In dogs, low dose of 5 mg/kg/day is used for sensitive organisms with MIC of 0.12 mcg/ml or less, or urinary tract infection; dose of 5–10 mg/kg/day is used for organisms with MIC of 0.12–0.5 mcg/ml; dose of 10–20 mg/kg/day is used for organisms with MIC of 0.5–1.0 mcg/ml. Solution is not approved for IV use but has been administered via this route safely if given slowly.	68, 22.7, and 5.7 mg tablets. Taste Tabs are 22.7 and 68 mg. 22.7 mg/ml injection.	Dog: 5–20 mg/kg/ q24h PO, IV, IM (see dosing information guidelines). Cat: 5 mg/kg q24h PO, IM Do not administer to cats at doses higher than 5 mg/kg and do not administer to cats IV.

(continues)

APPENDIX F. Drug Formulary (continued)

Drug Name (Trade or Other Names)	Pharmacology and Indications	Adverse Effects and Precautions	Dosing Information and Comments	Formulations	Dosage
Epsiprantel (Cestex)	Antehelmintic with activity against cat and dog tapeworms, including *Dipylidium caninum, Taenia taeniaformis, T. pisiformis,* and *T. hydatigena.*	No known contraindications. Very safe drug. Do not use in kittens or pups under age 7 wk.	A single oral dose is effective. Fasting is not necessary or recommended. Treatment of *D. caninum* should be coupled with an effective flea control program.	12.5, 25, 50, 100 mg film-coated tablets.	Dogs: 5.5 mg/kg PO once, repeat as necessary. Cats: 2.75 mg/kg PO once, repeat as necessary. Convenient dosing chart available.
Erythromycin (many brands and generic)	Macrolide antibiotic. Inhibits bacteria by binding to 50S ribosome and inhibiting protein synthesis. Spectrum of activity limited primarily to gram-positive aerobic bacteria. Used for skin and respiratory infections.	Most common side effect is vomiting (probably caused by cholinergic-like effect or motilin-induced motility). May cause diarrhea in some animals. Do not administer PO to rodents or rabbits.	There are several forms of erythromycin, including the ethylsuccinate and estolate esters, and stearate salt for oral administration. There are no convincing data to suggest that one form is absorbed better than another, and one dose is included for all. Only erythromycin gluceptate and lactate are to be administered IV. Motilin-like effect on GI motility occurs at low dose.	250 mg capsules or tablets.	10–20 mg/kg q8–12h PO; prokinetic effects at 0.5–1.0 mg/kg q8–12h PO.
Famotidine (Pepsid)	Histamine H_2-receptor antagonist. (See Cimetidine for details.)	See Cimetidine.	See Cimetidine. Clinical studies for famotidine have not been performed; therefore optimal dose for ulcer prevention and healing is not known.	10 mg tablet; 10 mg/ml injection.	0.1–0.2 mg/kg q12h PO, IV, SC, IM.

Drug	Description	Notes	Formulation	Dose
Febantel-praziquantel-pyrantel (Drontal Plus)	Broad-spectrum anthelmintic for dogs, with activity against tapeworms, hookworms, roundworms, and whipworms (label use) and *Giardia* spp. (off-label use). Febantel blocks parasites energy metabolism. See praziquantel and pyrantel for mechanism of action.	Febantel – metabolized to fenbendazole and oxfendazole by liver. Acute toxic dose in dogs is >10 g/kg. See praziquantel and pyrantel for adverse effects. Do not use in pregnant dogs, in dogs <1 kg, or puppies <3 wk of age.	Product formulated to deliver 25–30 mg of febantel, 5–7 mg of praziquantel, and 5–7 mg of pyrantel pomoate per kg. Tablets for small dogs contain: 22.7 mg praziquantel, 22.7 mg pyrantel, and 113.4 mg febantel. Tablets for medium and large dogs contain: 68 mg praziquantel, 68 mg pyrantel, and 340.2 mg febantel.	Single oral dose for on label use. Giardiasis: 1 tablet q24h PO for 3 consecutive days.
Fenbendazole (Panacur, Safe-Guard)	Benzimidazole antiparasite drugs. (See Albendazole). Effective for treatment of *Giardia* (Am J Vet Res 59:61–63, 1998).	Good safety margin, but vomiting and diarrhea have been reported. No known contraindication.	Dose recommendations based on clinical studies by manufacturer. Granules may be mixed with food. In studies for treatment of *Giardia*, it was safer than other treatments. Panacur granules 22.2% (222 mg/g); 100 mg/ml oral suspension.	50 mg/kg/day × 3 days PO
Fluconazole (Diflucan)	Azole antifungal drug. Similar mechanism as other azole antifungal agents. Inhibits ergosterol synthesis in fungal cell membrane. Fungistatic. Efficacious against dermatophytes and variety of systemic fungi.	Adverse effects have not been reported from fluconazole administration. Compared to ketoconazole, it has less effect on endocrine function. However, increased liver enzyme plasma concentrations and hepatopathy are possible. Compared with other oral azole antifungals, fluconazole is absorbed more predictably and completely, even on an empty stomach.	Doses for fluconazole are primarily based on studies performed in cats for treatment of cryptococcosis. Efficacy for other infections has not been reported. The primary difference between fluconazole and other azoles is that fluconazole attains higher concentrations in the CNS. 50, 100, 150, or 200 mg tablets; 10 or 40 mg/ml oral suspension; 2 mg/ml IV injection.	Dog: 10–12 mg/kg q24h, PO. Cat: 50 mg/cat q12h–24h.

(continues)

APPENDIX F. Drug Formulary (continued)				
Drug Name (Trade or Other Names)	Pharmacology and Indications	Adverse Effects and Precautions	Dosing Information and Comments	Formulations	Dosage
Flucytosine (Ancobon)	Antifungal drug. Used in combination with other antifungal drugs for treatment of cryptococcosis. Action is to penetrate fungal cells. Converted to fluorouracil, which acts as antimetabolite.	Adverse effects have not been reported in animals.	Flucytosine is used primarily to treat cryptococcosis in animals. Efficacy is based on flucytosine's ability to attain high concentrations in CSF. Flucytosine may be synergistic with amphotericin B.	250 mg capsule; 75 mg/ml oral suspension.	25–50 mg/kg q6–8h PO (up to a maximum dose of 100 mg/kg q12h PO).
Furazolidone (Furoxone)	Oral antiprotozoal drug with activity against *Giardia*. May have some activity against bacteria in intestine. Not used for systemic therapy	Adverse effects not reported in animals. In humans, mild anemia, hypersensitivity, and disturbance of intestinal flora have been reported.	Clinical studies have not been reported for animals. Doses and recommendations are based on extrapolation from humans. Other drugs, such as fenbendazole, may be preferred for *Giardia*.	100 mg tablets.	4 mg/kg q12h for 7–10 days PO.
Gentamicin sulfate (Gentocin)	Aminoglycoside antibiotic. Action is to inhibit bacteria protein synthesis via binding to 30S ribosome. Bactericidal. Broad spectrum of activity except streptococci and anaerobic bacteria	Nephrotoxicity is the most dose-limiting toxicity. Ensure that patients have adequate fluid and electrolyte balance during therapy. Ototoxicity and vestibulotoxicity also are possible. *Drug interactions:* When used with anesthetic agents, neuromuscular blockade is possible. Do not mix in vial or syringe with other antibiotics.	Dosing regimens are based on sensitivity of organisms. Some studies have suggested that once-daily therapy (combining multiple doses into a single daily dose) is as efficacious as multiple treatments. Activity against some bacteria (e.g., *Pseudomonas*) is enhanced when combined with a β-lactam antibiotic. Nephrotoxicity is increased with persistently high trough concentrations.	50 and 100 mg/ml solution for injection	Dog: 2–4 mg/kg q8h or 9–14 mg/kg q24h IV, IM, SC. Cat: 3 mg/kg q8h or 5–8 mg/kg q24h IV, IM, SC.

Griseofulvin (microsize) (Fulvicin U/F)	Antifungal drug. Incorporates into skin layers and inhibits mitosis of fungi. Antifungal activity is limited to dermatophytes.	Adverse effects in animals include teratogenicity in cats; anemia and leukopenia in cats; anorexia, depression, vomiting, and diarrhea. Do not administer to pregnant cats.	A wide range of doses has been reported. Doses listed here represent the current consensus. Griseofulvin should be administered with food to enhance absorption.	125, 250, 500 mg tablets; 25 mg/ml oral suspension; 125 mg/ml oral syrup.	50 mg/kg q24h PO (up to a maximum dose of 110–132 mg/kg/day in divided treatments).
Griseofulvin (ultramicrosize) (Fulvicin P/G, Gris-PEG)	Same as above.	Same as above.	Same as above. Ultramicrosize is absorbed to a greater extent, and doses should be less than microsize.	100, 125, 165, 250, 330 mg tablets.	30 mg/kg/day in divided treatments PO.
Imidocarb dipropionate (Imazol)	Injectable parasiticide with activity against *Babesia* (on label use), ehrlichiosis, and cytauxzoonosis (off-label use). Interferes with nucleic acid metabolism.	Pain/ulceration at injection site; periorbital edema, hypersalivation, lacrimation, shivering, diarrhea, vomiting, depression, or mental agitation (signs similar to organophosphate toxicity because it has anticholinesterase activity); posttreatment vomiting (consistent side effect). Preadminister atropine. Rarely, renal tubular necrosis develops. High doses (>10 mg/kg) toxic with cardiac effects and hepatic necrosis.	Reduce doses if renal or hepatic insufficiency present. Avoid use with preexisting pulmonary impairment. Not for IV use. May be synergistic with diminazene (which is not available in the United States).	12% (120 mg/ml) solution, in multidose 10 ml vial for SC or IM injection.	Babesiosis: 5–6.6 mg/kg IM or SC once, repeat in 14 days. Cytauxzoonosis (cats): 2 mg/kg IM once, repeat in 3–7 days. Ehrlichiosis (dogs and cats): 5 mg/kg IM once, repeat in 14 days.

(continues)

APPENDIX F. Drug Formulary (continued)

Drug Name (Trade or Other Names)	Pharmacology and Indications	Adverse Effects and Precautions	Dosing Information and Comments	Formulations	Dosage
Imipenem (Primaxin)	β-Lactam antibiotic with broad-spectrum activity. Action is similar to other β-lactam (see Amoxicillin). Imipenem is the ost active of all β-lactams. Used primarily for serious, multiple-resistant infections.	Allergic reactions may occur with β-lactam antibiotics. With rapid infusion or in patients with renal insufficiency, neurotoxicity may occur (seizures). Vomiting and nausea are possible. IM or SC injections may cause pain in dogs.	Doses and efficacy studies have not been determined in animals. Recommendations are based on studies performed in humans and extrapolation from humans. Reserve the use of this drug for only resistant, refractory infections. Observe manufacturer's instructions carefully for proper administration. For IV administration, add to IV fluids. For IM administration, add 2 ml lidocaine (1%); suspension is stable for only 1 hr.	250 or 500 mg vials for injection.	Dog: 5 mg/kg IV, IM, or SC q4h. Cat: Dose not established, but often used at same dose as in dogs.
Interferon (interferon-α, HuIFN-α) (Roferon)	Human interferon. Used to stimulate the immune system in patients.	Adverse effects have not been reported in animals.	Doses and indications for animals have primarily been based on extrapolation of human recommendations or limited experimental studies. (*J Am Vet Med Assoc* 199:1477, 1991.) To prepare, add 3 million U to 1 L sterile saline and divide into aliquots and freeze. Thaw as needed for 30 U/ml solution.	3 million U/vial.	Cat: 15–30 U per cat SC or IM q24h for 7 days and repeated every other week.

Drug	Description	Notes	Formulation	Dosage
Itraconazole (Sporanox)	Azole (triazole) antifungal drug. See Ketoconazole for mechanism of action. Active against dermatophytes and systemic fungi, such as *Blastomyces*, *Histoplasma*, and *Coccidioides*.	Itraconazole is better tolerated than ketoconazole. However, vomiting and hepatotoxicosis are possible, especially at high doses. In one study, hepatotoxicosis was more likely at high doses. 10%–15% of dogs will develop high liver enzyme levels. High doses in cats caused vomiting and anorexia.	Doses are based on studies in animals in which itraconazole has been used to treat blastomycosis in dogs. In cats, lower doses have been effective for dermatophytes (see dosage section). Other uses or doses are based on empiricism or extrapolation from the literature on humans.	100 mg capsules and 10 mg/ml oral liquid	Dog: 2.5 mg/kg q12h or 5 mg/kg q24h PO. *Malassezia* dermatitis: 5 mg/kg q24h PO for 2 days, repeated each week for 3 weeks. Cat: 5 mg/kg q12h PO. Dermatophyte infection in cats: 1.5–3.0 mg/kg (up to 5 mg/kg) q24h PO for 15 days.
Ivermectin (Heartgard, Ivomec, Eqvalan liquid)	Antiparasitic drug. Neurotoxic to parasites by potentiating effects of inhibitory neurotransmitter GABA.	Toxicity may occur at high doses and in breeds in which ivermectin crosses blood–brain barrier. Sensitive breeds include collies, Australian shepherds, shelties, and Old English sheepdogs. Toxicity is neurotoxic, and signs include depression, ataxia, difficulty with vision, coma, and death. Ivermectin appears to be safe for pregnant animals. Do not administer to animals under 6 wk of age. Animals with high microfilaremia may show adverse reactions to high doses.	Doses vary, depending on use. Heartworm prevention is lowest dose, other parasites require higher doses. Heartgard is only form approved for small animals; for other indications, large animal injectable products are often administered PO, IM, or SC to small animals. For demodectic therapy, it is advised to start with 100 mcg/kg/day and increase dose by 100 mcg/kg/day to 600 mcg/kg/day (*Compendium* 20:459–469, 1998).	1% (10 mg/ml) injectable solution; 10 mg/ml oral solution; 18.7 mg/ml oral paste; 68, 136, and 272 mcg tablets.	Heartworm preventive: 6 mcg/kg every 30 days PO in dogs and 24 mcg/kg every 30 days PO in cats. Microfilaricide: 50 mcg/kg PO 2 wks after adulticide therapy. Ectoparasite therapy (dogs and cats): 200–300 mcg/kg IM, SC, PO. Endoparasites (dogs and cats): 200–400 mcg/kg weekly SC, PO. *Demodex* therapy: start with 100 mcg/kg/day and increase dose by 100 mcg/kg/day to 600 mcg/kg/day for 60–120 days PO (*Compendium* 20:459–469, 1998).

(continues)

APPENDIX F. Drug Formulary (continued)

Drug Name (Trade or Other Names)	Pharmacology and Indications	Adverse Effects and Precautions	Dosing Information and Comments	Formulations	Dosage
Kanamycin (Kantrim)	Aminoglycoside antibiotic. (See Gentamicin, Amikacin for details.)	Shares same properties with other aminoglycosides (see Amikacin, Gentamicin).	See Gentamicin.	200, 500 mg/ml injection.	10 mg/kg q12h or 20 mg/kg q24h IV IM, SC.
Ketoconazole (Nizoral)	Azole (imidazole) antifungal drug. Similar mechanism of action as other azole antifungal agents. Inhibits ergosterol synthesis in fungal cell membrane. Fungistatic. Efficacious against dermatophytes and variety of systemic fungi, such as *Histoplasma*, *Blastomyces*, and *Coccidioides*.	Adverse effects in animals include dose-related vomiting, diarrhea, and hepatic injury. Enzyme elevations are common. Do not administer to pregnant animals. Ketoconazole causes endocrine abnormalities, most specifically, inhibition of cortisol synthesis. *Drug interactions:* Ketoconazole will inhibit metabolism of other drugs (anticonvulsants, cyclosporine, cisapride).	Oral absorption depends on acidity in stomach. Do not administer with anti-secretory drugs or antacids. Because of endocrine effects, ketoconazole has been used for short-term treatment of hyperadrenocorticism.	200 mg tablets; 100 mg/ml oral suspension (available only in Canada).	Dog: 10–15 mg/kg q8–12h PO. *Malassezia canis* infection: 5 mg/kg q24h PO. For hyperadrenocorticism: 15 mg/kg q12h PO. Cat: 5–10 mg/kg q8–12h PO.

Drug	Description	Comments	Adverse Effects	Supplied	Dosage
Levamisole (Levasole, Tramisol, Ergamisol)	Antiparasitic drug of the imidazothiazole class. Mechanism of action is neuromuscular toxicity to parasites. Levamisole has been used for endoparasites in dogs and as a microfilaricide. In humans, levamisole is used as immunostimulant to aid in treatment of colorectal carcinoma and malignant melanoma.	In heartworm-positive dogs, it may sterilize female adult heartworms. Levamisole has also been used as an immunostimulant; however, clinical reports of its efficacy are not available.	May produce cholinergic toxicity. May cause vomiting in some dogs.	0.184 g bolus; 11.7 g per 13-g packet; 50 mg tablet (Ergamisol).	Dog: Hookworms: 5–8 mg/kg once PO (up to 10 mg/kg PO for 2 days). Microfilaricide: 10 mg/kg q24h PO for 6–10 days. Immunostimulant: 0.5–2 mg/kg 3 times/week PO. Cat: Endoparasites: 4.4 mg/kg once PO. Lungworms: 20–40 mg/kg q48h for 5 treatments PO.
Lincomycin (Lincocin)	Lincosamide antibiotic, similar in mechanism to clindamycin and erythromycin. Spectrum includes primarily gram-positive bacteria. Used for pyoderma and other soft tissue infections.	Actions of lincomycin and clindamycin are similar enough that clindamycin can be substituted for lincomycin.	Adverse effects uncommon. Lincomycin has caused vomiting and diarrhea in animals. Do *not* administer orally to rodents and rabbits.	100, 200, 500 mg tablets.	15–25 mg/kg q12h PO. For pyoderma, doses as low as 10 mg/kg q12h have been used.
Lufenuron (Program)	Antiparasitic. Used for controlling fleas in animals. Inhibits development in hatching fleas. May be used for dermatophytes in dogs and cats, although efficacy has been questioned by some experts.	Lufenuron may control flea development with administration once every 30 days in animals.	Adverse effects have not been reported. Appears to be relatively safe during pregnancy and in young animals	45, 90, 135, 204.9, 409.8 mg tablets; 135 and 270 mg suspension per unit pack.	Dog: 10 mg/kg PO every 30 days. Antifungal: 80 mg/kg. Cat: 30 mg/kg PO every 30 days. Cat injection: 10 mg/kg SC every 6 months. Antifungal: 100 mg/kg. In endemic areas (e.g., catteries) treat cats once a month.

(continues)

APPENDIX F. Drug Formulary (continued)

Drug Name (Trade or Other Names)	Pharmacology and Indications	Adverse Effects and Precautions	Dosing Information and Comments	Formulations	Dosage
Lufenuron + milbemycin oxime (Sentinel tablets and Flavor Tabs)	Combination of two antiparasitic drugs. (See Lufenuron or Milbemycin oxime.) Used to protect against fleas, heartworms, roundworms, hookworms, and whipworms.	See Lufenuron or Milbemycin oxime.	See Lufenuron or Milbemycin oxime.	Milbemycin oxime/lufenuron ratio is as follows: 2.3/46 mg tablets; 5.75/115, 11.5/230, and 23/460 mg Flavor Tabs.	Dog: Administer 1 tablet every 30 days. Each tablet formulated for size of dog. Cat: This product is not registered for cats.
Marbofloxacin (Zeniquin)	Fluoroquinolone antimicrobial. Same mechanism as enrofloxacin and ciprofloxacin. Spectrum includes staphylococci, gram-negative bacilli, and some *Pseudomonas*.	Same precautions as enrofloxacin. May cause some nausea and vomiting at high doses. Avoid use in young animals. Safe for cats (ocular safety) at recommended dose.	Same dosing guidelines as for other fluoroquinolones. Higher doses are needed for organisms with higher MIC values. Safety data not available for cats. Doses published for European use may be lower than those U.S. approved for dogs.	25, 50, 100, and 200 mg tablets	2.75–5.55 mg/kg q24h PO
Meglumine antimonite (Glucantime)	Antiprotozoal pentavalent antimonial agent that interferes with energy metabolism in *Leishmania* spp.	Pain and swelling at injection site if given IM; SC preferred. Contraindications include renal and hepatic insufficiency, cardiac arrhythmias, and leukopenia.	May not always be available in the United States—contact CDC. Resistance to drug may develop during treatment. Use with allopurinol.	5 ml vials (300 mg/ml) for injection.	Multiple dosing regimens for leishmaniasis. 100 mg/kg q24h SC for 10 to 30 days. 200 mg/kg q48h SC or IV for 20–40 days. More effective if combined with oral allopurinol.

Drug	Description	Supplied	Dose
Melarsomine (Immiticide)	Organic arsenical compound used for heartworm therapy. Heartworm adulticide. Arsenicals alter glucose uptake and metabolism in heartworms.	Adverse effects: pulmonary thromboembolism (7–20 days after therapy), anorexia (13% incidence), injection site reaction (myositis) (32% incidence), lethargy or depression (15% incidence). Causes elevation of hepatic enzymes. High doses (3×) can cause pulmonary inflammation and death. If high doses are administered, dimercaprol (3 mg/kg IM) may be used as antidote.	25 mg/ml injection. After reconstitution, retains potency for 24 hr.	Dog: Administer via deep IM injection. Class I and II dogs: 2.5 mg/kg q24h for 2 consecutive days. Class III dogs: 2.5 mg/kg once, then in 1 month, two additional doses 24 hr apart.
Meropenem (Merrem IV)	Broad-spectrum carbapenem antibiotic; indicated primarily for resistant infections caused by bacteria resistant to other drugs. Bactericidal. More active than imipenem and ertapenem.	Risks similar to those of other β-lactam antibiotics. Meropenem does not cause seizures as frequently as imipenem. SC injections may cause slight hair loss at injection site.	500 mg/20 ml or 1 g/30 ml vial for injection.	8 mg/kg q12h SC up to 12 mg/kg q8h SC (for *Pseudomonas* infection); IV dose, 12 mg/kg q8h.

(continues)

APPENDIX F. Drug Formulary (continued)

Drug Name (Trade or Other Names)	Pharmacology and Indications	Adverse Effects and Precautions	Dosing Information and Comments	Formulations	Dosage
Metronidazole (Flagyl and generic)	Antibacterial and antiprotozoal drug. Disrupts DNA in organism via reaction with intracellular metabolite. Action is specific for anaerobic bacteria. Resistance is rare. Active against some protozoa, including *Giardia*; however, other drugs, such as fenbendazole, have been used for *Giardia*.	Most severe adverse effect is caused by toxicity to CNS. High doses have caused lethargy, CNS depression, ataxia, vomiting, and weakness. Metronidazole may be mutagenic. Fetal abnormalities have not been demonstrated in animals with recommended doses, but use cautiously during pregnancy. Cats may find broken tablets unpalatable.	Metronidazole is one of the most commonly used drugs for anaerobic infections. Although it is effective for giardiasis, other drugs used for giardiasis include albendazole, fenbendazole, and quinacrine. CNS toxicity is dose-related. Maximum dose that should be administered is 50–65 mg/kg/day in any species. Although tablets have been broken or crushed for oral administration to cats, they find these unpalatable.	250, 500 mg tablet; 50 mg/ml suspension; 5 mg/ml injection.	Dog: Anaerobes: 15 mg/kg q12h or 12 mg/kg q8h PO. *Giardia* spp.: 12–15 mg/kg q12h for 8 days PO. Cat: Anaerobes: 10–25 mg/kg q24h PO. *Giardia* spp.: 17 mg/kg (⅓ tablet per cat) q24h for 8 days.
Miconazole (Conifite, Candistat, Daktarin, Monistat)	Imidazole fungistatic agent, inhibits ergosterol biosynthesis and damages fungal cell wall with activity against *Candida albicans* (inhibits transformation of blastospores into invasive mycelial form).	Topical: may cause skin irritation (blistering, redness, irritation).	Available from human pharmacies as a cream, lotion, powder, spray liquid, and spray powder to be applied to the skin. Many preparations.	Topical creams: Monistat-derm 2%; Daktarin cream 2% (20 g); 2% Candistat (15 g)	Apply locally q12–24h for 3 wk.

Milbemycin oxime (Interceptor, Interceptor Flavor Tabs, and SafeHeart)	Antiparasitic drug. Action is similar to that of ivermectin. Acts as GABA agonist in nervous system of parasite. Used as heartworm preventive, miticide, and microfilaricide. Used to control hookworm, roundworm, and whipworm infections. At high doses, it has been used to treat Demodex infection in dogs.	In susceptible dogs (collie breeds), milbemycin may cross the blood–brain barrier and produce CNS toxicosis (depression, lethargy, coma). At doses used for heartworm prevention, this effect is less likely.	Doses vary, depending on parasite treated. Consult dose column. Treatment of Demodex requires high dose administered daily (*J Am Vet Med Assoc* 207:1581, 1995). (See also Lufenuron + milbemycin oxime.)	2.3, 5.75, 11.5, and 23 mg tablet.	Dog: Microfilaricide: 0.5 mg/kg; *Demodex:* 2 mg/kg q24h PO for 60–120 days. Heartworm prevention and control of endoparasites: 0.5 mg/kg every 30 days PO. Cat: Heartworm and endoparasite control: 2 mg/kg every 30 days PO.
Minocycline (Minocin)	Tetracycline antibiotic. Similar to doxycycline in pharmacokinetics. (See Doxycycline.)	See other tetracycline (Doxycycline). Adverse effects have not been reported for minocycline. Oral absorption is not affected by calcium products as with other tetracyclines.	Minocycline has received little attention for clinical use in North America. Clinical use has not been reported, but properties are similar to those of doxycycline.	50, 100 mg tablets; 10 mg/ml oral suspension.	5–12.5 mg/kg q12h PO.
Moxidectin (canine form: ProHeart; equine oral gel: Quest; cattle pour-on: Cydectin)	Antiparasitic drug. Neurotoxic to parasites by potentiating effects of inhibitory neurotransmitter GABA. Used for endo- and ectoparasites, as well as heartworm prevention.	Toxicity may occur at high doses and in species in which ivermectin crosses blood–brain barrier (collie breeds). Toxicity is neurotoxic, and signs include depression, ataxia, difficulty with vision, coma, and death.	Similar use as ivermectin. Extreme caution is recommended if equine formulation is considered for use in small animals. Toxic overdoses are likely because the equine formulation is highly concentrated.	30, 68, 136 mcg tablets for dogs; 20 mg/ml equine oral gel; and 5 mg/ml cattle pour-on.	Dog: Heartworm prevention: 3 mcg/kg q30d PO. Endoparasites: 25–300 mcg/kg *Demodex:* 500 mcg/kg/day for 21–22 wk.

(continues)

APPENDIX F. Drug Formulary (continued)				
Drug Name (Trade or Other Names)	Pharmacology and Indications	Adverse Effects and Precautions	Dosing Information and Comments	Formulations	Dosage
Moxifloxacin (Avelox)	Fluoroquinolone antibiotic of the new (4th) generation. Similar to other fluoroquinolones, except with greater activity against gram-positive and anaerobic bacteria.	Similar to those of other fluoroquinolones. Because of the increased spectrum of action on anaerobic bacteria, greater GI disturbance is expected from oral dose.	Doses and recommendations based primarily on limited clinical experience and extrapolation from human studies.	400 mg tablet.	10 mg/kg q24h PO.
Nandrolone decanoate (Deca-Durabolin)	Anabolic steroid. Derivative of testosterone. Anabolic agents are designed to maximize anabolic effects while minimizing androgenic action (see Methyltestosterone). Anabolic agents have been used for reversing catabolic conditions, increasing weight gain, increasing muscling in animals, and stimulating erythropoiesis.	Adverse effects from anabolic steroids can be attributed to the pharmacologic action of these steroids. Increased masculine effects are common. Increased incidence of some tumors has been reported in people. 17α-Methylated oral anabolic steroids (oxymetholone, stanozolol, and oxandrolone) are associated with hepatic toxicity.	Results of clinical studies in animals have not been reported. Use in animals (and doses) is based on experience in humans or anecdotal experience in animals.	50, 100, 200 mg/ml injection	Dog: 1–1.5 mg/kg/wk IM. Cat: 1 mg/kg/wk IM.

Drug	Description	Supply	Dosage
Neomycin (Biosol)	Aminoglycoside antibiotic. For mechanism, and other effects, see Gentamicin, Amikacin. Neomycin differs from other aminoglycosides because it is only administered topically or orally. Systemic absorption is minimal from oral absorption.	Although oral absorption is so small that systemic adverse effects are unlikely, some oral absorption has been demonstrated in young animals (calves). Alterations in intestinal bacterial flora from therapy may cause diarrhea.	Neomycin is primarily used for oral treatment of diarrhea. Efficacy for this indication (especially for nonspecific diarrhea) is questionable. Used also for treatment of hepatic encephalopathy.	500 mg bolus; 200 mg/ml oral liquid.	10–20 mg/kg q6–12h PO.
Nifurtimox (Lampit)	Antiprotozoal drug with activity against *Trypanosoma cruzi*. Experimental drug. Exact mechanism unknown.	Side effects are common and usually limit treatment to 3–4 wk; side effects include anorexia, vomiting, weight loss, CNS signs, polyneuritis, pulmonary infiltrates, and skin eruptions.	Available in United States only from the CDC. If side effects become too severe, stop treatment. May be given with glucocorticoids to treat acute myocarditis.	30 mg, 100 mg tablets.	2–7 mg/kg q6h PO for 3 to 5 months or until side effects become too severe.
Nitazoxanide (Alinia)	Antiprotozoal drug with activity against *Cryptosporidium*. Activity believed to be due to interference with the enzyme-dependent electron transfer reaction essential for energy metabolism.	Often causes vomiting in cats. Use with caution in hepatic or renal insufficiency. May also cause abdominal pain, diarrhea, and anorexia.	Has only been used in a few experimentally infected cats with mixed but promising results (*Am J Vet Res* 62:1690–1607, 2001).	100 mg/5 ml oral solution.	25 mg/kg q24h PO for 1–4 wk.

(continues)

APPENDIX F. Drug Formulary (continued)

Drug Name (Trade or Other Names)	Pharmacology and Indications	Adverse Effects and Precautions	Dosing Information and Comments	Formulations	Dosage
Nitrofurantoin (Macrodantin, Furalan, Furatoin, Furadantin, and generic)	Antibacterial drug. Urinary antiseptic. Action is via reactive metabolites that damage DNA. Therapeutic concentrations are reached only in the urine. Not to be used for systemic infections.	Adverse effects include nausea, vomiting, and diarrhea. Turns urine color rust-yellow brown. Do not administer during pregnancy.	Two dosing forms exist. Microcrystalline is rapidly and completely absorbed. Macrocrystalline (Macrodantin) is more slowly absorbed and causes less GI irritation. Urine should be at acidic pH for maximum effect. Administer with food to increase absorption.	Macrodantin and generic: 25, 50, 100 mg capsules; Furalan, Furatoin, and generic: 50, 100 mg tablets; Furadantin: 5 mg/ml oral suspension.	10 mg/kg/day divided into 4 daily treatments, then 1 mg/kg at night PO.
Norfloxacin (Noroxin)	Fluoroquinolone antibacterial drug. Same action as ciprofloxacin, except spectrum of activity is not as broad as with enrofloxacin or ciprofloxacin.	Adverse effects have not been reported in animals. Some effects are expected to be similar to those with cipro/enrofloxacin administration.	Use in animals (and doses) is based on pharmacokinetic studies in experimental animals, experience in humans, or anecdotal experience in animals.	400 mg tablets.	22 mg/kg q12h PO.
Nystatin (Nilstat, many others)	Fungistatic and fungicidal agent topically used to treat candidiasis. Binds to sterols in the fungal cell membrane; prevents membrane's inability to function as a selective barrier, allowing loss of essential intracellular constituents.	May cause mild skin irritation. If swallowed, can cause GI tract upsets with vomiting, diarrhea.	Can use oral products (Nystatin Oral Suspension) to swab out mouth ulcers caused by candidiasis (e.g., dogs post parvovirus infections).	Multiple topical cream preparations in 15, 30, and 540 g sizes (100,000 U/g); oral suspension (100,000 U/g).	Apply topically q6–12h for 2 wk.

Omeprazole (Prilosec [formerly Losec]; equine formulation (a paste:) GastroGard)	Proton pump inhibitor. Omeprazole inhibits gastric acid secretion by inhibiting the K^+/H^+ pump. Omeprazole is more potent and longer acting than most available antisecretory drugs. Used for treatment and prevention of GI ulcers.	Side effects have not been reported in animals. However, in humans, there is concern about hypergastrinemia with chronic use. *Drug interactions:* Do not administer with drugs that depend on stomach acid for absorption (e.g., ketoconazole).	Because of omeprazole's potency and accumulation in gastric cells, infrequent administration is possible. Lansoprazole is a newer drug of this class, but has not been used in animals.	20 mg capsules and equine paste.	Dog: 20 mg/dog q24h PO (or 0.7 mg/kg q24h). Cat: not recommended.
Orbifloxacin (Orbax)	Fluoroquinolone antimicrobial. Same mechanism as enrofloxacin and ciprofloxacin. Spectrum includes staphylococci, gram-negative bacilli, and some *Pseudomonas* spp.	Same precautions as enrofloxacin. May cause some nausea and vomiting at high doses. Avoid use in young animals. Blindness in cats has not been reported with doses ≤15 mg/kg/day.	Dose range is wide to account for susceptibility of bacteria. Most susceptible bacteria should be treated with low dose. More resistant bacteria, such as *Pseudomonas*, should be treated with high dose.	5.7, 22.7, and 68 mg tablets.	2.5–7.5 mg/kg q24h PO.
Ormetoprim + sulfadimethoxine	Trimethoprim-like drug used in combination with sulfadimethoxine. (See Primor.)				

(continues)

APPENDIX F. Drug Formulary (continued)

Drug Name (Trade or Other Names)	Pharmacology and Indications	Adverse Effects and Precautions	Dosing Information and Comments	Formulations	Dosage
Oxacillin (Prostaphlin and generic)	β-Lactam antibiotic. Inhibits bacterial cell wall synthesis. Spectrum is limited to gram-positive bacteria, especially staphylococci.	Use cautiously in animals allergic to penicillin-like drugs.	Doses based on empiricism or extrapolation from human studies. No clinical efficacy studies available for dogs or cats. Administer on empty stomach, if possible.	250, 500 mg capsules; 50 mg/ml oral solution.	22–40 mg/kg q8h PO.
Oxfendazole (Synanthic)	Benzimidazole anthelmintic for use in cattle and horses. Exclusively used in dogs to treat canine tracheal worm (Oslerus [Filaroides] osleri).	Good safety margin, but vomiting and diarrhea have been reported.	Available in the United States as a cattle deworming suspension (Synanthic). Oral LD_{50} is >1.6 g/kg for dogs.	9.06 % (90.6 mg/ml) oral suspension.	10 mg/kg q24h PO for 28 days. Couple with physical removal of nodules from the trachea and bifurcation using endoscopy.
Oxymetholone (Anadrol)	Anabolic steroid. See Nandrolone decanoate (there are no differences in efficacy among the anabolic steroids).	See Nandrolone decanoate.	See Nandrolone decanoate.	50 mg tablets.	1–5 mg/kg q24h PO.
Oxytetracycline (Terramycin)	Tetracycline antibiotic. (See Tetracycline). Same mechanism and spectrum as tetracycline. Oxytetracycline may be absorbed to higher extent.	Generally safe. Use cautiously in young animals. See precautions for tetracycline.	Oral dose forms are from large-animal use. Use of injectable long-acting forms has not been studied in small animals.	250 mg tablets; 100, 200 mg/ml injection.	7.5–10 mg/kg IV q12h; 20 mg/kg q12h PO.
Paromomycin (Humatin)	Aminoglycoside antibiotic with no absorption from the GI tract unless damaged. Activity against GI tract bacteria and Cryptosporidium spp.	Good safety margin in animals with intact GI tract. If absorbed (very young and patients showing blood in stool)—nephrotoxicity.	Careful assessment of patient is needed to determine if drug is likely to be absorbed from GI tract. Monitor for nephrotoxicity by examining urine for cast.	250 mg capsules.	125–165 mg/kg q12h PO for 5 days.

Penicillin G benzathine (Benza-Pen and other names)	All benzathine penicillin G is combined with procaine penicillin G in commercial formulation.	Same as for other penicillins (see Amoxicillin).	Benzathine is not recommended for therapy because concentrations are too low to be therapeutic.	150,000 U/ml combined with 150,000 U/ml of procaine penicillin G.	24,000 U/kg q48h IM.
Penicillin G potassium; Penicillin G sodium (many brands)	β-Lactam antibiotic. Action is similar to that of other penicillins (see Amoxicillin). Spectrum of penicillin G is limited to gram-positive bacteria and anaerobes.	Same as for other penicillins (see Amoxicillin).	See other penicillins (Amoxicillin).	5–20 million U vials.	20,000–40,000 U/kg q6–8h IV or IM.
Penicillin G procaine (generic)	Same as other forms of penicillin G, except procaine penicillin is absorbed slowly, producing concentrations for 12–24 hr after injection.	Same as for other penicillins (see Amoxicillin).	Same as for other penicillins (amoxicillin). Avoid SC injection with procaine penicillin G.	300,000 U/mL suspension.	20,000–40,000 U/kg q12–24h IM.
Penicillin V (Pen-Vee)	Oral penicillin. Otherwise, same as other penicillins. Not highly absorbed, and narrow spectrum in comparison with other penicillin derivatives.	Same as for other penicillins (see Amoxicillin).	Same as for other penicillins (amoxicillin). Penicillin V should be administered on an empty stomach for maximum absorption (250 mg = 400,000 U).	250, 500 mg tablets.	10 mg/kg q8h PO.
Pentamidine isethionate (Lomidine, Pentam)	An aromatic diamidine; interferes with synthesis of DNA, RNA, proteins, and phospholipids, with activity against *Pneumocystis* spp.	After systemic administration: hypotension, systemic anaphylaxis, nausea, vomiting, diarrhea, hypoglycemia, myelosuppression, renal failure, hypocalcemia, hypokalemia.	Pretreat with antihistamines to avoid allergic reactions. IM use can cause pain at injection site. Use sterile water or 5% dextrose for reconstitution because other solutions cause precipitation.	Lomidine: 20 ml vials (40 mg/ml) for injection. Pentam: 300 mg vials of powder (reconstitute with sterile water or 5% dextrose).	*Pneumocystis* infection: 4 mg/kg IM q24h for 2 weeks.

(continues)

APPENDIX F. Drug Formulary (continued)

Drug Name (Trade or Other Names)	Pharmacology and Indications	Adverse Effects and Precautions	Dosing Information and Comments	Formulations	Dosage
Piperacillin (Pipracil)	β-Lactam antibiotic of the acylureidopenicillin class. Similar to other penicillins, except with high activity against Pseudomonas aeruginosa. Also good activity against streptococci.	Same precautions as for other injectable penicillins (e.g., ampicillin).	Reconstituted solution should be used within 24 hr (or 7 days if refrigerated). Piperacillin is combined with tazobactam (β-lactamase inhibitor) in Zosyn.	2, 3, 4, 40 g vials for injection.	40 mg/kg IV or IM q6h.
Piperazine (many)	Antiparasitic compound. Produces neuromuscular blockade in parasite through inhibition of neurotransmitter, which causes paralysis of worms. Used primarily for treatment of helminth (ascarid) infections.	Remarkably safe in all species.	Used to treat all species for roundworms.	860 mg powder; 140 mg capsules; 170, 340, and 800 mg/ml oral solution.	44–66 mg/kg PO, administered once.
Potassium iodide (SSKI, Pima Syrup, many other generic).	Antifungal (exact mechanism unknown) with activity against Sporothrix spp.	Relatively safe in dogs. Cats may develop signs of iodism—vomiting, anorexia, muscle twitching, cardiomyopathy. Contraindicated in hyperthyroidism, iodine hypersensitivity, renal failure, and pregnancy.	Concurrent use with potassium-containing medications may cause hyperkalemia. Can formulate own super saturated solution of KI by dissolving 1 g/ml in water.	Oral solutions: SSKI, many other generic (1 g/ml in 300 ml bottles). Pima Syrup (325 mg/5 ml).	Dogs: 40 mg/kg q8h PO for at least 30 days, usually >60 days. Cats: 20 mg/kg q12h PO for at least 30 days, usually >60 days.

Drug	Action	Adverse effects / Contraindications	Special considerations	Supplied	Dosage
Praziquantel (Droncit)	Antiparasitic drug. Action on parasites related to neuromuscular toxicity and paralysis via altered permeability to calcium. Used primarily to treat infection caused by tapeworms.	Vomiting occurs at high doses. Anorexia and transient diarrhea have been reported. Safe in pregnant animals.	Dose recommendations based on label dose supplied by manufacturer.	23, 34 mg tablet; 56.8 mg/ml injection	Dog: Oral dose—<6.8 kg: 7.5 mg/kg PO, once; >6.8 kg: 5 mg/kg PO, once. Injection—≤2.3 kg: 7.5 mg/kg IM or SC, once; 2.7–4.5 kg: 6.3 mg/kg IM or SC, once; ≤5 kg: 5 mg/kg IM or SC, once. Cat: Oral dose—<1.8 kg: 6.3 mg/kg PO, once; >1.8 kg: 5 mg/kg PO, once. *Paragonimus* infection: 25 mg/kg q8h PO for 2–3 days. Injection: 5 mg/kg IM or SC.
Primaquine phosphate	Antiprotozoal agent that binds DNA and alters mitochondria with activity against *Babesia* spp.	Methemoglobinemia, hemolysis, myelosuppression. Contraindicated when concurrent hemolysis or bone marrow suppression, or when other myelosuppressive drugs are used.	Check CBC once weekly while treating (monitor for myelosuppression). Give with food to avoid GI side effects.	26.3 mg (15 mg active base) tablets.	*Babesia* infection: 0.3 mg/kg q24h PO for 14 days.

(continues)

APPENDIX F. Drug Formulary (continued)					
Drug Name (Trade or Other Names)	Pharmacology and Indications	Adverse Effects and Precautions	Dosing Information and Comments	Formulations	Dosage
Primor (ormetoprim + sulfadimethoxine) (Primor)	Antibacterial drug. Ormetoprim inhibits bacterial dihydrofolate reductase, sulfonamide competes with p-aminobenzoic acid (PABA) for synthesis of nucleic acids. Bactericidal/bacteriostatic. Broad antibacterial spectrum and active against some coccidia.	Several adverse effects have been reported from sulfonamides (see Trimethoprim/sulfonamides). No adverse effects reported from ormetoprim.	Doses listed are based on manufacturer's recommendations. Controlled trials have demonstrated efficacy for treatment of pyoderma on once-daily schedule.	Combination tablet (ormetoprim + sulfadimethoxine).	27 mg/kg on first day, followed by 13.5 mg/kg q24h PO.
Pyrantel pamoate (Nemex, Strongid)	Antiparasitic drug. Acts to block ganglionic neurotransmission via cholinergic action.	No adverse effects reported.	Dose recommendations based on manufacturer's recommendations.	180 mg/ml paste; 50 mg/ml suspension.	Dog: 5 mg/kg once PO and repeat in 7–10 days. Cat: 20 mg/kg once PO.
Pyrimethamine (Daraprim)	Antibacterial, antiprotozoal drug. Blocks dihydrofolate reductase enzyme, which inhibits synthesis of reduced folate and nucleic acids. Activity of pyrimethamine is more specific against protozoa than bacteria.	When administered with trimethoprim-sulfonamide combinations, anemia has been observed. Folic or folinic acid has been supplemented to prevent anemia, but benefit of this treatment is unclear.	Used either alone or in combination with sulfonamides.	25 mg tablets.	Dog: 1 mg/kg q24h PO for 14–21 days (5 days for *Neosporum caninum*). Cat: 0.5–1 mg/kg q24h PO for 14–28 days.

| Ranitidine (Zantac) | Histamine H$_2$-antagonist. See Cimetidine for details. Same as cimetidine except 4–10× more potent and longer acting. | See Cimetidine. Ranitidine may have fewer effects on endocrine function and drug interactions, compared to cimetidine. | See Cimetidine. Pharmacokinetic information in dogs suggests that ranitidine may be administered less often than cimetidine to achieve continuous suppression of stomach acid secretion. Ranitidine may stimulate stomach emptying and colon motility via anticholinesterase action. | 75, 150, 300 mg tablets; 150, 300 mg capsules; 25 mg/ml injection. | Dog: 2 mg/kg q8h IV, PO. Cat: 2.5 mg/kg q12h IV; 3.5 mg/kg q12h PO. |
| Rifampin (Rifadin) | Antibacterial. Action is to inhibit bacterial RNA synthesis. Spectrum of action includes staphylococci and mycobacteria. Other susceptible bacteria include streptococci. Used in humans primarily for treatment of tuberculosis. | Adverse effects not reported in animals, but in humans, hypersensitivity and flulike symptoms are reported. *Drug interactions:* Multiple drug interactions are possible. Induces cytochrome P-450 enzymes. Drugs affected include barbiturates, chloramphenicol, and corticosteroids. | Results of clinical studies in animals have not been reported. Use in animals (and doses) is based on experience in humans or anecdotal experience in animals. Rifampin is highly lipid soluble and has been used to treat intracellular infections. Administer on an empty stomach. | 150, 300 mg capsules; injection solution: 600 mg Rifadin IV. | 5 mg/kg q12–24h PO. |

(continues)

APPENDIX F. Drug Formulary (continued)

Drug Name (Trade or Other Names)	Pharmacology and Indications	Adverse Effects and Precautions	Dosing Information and Comments	Formulations	Dosage
Selamectin (Revolution)	Topical parasiticide and heartworm prevention.	Transient localized alopecia with or without inflammation at or near the site of application was observed in approximately 1% of 691 treated cats. Other signs observed rarely included GI signs, anorexia, lethargy, salivation, tachypnea, and muscle tremors.	Recommended for use in dogs 6 wk of age or older and in cats 8 wk of age or older.	Available in six separate dose strengths.	The recommended minimum dose is 6 mg/kg topically; see insert.
Septra (sulfamethoxazole + trimethoprim)	See Trimethoprim + sulfadiazine.				
Sodium stibogluconate (Pentostam)	Antiprotozoal pentavalent antimonial agent that interferes with energy metabolism in *Leishmania* spp.	Muscle pain at injection site, pancreatitis, myocardial injury, hemolytic anemia, leukopenia, vomiting, diarrhea, cardiac arrhythmias, renal dysfunction, shock, sudden death, thrombophlebitis (if given IV), elevated ALT.	May not always be available in the United States—contact CDC. Resistance to drug may develop during treatment. Use with allopurinol.	100 ml multidose vials (100 mg/ml).	30–50 mg/kg q24h SC or IV for 30 days. More effective if combined with oral allopurinol.

Drug	Mechanism / Spectrum	Adverse Effects	Comments	How Supplied	Dosage
Sulfadiazine (generic, combined with trimethoprim in Tribrissen)	Sulfonamides compete with PABA for enzyme that synthesizes dihydrofolic acid in bacteria. Synergistic with trimethoprim. Broad spectrum of activity, including some protozoa. Bacteriostatic.	Adverse effects associated with sulfonamides include allergic reactions, type II and III hypersensitivity, hypothyroidism (with prolonged therapy), keratoconjunctivitis sicca, and skin reactions.	Usually, sulfonamides are combined with trimethoprim or ormetoprim in 5:1 ratio. There is no clinical evidence that one sulfonamide is more or less toxic or efficacious than another.	500 mg tablets.	100 mg/kg IV, PO (loading dose), followed by 50 mg/kg q12h IV, PO (see also Trimethoprim + sulfadiazine).
Sulfadimethoxine (Albon, Bactrovet, and generic)	See Sulfadiazine.		See Sulfadiazine. Sulfadimethoxine is combined with ormetoprim in Primor.	125, 250, 500 mg tablets; 400 mg/ml injection; 50 mg/ml suspension.	55 mg/kg PO (loading dose), followed by 27.5 mg/kg q12h PO.
Sulfamethazine (many brands [e.g., Sulmet])	See Sulfadiazine.		See Sulfadiazine.	30 g bolus.	100 mg/kg PO (loading dose), followed by 50 mg/kg q12h PO.
Sulfamethoxazole (Gantanol)	See Sulfadiazine.		See Sulfadiazine.	500 mg tablets.	100 mg/kg PO (loading dose), followed by 50 mg/kg q12h PO.
Sulfisoxazole (Gantrisin)	See Sulfadiazine. Sulfisoxazole is primarily used only for treating urinary tract infections.		See Sulfadiazine.	500 mg tablets; 500 mg/5 ml syrup.	50 mg/kg q8h PO (urinary tract infections).
Terbinafine (Lamisil)	Fungicidal agent that interferes with ergosterol biosynthesis by inhibiting squalene epoxidase in the fungal cell membrane.	High margin of safety. May cause GI tract disturbances (vomiting, diarrhea). Hepatic failure, pancytopenia, toxic epidermal necrolysis reported in humans.	Used for the systemic treatment of pythiosis and cryptococcosis.	125, 250 mg tablets.	5–10 mg/kg q24h PO for 4–6 months.

(continues)

APPENDIX F. Drug Formulary (continued)

Drug Name (Trade or Other Names)	Pharmacology and Indications	Adverse Effects and Precautions	Dosing Information and Comments	Formulations	Dosage
Tetracycline (Panmycin)	Tetracycline antibiotic. Mechanism of action of tetracyclines is to bind to 30S ribosomal subunit and inhibit protein synthesis. Usually bacteriostatic. Broad spectrum of activity, including bacteria, some protozoa, *Rickettsia* spp., and *Ehrlichia* spp.	Tetracyclines in general may cause renal tubular necrosis at high doses. Tetracyclines can affect bone and teeth formation in young animals. Tetracyclines have been implicated in drug fever in cats. Hepatotoxicity may occur at high doses in susceptible individuals. *Drug interactions*: Tetracyclines bind to calcium-containing compounds, which decreases oral absorption.	Pharmacokinetic and experimental studies have been conducted in small animals, but no clinical studies. Do not use outdated solutions.	250, 500 mg capsules; 100 mg/ml suspension.	15–20 mg/kg q8h PO; or 4.4–11 mg/kg q8h IV, IM.
Tetramizole hydrochloride (Nilverm)	A broad-spectrum imidazothiazole anthelmintic. Mechanism of action is neuromuscular toxicity to parasites. In humans, used as an immunostimulant to aid in the treatment of colorectal carcinoma.	Similar side effects of levamisole (potentiates cholinergic toxicity). May cause vomiting.	Rarely used in small animals. Still recommended for treatment of *Ollulanus* infections in cats. Available in Australia and New Zealand as a cattle and sheep drench (Nilverm).	Nilverm Oral drench: 32 g/L.	5 mg/kg PO once administer as a 2.5% (25 mg/ml) solution.

Drug	Action / Indications	Adverse Effects / Interactions	Comments	Supplied	Dosage
Thiabendazole (Omnizole, Equizole)	Benzimidazole anthelmintic. (See Fenbendazole, Albendazole.)	Adverse effects uncommon.	Ordinarily administered to horses and cattle. Experience in small animals is limited.	2 or 4 g per oz (30 ml) suspension or liquid.	Dog: 50 mg/kg q24h for 3 days, repeat in 1 month. Respiratory parasites: 30–70 mg/kg q12h PO. Cat: *Strongyloides* spp.: 125 mg/kg q24h for 3 days.
Ticarcillin (Ticar, Ticillin)	β-Lactam antibiotic. Action similar to ampicillin/amoxicillin. Spectrum similar to that of carbenicillin. Ticarcillin is primarily used for gram-negative infections, especially those caused by *Pseudomonas* spp.	Adverse effects are uncommon. However, allergic reactions are possible. High doses can produce seizures and decreased platelet function. *Drug interactions*: Do not combine in same syringe or in vial with aminoglycosides.	Ticarcillin is synergistic and often combined with aminoglycosides (e.g., amikacin, gentamicin). 1% lidocaine may be used for reconstitution to decrease pain from IM injection.	6 g/50 ml vial; vials containing 1, 3, 6, 20, and 30 g.	33–50 mg/kg q4–6h IV, IM.
Ticarcillin + clavulanate (Timentin)	Same as ticarcillin, except clavulanic acid has been added to inhibit bacterial β-lactamase and increase spectrum. Clavulanate does not increase activity against *Pseudomonas* spp., however.	Same as for ticarcillin.	Same as for ticarcillin.	3 g per vial for injection.	Dose according to rate for ticarcillin.
Tobramycin (Nebcin)	Aminoglycoside antibacterial drug. Similar mechanism of action and spectrum as amikacin and gentamicin.	Adverse effects similar to those of amikacin, gentamicin.	Dosing requirements vary depending on bacterial susceptibility. See dose schedules for gentamicin and amikacin.	40 mg/ml injection.	Dog: 2–4 mg/kg q8h IV, IM, SC or 9–14 mg/kg q24h IV, IM, SC. Cat: 3 mg/kg q8h IV, IM, SC or 5–8 mg/kg q24h, IV, IM, SC.

(continues)

APPENDIX F. Drug Formulary (continued)

Drug Name (Trade or Other Names)	Pharmacology and Indications	Adverse Effects and Precautions	Dosing Information and Comments	Formulations	Dosage
Trimethoprim + sulfadiazine (Tribrissen, Tucoprim, and others)	Combines the antibacterial drug action of trimethoprim and a sulfonamide. Together, the combination is synergistic, with a broad spectrum of activity.	Adverse effects primarily caused by sulfonamide component. (See Sulfadiazine.)	Dosage recommendations vary. There is evidence that 30 mg/kg/day is efficacious for pyoderma; for other infections, 30 mg/kg twice daily has been recommended.	30, 120, 240, 480, 960 mg tablet (all formulations have ratio of 5:1 sulfa:trimethoprim).	15 mg/kg q12h PO or 30 mg/kg q12–24h PO. *Toxoplasma*: 30 mg/kg q12h PO.
Trimethoprim + sulfamethoxazole (Bactrim, Septra, and generic forms)	Combines the antibacterial drug action of trimethoprim and a sulfonamide. Together, the combination is synergistic, with a broad spectrum of activity.	Adverse effects primarily caused by sulfonamide component. (See Sulfadiazine.)	Dosage recommendations vary. There is evidence that 30 mg/kg/day is efficacious for pyoderma; for other infections, 30 mg/kg twice daily has been recommended.	480, 960 mg tablet; 240 mg/5 ml oral suspension (all formulations have ratio of 5:1 sulfa:trimethoprim).	15 mg/kg q12h PO or 30 mg/kg q12–24h PO.
Tylosin (Tylocine, Tylan, Tylosin tartrate)	Macrolide antibiotic. (See Erythromycin for mechanisms of action and spectrum of activity.)	May cause diarrhea in some animals. Do not administer orally to rodents or rabbits.	Tylosin is rarely used in small animals. Powdered formulation (tylosin tartrate) has been administered on food for control of signs of colitis in dogs. Tablets are approved in Canada for treatment of colitis.	Available as soluble powder 2.2 tylosin per tsp (tablets for dogs in Canada)	Dog and cat: 7–15 mg/kg q12–24h PO Dog (for colitis): 10–20 mg/kg q8h with food; if there is a response, increase the interval to q12–24h

| Vancomycin (Vancocin, Vancoled) | Antibacterial drug. Mechanism of action is to inhibit cell wall and cause bacterial cell lysis (via mechanism different from that of β-lactams). Spectrum includes staphylococci, streptococci, and enterococci (but not gram-negative bacteria). Used primarily for treatment of resistant staphylococci and enterococci. | Adverse effects have not been reported in animals. Administer IV; causes severe pain and tissue injury if administered IM or SC. Do not administer rapidly; use slow infusion, if possible (e.g., over 30 min). Adverse effects in humans include renal injury (more common with older products that contained impurities) and histamine release. | Vancomycin use is not common in animals, but is valuable for treatment of enterococci or staphylococci that are resistant to other antibiotics. Doses are derived from pharmacokinetic studies in dogs. Monitoring of trough plasma concentrations is recommended to ensure proper dose. Maintain trough concentration above 5 mcg/ml. Infusion solution can be prepared in 0.9% saline or 5% dextrose, but not alkalinizing solutions. | Vials for injection (0.5 to 10 g). | Dog: 15 mg/kg q6–8h IV infusion. Cat: 12–15 mg/kg q8h IV Infusion. |

Modified from Papich MG: Drug formulary. In Tilley LP, Smith FWK Jr. *The 5-Minute Veterinary Consult: Canine and Feline*, 3rd ed. Baltimore: Lippincott Williams & Wilkins, 2004.

Abbreviations: ALT, alanine aminotransferase; CDC, Centers for Disease Control and Prevention; CNS, central nervous system; CSF, cerebrospinal fluid; DNA, deoxyribonucleic acid; GABA, γ-aminobutyric acid; GI, gastrointestinal; IM, intramuscular; IV, intravenous; MIC, minimum inhibitory concentration; PO, per os (oral), PU/PD, polyuria/polydipsia; q, every, as in q8h = every 8 hours; SC, subcutaneous; U, units.

Disclaimer for Dose Tables: Doses listed are for dogs *and* cats, unless otherwise listed. Many of the doses listed are extra-label or are human drugs not approved for animals administered in an extra-label manner. Doses listed are based on best available information at the time of table editing. The author cannot ensure efficacy or absolute safety of drugs used according to recommendations in this table. Adverse effects may be possible from drugs listed in this table of which authors were not aware at the time of table preparation. Veterinarians using this table are encouraged to consult current literature, product labels and inserts, and the manufacturer's disclosure information for additional information on adverse effects, interactions, and efficacy that were not identified at the time these tables were prepared.

Index

Pages in italics denote figures; those followed by a "t" denote tables

A

A. fumigatus, 67
A. maculatum, 499
A. platys, ehrlichiosis concurrent with, 202
A. terreus, 67
A. vasorum larva, Angiostrongylus infection v., 11, *11*
Acanthamoeba castellani, 1
   Amebiasis and, 2
Acaricides, ticks and, 505
Acemannan, 562
   FeLV and, 230
   FIV and, 215, 216t
ACTH response test, whipworms and, 545
Acute hepatitis, Tyzzer's disease and, 536
Acute myocarditis, Chagas' disease and, 113, 114
Adult larvae dewormer, hookworms and, 305
Adulticide treatment
   dog heartworm and, 281
   interactions of, cat heartworm disease and, 274
   roundworms and, 450–451
Advantage. *See* Imidacloprid
Aelurostrongylus abstrusus. See Feline lungworm
Aged animals, salmonellosis and, 458
AGID, blastomycosis and, 47
Alanine aminotransferase (ALT), trichosporonosis
   and, 529
Albendazole (Valbazen), 562
   encephalitozoonosis and, 204, 205t
   giardiasis, 263
   myelosuppression and, 204, 205t
   precautions for, 263, 263t
   trichinosis and, 520
Allergy, ear mites and, 193
Allopurinol, 562
   leishmaniasis and, 326, 327t
ALT. *See* Alanine aminotransferase
Amblyomma americanum, 499
Amebiasis, 1–4
   clinical features of, 2
   diagnostics of, 3
   differential diagnosis of, 2
   etiology of, 1
   pathophysiology of, 1
   therapeutics for, 3–4
American trypanosomiasis. *See* Chagas' disease
Amikacin, 563
   nocardiosis and, 383, 384t

Aminoglycosides
   anaerobic infections and, 7
   botulism and, 59
   precautions for, 384
Amitraz (Mitaban), 563
   cheyletiellosis and, 123
   demodicosis and, 177
   ear mites and, 193
   side effects of, 178
Amoxicillin, 563
   anaerobic infections and, 7
   bordetellosis and, 56
   colibacillosis and, 147
   dermatophilosis and, 183
   feline calicivirus infection and, 211
   feline rhinotracheitis virus infection and, 247
   Lyme disease and, 353
   nocardiosis and, 383, 384t
   salmonellosis and, 459
   tularemia and, 533
Amoxicillin + clavulanate potassium (Clavamox), 564
Amoxicillin trihydrate, 564
Amoxicillin/clavulanic acid, bordetellosis and, 55, 55t
Amphotericin B (Fungizone), 564
   blastomycosis and, dogs and, 49
   coccidioidomycosis and, 139
   cryptococcosis and, 153–154, 153t
   histoplasmosis and, 298
   leishmaniasis and, 327, 327t
   protothecosis and, 407, 407t
   pythiosis and, 415–416, 416t
Amphotericin B liposomal formulation, 565
Ampicillin, 565
   dermatophilosis and, 183
   nocardiosis and, 383, 384t
   streptococcal infections and, 482, 482t
Ampicillin + sulbactam (Unasyn), 565
Ampicillin trihydrate (Polyflex), 565
Amproline, 566
Amprolium, coccidiosis and, 143
Anabolic steroids, FIV and, 215, 216t
Anaerobes, anaerobic infections and, 5
Anaerobic infections, 5–8
   clinical features of, 5
   diagnostics for, 6
   differential diagnosis for, 6
   drugs for, 7, 7t

T